Activation and Modulation of Mast Cells

Activation and Modulation of Mast Cells

Special Issue Editor
Satoshi Tanaka

MDPI • Basel • Beijing • Wuhan • Barcelona • Belgrade • Manchester • Tokyo • Cluj • Tianjin

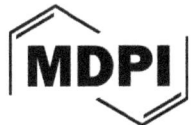

Special Issue Editor
Satoshi Tanaka
Kyoto Pharmaceutical University
Japan

Editorial Office
MDPI
St. Alban-Anlage 66
4052 Basel, Switzerland

This is a reprint of articles from the Special Issue published online in the open access journal *International Journal of Molecular Sciences* (ISSN 1422-0067) (available at: https://www.mdpi.com/journal/ijms/special_issues/mast_activation).

For citation purposes, cite each article independently as indicated on the article page online and as indicated below:

LastName, A.A.; LastName, B.B.; LastName, C.C. Article Title. *Journal Name* **Year**, *Article Number*, Page Range.

ISBN 978-3-03936-563-0 (Hbk)
ISBN 978-3-03936-564-7 (PDF)

© 2020 by the authors. Articles in this book are Open Access and distributed under the Creative Commons Attribution (CC BY) license, which allows users to download, copy and build upon published articles, as long as the author and publisher are properly credited, which ensures maximum dissemination and a wider impact of our publications.

The book as a whole is distributed by MDPI under the terms and conditions of the Creative Commons license CC BY-NC-ND.

Contents

About the Special Issue Editor vii

Preface to "Activation and Modulation of Mast Cells" ix

Satoshi Tanaka
Phenotypic and Functional Diversity of Mast Cells
Reprinted from: *Int. J. Mol. Sci.* **2020**, *21*, 3835, doi:10.3390/ijms21113835 1

Chalatip Chompunud Na Ayudhya, Saptarshi Roy, Ibrahim Alkanfari, Anirban Ganguly and Hydar Ali
Identification of Gain and Loss of Function Missense Variants in MRGPRX2's Transmembrane and Intracellular Domains for Mast Cell Activation by Substance P
Reprinted from: *Int. J. Mol. Sci.* **2019**, *20*, 5247, doi:10.3390/ijms20215247 5

Kazuki Yoshida, Makoto Tajima, Tomoki Nagano, Kosuke Obayashi, Masaaki Ito, Kimiko Yamamoto and Isao Matsuoka
Co-Stimulation of Purinergic P2X4 and Prostanoid EP3 Receptors Triggers Synergistic Degranulation in Murine Mast Cells
Reprinted from: *Int. J. Mol. Sci.* **2019**, *20*, 5157, doi:10.3390/ijms20205157 21

Erica Arriaga-Gomez, Jaclyn Kline, Elizabeth Emanuel, Nefeli Neamonitaki, Tenzin Yangdon, Hayley Zacheis, Dogukan Pasha, Jinyoung Lim, Susan Bush, Beebie Boo, Hanna Mengistu, Ruby Kinnamon, Robin Shields-Cutler, Elizabeth Wattenberg and Devavani Chatterjea
Repeated Vaginal Exposures to the Common Cosmetic and Household Preservative Methylisothiazolinone Induce Persistent, Mast Cell-Dependent Genital Pain in ND4 Mice
Reprinted from: *Int. J. Mol. Sci.* **2019**, *20*, 5361, doi:10.3390/ijms20215361 37

Kayoko Ishimaru, Shotaro Nakajima, Guannan Yu, Yuki Nakamura and Atsuhito Nakao
The Putatively Specific Synthetic REV-ERB Agonist SR9009 Inhibits IgE- and IL-33-Mediated Mast Cell Activation Independently of the Circadian Clock
Reprinted from: *Int. J. Mol. Sci.* **2019**, *20*, 6320, doi:10.3390/ijms20246320 55

Aya Kakinoki, Tsuyoshi Kameo, Shoko Yamashita, Kazuyuki Furuta and Satoshi Tanaka
Establishment and Characterization of a Murine Mucosal Mast Cell Culture Model
Reprinted from: *Int. J. Mol. Sci.* **2020**, *21*, 236, doi:10.3390/ijms21010236 67

Yuka Gion, Mitsuhiro Okano, Takahisa Koyama, Tokie Oura, Asami Nishikori, Yorihisa Orita, Tomoyasu Tachibana, Hidenori Marunaka, Takuma Makino, Kazunori Nishizaki and Yasuharu Sato
Clinical Significance of Cytoplasmic IgE-Positive Mast Cells in Eosinophilic Chronic Rhinosinusitis
Reprinted from: *Int. J. Mol. Sci.* **2020**, *21*, 1843, doi:10.3390/ijms21051843 81

Zhirong Fu, Srinivas Akula, Michael Thorpe and Lars Hellman
Highly Selective Cleavage of TH2-Promoting Cytokines by the Human and the Mouse Mast Cell Tryptases, Indicating a Potent Negative Feedback Loop on TH2 Immunity
Reprinted from: *Int. J. Mol. Sci.* **2019**, *20*, 5147, doi:10.3390/ijms20205147 95

Kinuko Ohneda, Shin'ya Ohmori and Masayuki Yamamoto
Mouse Tryptase Gene Expression is Coordinately Regulated by GATA1 and GATA2 in Bone Marrow-Derived Mast Cells
Reprinted from: *Int. J. Mol. Sci.* **2019**, *20*, 4603, doi:10.3390/ijms20184603 113

Ryota Uchida, Michiko Kato, Yuka Hattori, Hiroko Kikuchi, Emi Watanabe, Katsuumi Kobayashi and Keigo Nishida
Identification of 5-Hydroxymethylfurfural (5-HMF) as an Active Component Citrus Jabara That Suppresses FcεRI-Mediated Mast Cell Activation
Reprinted from: *Int. J. Mol. Sci.* **2020**, *21*, 2472, doi:10.3390/ijms21072472 131

Tatsuki R. Kataoka, Chiyuki Ueshima, Masahiro Hirata, Sachiko Minamiguchi and Hironori Haga
Killer Immunoglobulin-Like Receptor 2DL4 (CD158d) Regulates Human Mast Cells both Positively and Negatively: Possible Roles in Pregnancy and Cancer Metastasis
Reprinted from: *Int. J. Mol. Sci.* **2020**, *21*, 954, doi:10.3390/ijms21030954 143

David O. Lyons and Nicholas A. Pullen
Beyond IgE: Alternative Mast Cell Activation Across Different Disease States
Reprinted from: *Int. J. Mol. Sci.* **2020**, *21*, 1498, doi:10.3390/ijms21041498 159

About the Special Issue Editor

Satoshi Tanaka Ph.D., Professor of Pharmacology at Kyoto Pharmaceutical University, is engaged in the basic research of mast cells. He was awarded the degree of Ph.D. for his thesis entitled "Regulation of Histidine Decarboxylase" from Kyoto University in 1999. From 1997 to 2005, he studied the physiological roles of histamine using gene-targeted mice lacking histidine decarboxylase as a Research Associate at the Graduate School of Pharmaceutical Sciences, Kyoto University. During this period, he began his research on mast cells, which are the major source of histamine and one of the essential players of immediate allergic responses. He moved to Mukogawa Women's University in 2005 as Associate Professor and joined Okayama University in 2009. He was appointed Professor of Department of Immunobiology, Okayama University Graduate School of Medicine, Dentistry, and Pharmaceutical Sciences in 2012, where he focused attention on the heterogeneity of tissue mast cells and established a culture model of murine cutaneous mast cells. In 2018, he moved to Kyoto Pharmaceutical University. He has focused on functional changes of tissue mast cells during their differentiation and maturation, in particular, the GPCR-mediated regulation of mast cell functions. He is also engaged in the promotion of research integrity. He is a regular member of the American Society for Biochemistry and Molecular Biology (ASBMB) and an associate member of the Committee of Publication Ethics (COPE). ORCID ID: 0000-0002-3468-7694.

Preface to "Activation and Modulation of Mast Cells"

Preface to "Activation and Modulation of Mast Cells"Mast cells originate from hematopoietic stem cells in bone marrow, although the process of differentiation and maturation remains to be clarified. How mast cell precursors infiltrate into peripheral tissues and follow the intrinsic program of differentiation it is both fascinating and a mystery. The specific characteristics of tissue mast cells are largely determined by their microenvironment. Mast cells serve as local sources of a wide variety of chemical mediators, such as biogenic amines, neutral proteases, lipid mediators, cytokines, chemokines, and growth factors, all of which are released in a timely manner in response to environmental changes, and are then involved in shaping the appropriate immune responses. Early studies in the field of mast cell research have focused on the pathophysiological roles of mast cells during IgE-mediated immediate responses. They have provided us with a great deal of knowledge regarding the biology of mast cells. Recent progress in the gene-targeting techniques has enabled us to unravel the pathophysiological roles of tissue mast cells, a significant part of which has been found in IgE-independent immune responses. I believe that this frontier in the field of mast cell research should be further explored. Accumulating evidence strongly suggests that the discovery of novel functions of tissue mast cells should lead to the development of novel therapeutic approaches of a series of chronic inflammatory diseases. I hope that this Special Issue will become a significant part of the everlasting story of mast cell research. I present my sincere appreciation to all the contributors and the editorial staff of the International Journal of Molecular Sciences.

Satoshi Tanaka
Special Issue Editor

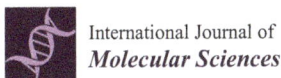

Editorial

Phenotypic and Functional Diversity of Mast Cells

Satoshi Tanaka

Department of Pharmacology, Division of Pathological Sciences, Kyoto Pharmaceutical University, Misasagi Nakauchi-cho 5, Yamashina-ku, Kyoto 607-8414, Japan; tanaka-s@mb.kyoto-phu.ac.jp; Tel.: +81-75-595-4667

Received: 14 May 2020; Accepted: 27 May 2020; Published: 28 May 2020

Mast cells, which originate from hematopoietic stem cells, are distributed in nearly all vascularized tissues. As no leukocytes that are categorized as mast cells could be found in the circulation, it is considered that the terminal differentiation of mast cells occurs under the strong influence of their microenvironment [1–3]. Recent studies shed light on the origin and heterogeneity of tissue human and murine mast cells [4–6]. The microenvironment might regulate the expression profiles of both the receptors and mediators of tissue mast cells. The sensor molecules, including the cell surface receptors expressed in tissue mast cells, determine to which types of environmental changes they should respond, while the capacity of the mediators' release determine how they should act on these changes (Figure 1). Accumulating evidence indicates that mast cells could exert a wide variety of physiological and pathological effects in the context of spatiotemporal immune responses. Recent progress in the field of mast cell research has provided us with many powerful tools, such as a variety of gene-targeted mice lacking tissue mast cells, primary mast cell cultures, and various "omics" approaches to clarify this complexity [7], thereby enabling a comprehensive update of our knowledge about mast cell functions. The studies found in this Special Issue "Activation and Modulation of Mast Cells" are involved in this new tide of research.

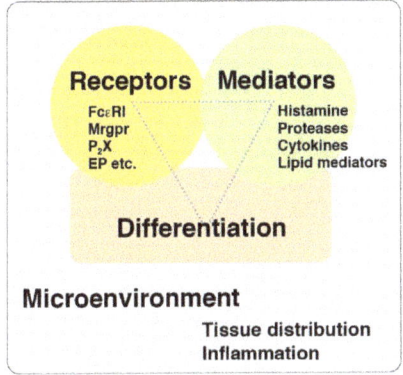

Figure 1. A viewpoint of mast cell research. Three viewpoints, such as differentiation states, expression patterns of the receptors, and capacities of the mediator release, might be useful for the comprehensive understanding of functions of tissue mast cells. Mrgpr, Mas-related G protein-coupled receptor; P_2X, purine ionotropic receptor; EP, prostaglandin E receptor.

IgE-mediated activation of mast cells has been intensively studied because mast cells play an essential role in IgE-mediated immediate allergic responses. Mast cells were also found to undergo degranulation in an IgE-independent manner, although it remains largely unknown how mast cells are activated by various secretagogues, such as compound 48/80 and several bioactive peptides including neuropeptides and antibacterial peptides because no suitable culture models have been developed for the in-depth investigation of IgE-independent degranulation. Recently, Staphylococcus δ-toxin was found to induce degranulation of murine mast cells, implying the important role of degranulation induced by the bacterial peptide toxin in atopic dermatitis [8]. Tatemoto et al. first proposed that a Mas-related G protein-coupled receptor subtype, MRGPRX2, should be involved in secretagogue-induced degranulation of mast cells [9]. McNeil et al. recently demonstrated that one of the murine MRGPRX2 orthologues, MrgprB2, should be responsible for IgE-independent degranulation of mast cells and various pseudo allergic responses in mice [10]. In this issue, Chompunud Na Ayudhya et al. demonstrated the functional roles of some key amino acid residues of MRGPRX2 using molecular biochemical approaches [11]. Apart from the Mrgpr family, Yoshida et al. also investigated IgE-independent degranulation of murine mast cells. They revealed that prostaglandin E_2 and ATP could synergistically induce degranulation by acting on EP3 and P_2X_4 receptors, respectively [12]. Arriaga-Gomez et al. demonstrated that methylisothiazolinone could induce persistent tactile sensitivity and mast cell accumulation in female genital skin tissues [13]. Although the target molecules of methylisothiazolinone remain to be identified, it is likely that cutaneous mast cells could be directly activated by several contact allergens. Indeed, Dudeck et al. demonstrated the activation of cutaneous mast cells in the presence of several conventional contact allergens [14]. IL-33 and thymic stromal lymphopoietin were found to be potential modulators of mast cell functions [15]. Ishimaru et al. unexpectedly found that a synthetic REV-ERB agonist, SR9009, could suppress the activation of murine mast cells induced by the IgE/antigen complex or IL-33 and these effects were independent of disturbance of the circadian clock [16]. Lyons and Pullen reviewed the recent findings of IgE-independent activation of mast cells, with a focus on the context-dependent actions of TGF-β and IL-10 [17].

Diversity of phenotype and function of tissue mast cells needs more attention for a better understanding of their function. Although the concept that tissue mast cells can be categorized into two subtypes—connective tissue type and mucosal type—is commonly recognized, more detailed characterization in the context of spatiotemporal localization should be useful for elucidation of the roles of tissue mast cells. In this issue, Kakinoki et al. characterized the phenotypic changes of murine mast cells induced by IL-9, which might be essential for the development of the intestinal mast cell population [18]. Gion et al. characterized a unique population of mast cells, which may uptake IgE molecules in human eosinophilic chronic rhinosinusitis [19]. Mast cells are well known for their potential to produce a wide variety of mediators, such as biogenic amines, lipid mediators, cytokines/chemokines, and growth factors [20]. Among them, the physiological and pathological roles of mast cell proteases have emerged in recent studies using various gene-targeted mouse models [21]. Accumulating evidence suggests that the expression profiles of mast cell proteases should reflect the heterogeneity of tissue mast cells [22,23]. In this issue, Fu et al. demonstrated the specific in vitro cleavages of a series of cytokines and chemokines by mast cell proteases including human tryptase, raising the possibility that mast cell proteases modulate the direction of immune responses [24]. Ohneda et al. clarified the functional roles of GATA1 and GATA2 in transcriptional regulation of the Tpsb2 gene that encodes mouse mast cell protease 6 in murine mast cells [25].

It will be of great help for novel therapeutic approaches of inflammatory diseases to identify endogenous target molecules and synthetic compounds that could modulate the activity of tissue mast cells. Kataoka et al. summarized the modulatory roles and therapeutic potential of killer immunoglobulin-like receptor 2DL4 (CD158d) in human mast cells [26]. Uchida et al. identified a natural compound from a citrus fruit, Jabara, which could suppress degranulation and IL-6 production of murine mast cells upon IgE-mediated antigen stimulation [27].

The contents of this Special Issue reflect the diverse aspects of mast cell research. I hope that these studies will stimulate researchers and encourage further exploration in the field of mast cell research.

Conflicts of Interest: The author declares no conflict of interest.

References

1. Kitamura, Y. Heterogeneity of mast cells and phenotypic change between subpopulations. *Annu. Rev. Immunol.* **1989**, *7*, 59–76. [CrossRef] [PubMed]
2. Cildir, G.; Pant, H.; Lopez, A.F.; Tergaonkar, V. The transcriptional program, functional heterogeneity, and clinical targeting of mast cells. *J. Exp. Med.* **2017**, *214*, 2491–2506. [CrossRef] [PubMed]
3. Frossi, B.; Mion, F.; Sibilano, R.; Danelli, L.; Pucillo, C.E.M. Is it time for a new classification of mast cells? What do we know about mast cell heterogeneity? *Immunol. Rev.* **2018**, *282*, 35–46. [CrossRef] [PubMed]
4. Dwyer, D.F.; Barrett, N.A.; Austen, K.F. Immunological Genome Project Consortium. Expression profiling of constitutive mast cells reveals a unique identity within the immune system. *Nat. Immunol.* **2016**, *17*, 878–887. [CrossRef]
5. Gentek, R.; Ghigo, C.; Hoeffel, G.; Bulle, M.J.; Msallam, R.; Gautier, G.; Launay, P.; Chen, J.; Ginhoux, F.; Bajénoff, M. Hemogenic endothelial fate mapping reveals dual developmental origin of mast Cells. *Immunity* **2018**, *48*, 1160–1171.e5. [CrossRef]
6. Plum, T.; Wang, X.; Rettel, M.; Krijgsveld, J.; Feyerabend, T.B.; Rodewald, H.R. Human mast cell proteome reveals lineage, putative functions, and structural basis for cell ablation. *Immunity* **2020**, *18*, 404–416.e5. [CrossRef]
7. Reber, L.L.; Marichal, T.; Galli, S.J. New models for analyzing mast cell functions in vivo. *Trends Immunol.* **2012**, *33*, 613–625. [CrossRef]
8. Nakamura, Y.; Oscherwitz, J.; Cease, K.B.; Chan, S.M.; Muñoz-Planillo, R.; Hasegawa, M.; Villaruz, A.E.; Cheung, G.Y.C.; McGavin, M.J.; Travers, J.B.; et al. Staphylococcus δ-toxin induces allergic skin disease by activating mast cells. *Nature* **2013**, *503*, 397–401. [CrossRef]
9. Tatemoto, K.; Nozaki, Y.; Tsuda, R.; Konno, S.; Tomura, K.; Furuno, M.; Ogasawara, H.; Edamura, K.; Takagi, H.; Iwamura, H.; et al. Immunoglobulin E-independent activation of mast cell is mediated by Mrg receptors. *Biochem. Biophys. Res. Commun.* **2006**, *349*, 1322–1328. [CrossRef]
10. McNeil, B.D.; Pundir, P.; Meeker, S.; Han, L.; Undem, B.J.; Kulka, M.; Dong, X. Identification of a mast-cell-specific receptor crucial for pseudo-allergic drug reactions. *Nature* **2015**, *519*, 237–241. [CrossRef] [PubMed]
11. Chompunud Na Ayudhya, C.; Roy, S.; Alkanfari, I.; Ganguly, A.; Ali, H. Identification of Gain and Loss of Function Missense Variants in MRGPRX2's Transmembrane and Intracellular Domains for Mast Cell Activation by Substance P. *Int. J. Mol. Sci.* **2019**, *20*, 5247. [CrossRef] [PubMed]
12. Yoshida, K.; Tajima, M.; Nagano, T.; Obayashi, K.; Ito, M.; Yamamoto, K.; Matsuoka, I. Co-Stimulation of Purinergic P2X4 and Prostanoid EP3 Receptors Triggers Synergistic Degranulation in Murine Mast Cells. *Int. J. Mol. Sci.* **2019**, *20*, 5157. [CrossRef] [PubMed]
13. Arriaga-Gomez, E.; Kline, J.; Emanuel, E.; Neamonitaki, N.; Yangdon, T.; Zacheis, H.; Pasha, D.; Lim, J.; Bush, S.; Boo, B.; et al. Repeated Vaginal Exposures to the Common Cosmetic and Household Preservative Methylisothiazolinone Induce Persistent, Mast Cell-Dependent Genital Pain in ND4 Mice. *Int. J. Mol. Sci.* **2019**, *20*, 5361. [CrossRef] [PubMed]
14. Dudeck, A.; Dudeck, J.; Scholten, J.; Petzold, A.; Surianarayanan, S.; Köhler, A.; Peschke, K.; Vöhringer, D.; Waskow, C.; Krieg, T.; et al. Mast cells are key promoters of contact allergy that mediate the adjuvant effects of haptens. *Immunity* **2011**, *34*, 973–984. [CrossRef] [PubMed]
15. Saluja, R.; Zoltowska, A.; Ketelaar, M.E.; Nilsson, G. IL-33 and Thymic Stromal Lymphopoietin in mast cell functions. *Eur. J. Pharmacol.* **2016**, *778*, 68–76. [CrossRef]
16. Ishimaru, K.; Nakajima, S.; Yu, G.; Nakamura, Y.; Nakao, A. The Putatively Specific Synthetic REV-ERB Agonist SR9009 Inhibits IgE–and IL-33-Mediated Mast Cell Activation Independently of the Circadian Clock. *Int. J. Mol. Sci.* **2019**, *20*, 6320. [CrossRef]
17. Lyons, D.O.; Pullen, N.A. Beyond IgE: Alternative Mast Cell Activation Across Different Disease States. *Int. J. Mol. Sci.* **2020**, *21*, 1498. [CrossRef]
18. Kakinoki, A.; Kameo, T.; Yamashita, S.; Furuta, K.; Tanaka, S. Establishment and Characterization of a Murine Mucosal Mast Cell Culture Model. *Int. J. Mol. Sci.* **2020**, *21*, 236. [CrossRef]
19. Gion, Y.; Okano, M.; Koyama, T.; Oura, T.; Nishikori, A.; Orita, Y.; Tachibana, T.; Marunaka, H.; Makino, T.; Nishizaki, K.; et al. Clinical Significance of Cytoplasmic IgE-Positive Mast Cells in Eosinophilic Chronic Rhinosinusitis. *Int. J. Mol. Sci.* **2020**, *21*, 1843. [CrossRef]

20. Mukai, K.; Tsai, M.; Saito, H.; Galli, S.J. Mast cells as sources of cytokines, chemokines, and growth factors. *Immunol. Rev.* **2018**, *282*, 121–150. [CrossRef]
21. Caughey, G.H. Mast cell proteases as pharmacological targets. *Eur. J. Pharmacol.* **2016**, *778*, 44–55. [CrossRef] [PubMed]
22. Reynolds, D.S.; Stevens, R.L.; Lane, W.S.; Carr, M.H.; Austen, K.F.; Serafin, W.E. Different mouse mast cell populations express various combinations of at least six distinct mast cell serine proteases. *Proc. Natl. Acad. Sci. USA* **1990**, *87*, 3230–3234. [CrossRef]
23. Lutzelschwab, C.; Pejler, G.; Aveskogh, M.; Hellman, L. Secretory granule proteases in rat mast cells. Cloning of 10 different serine proteases and a carboxypeptidase A from various rat mast cell populations. *J. Exp. Med.* **1997**, *185*, 13–29. [CrossRef] [PubMed]
24. Fu, Z.; Akula, S.; Thorpe, M.; Hellman, L. Highly Selective Cleavage of TH2-Promoting Cytokines by the Human and the Mouse Mast Cell Tryptases, Indicating a Potent Negative Feedback Loop on TH2 Immunity. *Int. J. Mol. Sci.* **2019**, *20*, 5147. [CrossRef] [PubMed]
25. Ohneda, K.; Ohmori, S.; Yamamoto, M. Mouse Tryptase Gene Expression is Coordinately Regulated by GATA1 and GATA2 in Bone Marrow-Derived Mast Cells. *Int. J. Mol. Sci.* **2019**, *20*, 4603. [CrossRef] [PubMed]
26. Kataoka, T.R.; Ueshima, C.; Hirata, M.; Minamiguchi, S.; Haga, H. Killer Immunoglobulin-Like Receptor 2DL4 (CD158d) Regulates Human Mast Cells Both Positively and Negatively: Possible Roles in Pregnancy and Cancer Metastasis. *Int. J. Mol. Sci.* **2020**, *21*, 954. [CrossRef] [PubMed]
27. Uchida, R.; Kato, M.; Hattori, Y.; Kikuchi, H.; Watanabe, E.; Kobayashi, K.; Nishida, K. Identification of 5-Hydroxymethylfurfural (5-HMF) as an Active Component Citrus Jabara That Suppresses FcεRI-Mediated Mast Cell Activation. *Int. J. Mol. Sci.* **2020**, *21*, 2472. [CrossRef]

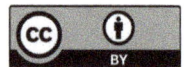

© 2020 by the author. Licensee MDPI, Basel, Switzerland. This article is an open access article distributed under the terms and conditions of the Creative Commons Attribution (CC BY) license (http://creativecommons.org/licenses/by/4.0/).

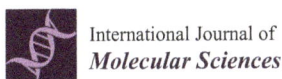

Article

Identification of Gain and Loss of Function Missense Variants in MRGPRX2's Transmembrane and Intracellular Domains for Mast Cell Activation by Substance P

Chalatip Chompunud Na Ayudhya, Saptarshi Roy, Ibrahim Alkanfari [†], Anirban Ganguly and Hydar Ali *

Department of Basic and Translational Sciences, University of Pennsylvania, School of Dental Medicine, Philadelphia PA-19104, USA; chalatip@upenn.edu (C.C.N.A.); roysapta@upenn.edu (S.R.); ibrahim.alkanfari@gmail.com (I.A.); anirban711@aol.com (A.G.)
* Correspondence: alih@upenn.edu; Tel.: +1-21-5573-1993
† Current Address: Faculty of Dentistry, King AbdulAziz University, Jeddah 21589, Saudi Arabia; ibrahim.alkanfari@gmail.com

Received: 2 October 2019; Accepted: 22 October 2019; Published: 23 October 2019

Abstract: The neuropeptide substance P (SP) contributes to neurogenic inflammation through the activation of human mast cells via Mas-related G protein-coupled receptor-X2 (MRGPRX2). Using pertussis toxins and YM-254890, we demonstrated that SP induces Ca^{2+} mobilization and degranulation via both the Gαi and Gαq family of G proteins in rat basophilic leukemia (RBL-2H3) cells stably expressing MRGPRX2. To determine the roles of MRGPRX2's transmembrane (TM) and intracellular domains on SP-induced responses, we utilized information obtained from both structural modeling and naturally occurring MRGPRX2 missense variants. We found that highly conserved residues in TM6 (I225) and TM7 (Y279) of MRGPRX2 are essential for SP-induced Ca^{2+} mobilization and degranulation in transiently transfected RBL-2H3 cells. Cells expressing missense variants in the receptor's conserved residues (V123F and V282M) as well as intracellular loops (R138C and R141C) failed to respond to SP. By contrast, replacement of all five Ser/Thr residues with Ala and missense variants (S325L and L329Q) in MRGPRX2's carboxyl-terminus resulted in enhanced mast cell activation by SP when compared to the wild-type receptor. These findings suggest that MRGPRX2 utilizes conserved residues in its TM domains and intracellular loops for coupling to G proteins and likely undergoes desensitization via phosphorylation at Ser/Thr residues in its carboxyl-terminus. Furthermore, identification of gain and loss of function MRGPRX2 variants has important clinical implications for SP-mediated neurogenic inflammation and other chronic inflammatory diseases.

Keywords: mast cells; MRGPRX2; missense variants; substance P; neurogenic inflammation

1. Introduction

Mast cells (MCs) are tissue-resident granulocytes of hematopoietic origin that play a pivotal role in the inflammatory processes due to their ability to release a wide array of proinflammatory mediators and recruit various immune cells upon stimulation [1–3]. MCs are widely distributed throughout the body and are found in close proximity to peripheral nerve endings in various tissues including skin, gastrointestinal mucosa, and respiratory tract [4]. In addition to close anatomic localization, accumulating evidence suggests bidirectional functional communication between MCs and neurons, providing a significant link between the immune and nervous systems [4,5]. MC-derived mediators such as histamine and tryptase activate receptors on sensory nerve endings, resulting in the release of neuropeptides including substance P (SP) which, in turn, evokes further MC activation [5–8].

Activation of MCs by SP leads to their degranulation, resulting in vasodilation, plasma extravasation, and the recruitment of immune cells including lymphocytes, neutrophils, and macrophages [5,9,10]. Immune cell recruitment further amplifies local inflammatory responses and facilitates peripheral nerve sensitization, which are critical characteristics of neurogenic inflammation [10]. SP-induced MC activation has been implicated in the pathogenesis of pain and many chronic inflammatory diseases such as sickle cell disease [11], atopic dermatitis [12], and chronic idiopathic urticaria [13].

The biological effects of SP were previously thought to be mediated via its canonical neurokinin-1 receptor (NK-1R) [9,14,15]. Several antagonists of this receptor have been developed as potential therapies for a variety of conditions including chemotherapy-induced nausea, inflammation, and pain. While NK-1R antagonists are effective in the treatment of chemotherapy-induced nausea and vomiting, they fail to demonstrate significant anti-inflammatory and analgesic effects [14,15]. This raises the interesting possibility that the nociceptive and proinflammatory actions of SP may be mediated via alternative mechanisms. Recent studies have demonstrated that SP activates human and murine MCs via Mas-related G protein-coupled receptor-X2 (MRGPRX2) and Mrgprb2, respectively [16,17]. Expression of MRGPRX2 is upregulated in human skin MCs of patients with chronic idiopathic urticaria when compared to healthy individuals [13]. A recent study by Serhan et al. [12] demonstrated that SP released from sensory neurons activates murine skin MCs via Mrgprb2 and contributes to the development of atopic dermatitis. Furthermore, Green et al. [18] showed that inflammatory and thermal hyperalgesia requires Mrgprb2-mediated recruitment of immune cells at the injury site. They also demonstrated that SP promotes the release of multiple pro-inflammatory cytokines and chemokines from human MCs via activation of MRGPRX2 [18]. Taken together, these findings suggest that MRGPRX2/Mrgprb2 participate in neurogenic inflammation, chronic urticaria, atopic dermatitis, and pain [12,13,18,19]. However, the molecular mechanism by which MRGPRX2 is activated in response to SP has not been determined.

All G protein-coupled receptors (GPCRs) are structurally similar containing seven transmembrane (TM) α-helices. Binding of ligands to the receptor from the extracellular site promotes the opening of TM6, which results in conformational changes in the cytoplasmic side of membrane, leading to allosteric activation of G proteins [20–22]. Venkatakrishnan et al. [22] analyzed the pattern of contact between structurally equivalent residues from the crystal structures of 27 class A GPCRs. From this analysis, it became clear that, upon receptor activation, there is a highly conserved reorganization of residue contacts in TM3 (3x46), TM6 (6x37), and TM7 (7x53) [22]. In this GPCR numbering scheme, the first number denotes the TM domains (1–7) and the second number indicates the residue position relative to the most conserved position, which is assigned the number 50 [23,24]. Thus, 3x46 denotes a residue in TM3, which is at four positions before the most conserved residue (3x50). Similarly, 7x53 denotes a residue in TM7, which is at three positions after the most conserved residue (7x50). Mutations of residues 3x46, 6x37, and 7x53 in a number of class A GPCRs result in significant reduction of G protein activation and downstream signaling, confirming the roles of these positions for the activation of different G proteins [22,25]. In addition to TM domains, conserved residues present in the second intracellular loop (ICL2) of a number of class A GPCRs are involved in coupling to G proteins [26,27]. MRGPRX2 is a member of the class A GPCR family, but the possibility that residues 3x46, 6x37, and 7x53 and conserved residues present in its ICL2 couple to G proteins to cause MC activation has not been tested.

In addition to G proteins, most class A GPCRs signal via another pathway that involves phosphorylation of the receptors at Ser/Thr residues in their carboxyl-terminus by GPCR kinases and the recruitment of adapter proteins known as β-arrestins [28–31]. This pathway has been implicated in the regulation of GPCR desensitization (uncoupling of the G protein from the receptor), endocytosis, and internalization [30]. GPCR agonists that preferentially activate G proteins are known as G protein-biased and those activate β-arrestin are known as β-arrestin-biased agonists. However, agonists that activate both pathways are known as balanced agonists [32]. Our original studies using host defense peptide LL-37 as a ligand for MRGPRX2 demonstrated that the receptor is resistant to agonist-induced phosphorylation and desensitization, indicating that it acts as a G protein-biased agonist for the receptor [33]. However, our more recent studies demonstrated that distinct ligands act as balanced or G protein-biased agonists for MRGPRX2 [32]. The carboxyl terminus of MRGPRX2 contains five Ser/Thr residues. However, the possibility that these potential phosphorylation sites contribute to receptor regulation by SP has not been determined.

Molecular modeling and mutagenesis studies led to the identification of a ligand binding pocket for a number of MRGPRX2 agonists [34–36]. We recently demonstrated that naturally occurring missense variants in MRGPRX2's predicted ligand binding pocket result in loss of function phenotype of MC activation in response to a diverse group of ligands including the neuropeptide SP [36]. The goal of the present study was to utilize both structural information derived crystal structures of other GPCRs and naturally occurring MRGPRX2 missense variants to determine the roles of MRGPRX2's TM and intracellular (IC) domains on MC activation by SP. The data presented herein identify a number of gain and loss of function of missense variants of MRGPRX2. These findings have important clinical implications with regard to resistance and susceptibility for developing MC-mediated neurogenic inflammation, pain, atopic dermatitis, and chronic urticaria [12,13,18,19].

2. Results

2.1. MRGPRX2 Mediates SP-Induced MC Activation via Both Gαi and Gαq

In addition to SP, amphipathic peptides such as the cathelicidin LL-37 and human β-defensin-3 activate human MCs via MRGPRX2 [33,37]. We previously showed that while degranulation in response to these agonists is blocked by pertussis toxin (PTx), Ca^{2+} mobilization is not [33,37]. These findings suggest that MRGPRX2 may couple to both PTx-sensitive (Gαi) and insensitive (Gαq) G proteins. To determine the G protein specificity for SP-induced MRGPRX2-mediated responses, we utilized a pharmacological approach using a Gαi-specific inhibitor (PTx) and a Gαq-specific inhibitor (YM-254890) [38]. Rat basophilic leukemia (RBL-2H3), a commonly used model for MC activation, does not endogenously express MRGPRX2. We therefore utilized RBL-2H3 cells stably expressing MRGPRX2 (RBL-MRGPRX2) to determine the effects of SP on MC activation [33,37,39].

SP has been shown to induce MRGPRX2-mediated MC degranulation in a dose-dependent manner [16]. We found that at a low concentration of SP (0.1 μM), PTx caused substantial inhibition of MC degranulation. However, at higher concentrations of SP, only about 50% of MC degranulation was inhibited by PTx (Figure 1A). A similar inhibitory profile was also observed for the Gαq inhibitor, YM-254890, but the extent of inhibition was lower at high concentrations of SP (1 and 10 μM) (Figure 1A). However, SP-induced degranulation was abolished in cells treated with both PTx and YM-254890 (Figure 1A). We also tested the effects of PTx and YM-254890 alone and in combination on SP-induced Ca^{2+} mobilization. Similar to degranulation, we found that PTx or YM-254890 caused partial inhibition of the SP response but a combination of both inhibitors resulted in almost complete inhibition of SP-induced Ca^{2+} response (Figure 1B). Taken together, these findings suggest that MRGPRX2 utilizes both the Gαi and Gαq families of G proteins for SP-induced MC degranulation.

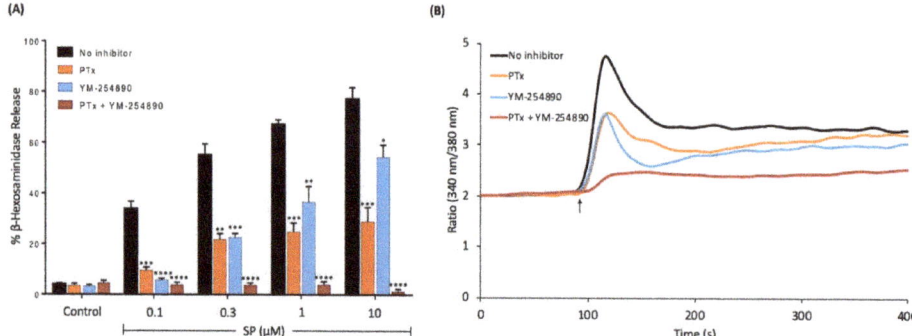

Figure 1. Effects of pertussis toxin (PTx) and YM-254890 on substance P (SP)-induced degranulation and Ca^{2+} mobilization in RBL-2H3 cells stably expressing MRGPRX2, (RBL-MRGPRX2). (**A**) Cells were cultured overnight in the absence or presence of PTx (100 ng/mL, 16 h), washed and incubated with or without YM-254890 (10 μM) for 5 min. Cells were then exposed to a buffer (control) or different concentrations of SP for 30 min, and β-hexosaminidase release was determined. All data points are the mean ± SEM of at least three experiments performed in triplicate. (**B**) Cells were cultured overnight in the absence or presence of PTx (100 ng/mL, 16 h), then loaded with Fura-2 and intracellular Ca^{2+} mobilizations in response to SP (1 μM) were determined. To determine the effect of Gαq, cells were incubated with YM-254890 (10 μM) for 5 min before stimulating with SP. Data shown are representative of three independent experiments. Statistical significance was determined by the nonparametric *t*-test and two-way ANOVA. * $p \leq 0.05$, ** $p \leq 0.01$, *** $p \leq 0.001$, and **** $p \leq 0.0001$.

2.2. Mutations of the Highly Conserved Residues 3x46, 6x37, and 7x53 in MRGPRX2 Lead to a Significant Reduction in SP-Induced MC Activation

Based on structural and computational studies, it was proposed that positions 3x46, 6x37, and 7x53 are conserved among class A GPCRs and likely participate in G protein coupling [22]. Amino acids at these positions in MRGPRX2 were identified from the GPCR database (GPCRdb) [24]. Residues at positions 3x46, 6x37, and 7x53 in MRGPRX2 are Val, Ile, and Tyr, respectively. Notably, these residues are either large hydrophobic or aromatic residues which are likely to fulfill the van der Waals criterion and facilitate contact formation during the receptor conformational rearrangement [22].

To determine if these residues in MRGPRX2 contribute to SP-induced MC activation, we first constructed single Ala substitution mutations at these positions, namely V123A, I225A, and Y279A, respectively (Figure 2A,B). We then generated transient transfectants in RBL-2H3 cells. Flow cytometry analysis using phycoerythrin (PE)-conjugated anti-MRGPRX2 antibody showed that these point mutations did not adversely affection cell surface receptor expression (Figure 2C). Interestingly, cells expressing V123A mutant responded normally to SP for Ca^{2+} mobilization but degranulation was inhibited by ~50% when compared to the wild-type (WT) receptor (Figure 2D,E). Although the mutants I225A and Y279A expressed normally on the cell surface (Figure 2C), they did not respond to SP for Ca^{2+} mobilization or degranulation (Figure 2D,E).

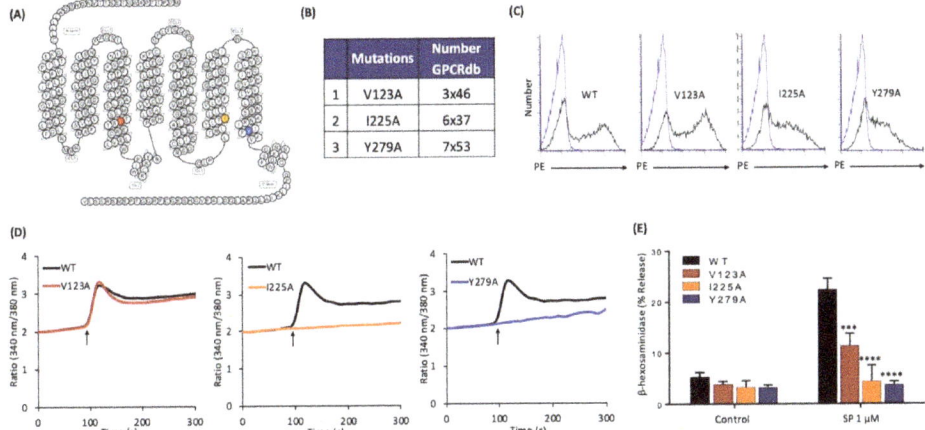

Figure 2. Effects of mutations at MRGPRX2's highly conserved positions within transmembrane domains (V123A, I225A, and Y279A) on cell surface expression, SP-induced Ca^{2+} mobilization, and degranulation in transiently transfected RBL-2H3 cells. (**A**) Snake diagram of secondary structure of MRGPRX2. Each circle represents amino acid residue with one letter code. Solid red, yellow, and blue backgrounds denote the residues at positions 3x46 (V123), 6x37 (I225), and 7x53 (Y279), respectively; (**B**) amino acid change for each MRGPRX2 mutant.; (**C**) RBL-2H3 cells transiently expressing wild-type (WT)-MRGPRX2 and its mutants were incubated with phycoerythrin (PE)-anti-MRGPRX2 antibody and cell surface receptor expression was determined by flow cytometry. Representative histograms for WT/mutant (black line) and control untransfected cells (blue line) are shown; (**D**) cells expressing WT-MRGPRX2 and its mutants were loaded with Fura-2 and intracellular Ca^{2+} mobilization in response to SP (1 μM) was determined. Data shown are representative of three independent experiments; (**E**) cells were exposed to a buffer (control) or SP (1 μM) for 30 min, and β-hexosaminidase release was determined. All data points are the mean ± SEM of at least three experiments performed in triplicate. Statistical significance was determined by a nonparametric *t*-test. *** $p \leq 0.001$ and **** $p \leq 0.0001$.

2.3. Naturally Occurring Missense MRGPRX2 Variants at or Near the Conserved Residues, V123F and V282M, Display Loss of Function Phenotype for SP-Induced MC Activation

Next, we searched the GPCRdb [24] to determine if there were any missense MRGPRX2 variants present in the human population with mutations at or near position 3x46, 6x36, or 7x53. We identified three MRGPRX2 variants, namely V123F (3x46), T224A (6x36), and V282M (7x56) (Figure 3A,B). Allele frequency for each variant is shown in Figure 3B. We used the site-directed mutagenesis approach to generate cDNAs encoding each of these variants, which were then transiently transfected in RBL-2H3 cells. Flow cytometry analysis demonstrated that MRGPRX2 and all its variants were expressed on the cell surface (Figure 3C). SP-induced Ca^{2+} mobilization was partially reduced in cells expressing the variant V123F when compared to the WT receptor, but degranulation was completely inhibited (Figure 3D,E). However, cells expressing the variant T224A responded normally to SP for Ca^{2+} mobilization and degranulation (Figure 3B,D,E). By contrast, V282M variant was resistant to both SP-induced Ca^{2+} mobilization and degranulation (Figure 3B,D,E).

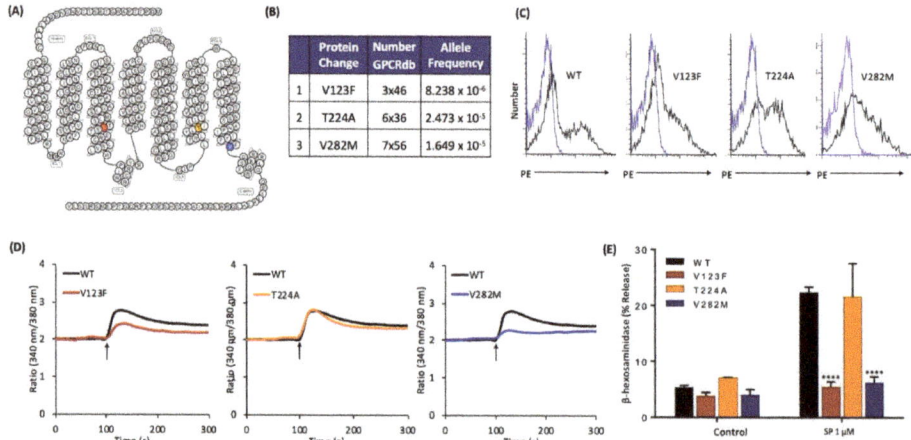

Figure 3. Effects of naturally occurring MRGPRX2 variants at the receptor's conserved transmembrane domains (V123F, T224A, and V282M) on SP-induced responses in transiently transfected RBL-2H3 cells. (**A**) Snake diagram of secondary structure of MRGPRX2. Each circle represents amino acid residue with one letter code. Solid red, yellow, and blue backgrounds denote the naturally occurring MRGPRX2 variants V123F, T224A, and V282M, respectively; (**B**) amino acid change for each MRGPRX2 variant with allele frequency; (**C**) cell surface expression of WT-MRGPRX2 and its variants was determined by flow cytometry using PE-anti-MRGPRX2 antibody. Representative histograms for WT/variant (black line) and control untransfected cells (blue line) are shown; (**D**) cells expressing WT-MRGPRX2 and its variants were loaded with Fura-2 and intracellular Ca^{2+} mobilization in response to SP (1 μM) was determined. Data shown are representative of three independent experiments; (**E**) cells were exposed to a buffer (control) or SP (1 μM) for 30 min, and β-hexosaminidase release was determined. All data points are the mean ± SEM of at least three experiments performed in triplicate. Statistical significance was determined by nonparametric t test. **** $p \leq 0.0001$.

2.4. Naturally Occurring Missense MRGPRX2 Variants at the Second Intracellular Loop, R138C and R141C, Display Loss of Function Phenotype for SP-Induced MC Activation

Apart from conformational changes in TM helices, recent crystallography and spectroscopy studies on GPCR-heterotrimeric G protein complexes have shown that intracellular loops of the receptors also interact with G proteins and are important for G protein activation [27,40]. Thus, we further searched for naturally occurring missense MRGPRX2 variants in the receptor's intracellular loops and were able to identify four missense variants within ICL2 (Figure 4A,B). cDNAs encoding these variants were generated and transiently transfected in RBL-2H3 cells. Flow cytometry analysis demonstrated that all four variants expressed on the cell surface (Figure 4C). We found that Y137H and R140C variants responded to SP for Ca^{2+} mobilization and degranulation similar to the WT receptor (Figure 4D,E). By contrast, SP failed to activate these responses in cells expressing R138C and R141C variants (Figure 4D,E).

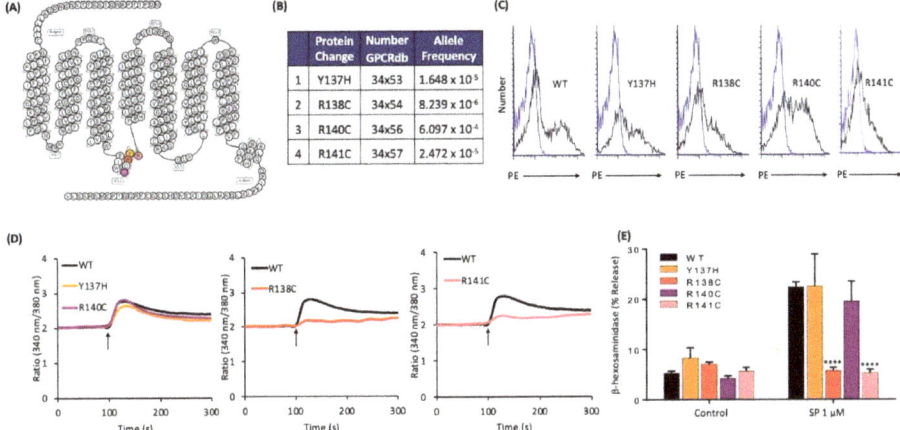

Figure 4. Effects of naturally occurring MRGPRX2 variants at the receptor's intracellular loops (Y137H, R138C, R140C, and R141C) on SP-induced responses in transiently transfected RBL-2H3 cells. (**A**) Snake diagram of secondary structure of MRGPRX2. Each circle represents amino acid residue with one letter code. Solid yellow, red, purple, and pink backgrounds denote the naturally occurring MRGPRX2 variants; (**B**) amino acid change for each MRGPRX2 variant with allele frequency; (**C**) cell surface expression of WT-MRGPRX2 and its variants was determined by flow cytometry using PE-anti MRGPRX2 antibody. Representative histograms for WT/variant (black line) and control untransfected cells (blue line) are shown; (**D**) cells expressing WT-MRGPRX2 and its variants were loaded with Fura-2 and intracellular Ca^{2+} mobilization in response to SP (1 µM) was determined. Data shown are representative of three independent experiments; (**E**) cells were exposed to a buffer (control) or SP (1 µM) for 30 min, and β-hexosaminidase release was determined. All data points are the mean ± SEM of at least three experiments performed in triplicate. Statistical significance was determined by a nonparametric *t*-test. **** $p \leq 0.0001$.

2.5. Mutations in Potential Phosphorylation Sites of MRGPRX2 Leads to Enhanced MC Activation in Response to SP

Phosphorylation of GPCRs by GPCR kinases provides an important mechanism for their desensitization [28,29,31]. Human MRGPRX2 possesses five potential phosphorylation sites at its carboxyl-terminus. To determine the role of MRGPRX2 phosphorylation on SP-induced responses, we generated cDNAs encoding an MRGPRX2 mutant in which all Ser/Thr residues were replaced with alanine (ΔST-MRGPRX2) (Figure 5A,B). Transiently transfected RBL-2H3 cells demonstrated reduced cell surface expression of ΔST-MRGPRX2, when compared to the WT receptor (Figure 5C). Despite this, SP induced greater Ca^{2+} mobilization and degranulation in cells expressing ΔST-MRGPRX2 when compared to the WT receptor (Figure 5D,E).

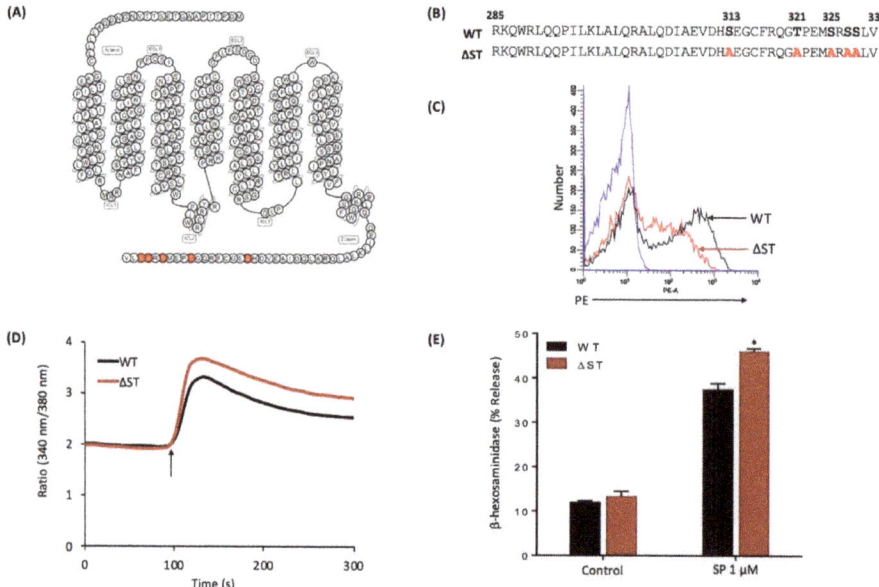

Figure 5. Effects of Ser/Thr residues on MRGPRX2's carboxyl-terminus on cell surface expression, SP-induced Ca^{2+} mobilization, and degranulation in transiently transfected RBL-2H3 cells. (**A**) Snake diagram of secondary structure of MRGPRX2. Each circle represents amino acid residue with one letter code. Solid red backgrounds denote Ser/Thr residues; (**B**) schematic representation of the carboxyl-terminus of MRGPRX2 (WT) and a phosphorylation-deficient mutant in which all Ser/Thr were replaced with Ala (ΔST-MRGPRX2); (**C**) cell surface expression of WT and ΔST-MRGPRX2 was determined by flow cytometry using PE-anti-MRGPRX2 antibody. Representative histograms for WT-MRGPRX2 (black line), ΔST-MRGPRX2 (red line), and control untransfected cells (blue line) are shown; (**D**) cells expressing WT and ΔST-MRGPRX2 were loaded with Fura-2 and intracellular Ca^{2+} mobilization in response to SP (1 μM) was determined. Data shown are representative of three independent experiments; (**E**) cells were exposed to a buffer (control) or SP (1 μM) for 30 min, and β-hexosaminidase release was determined. All data points are the mean ± SEM of at least three experiments performed in triplicate. Statistical significance was determined by a nonparametric *t*-test. * $p \leq 0.05$.

2.6. Naturally Occurring Missense MRGPRX2 Variants at its Carboxyl-Terminus, S325L and L329Q, Display Gain of Function Phenotype for SP-Induced MC Activation

Search of the GPCRdb [24] led to the identification of four missense variants in the carboxyl-terminus of MRGPRX2 (Figure 6A,B), of which one variant results in the replacement of Ser with Leu (S325L). Flow cytometry analysis of transfected RBL-2H3 cells demonstrated equivalent cell surface expression of all variants (Figure 6C). Cells expressing Q305R and D311H variants responded similarly to SP for Ca^{2+} mobilization and degranulation when compared to the WT receptor (Figure 6D,E). By contrast, S325L and L329Q variants displayed higher responses to SP for both Ca^{2+} mobilization and degranulation (Figure 6D,E).

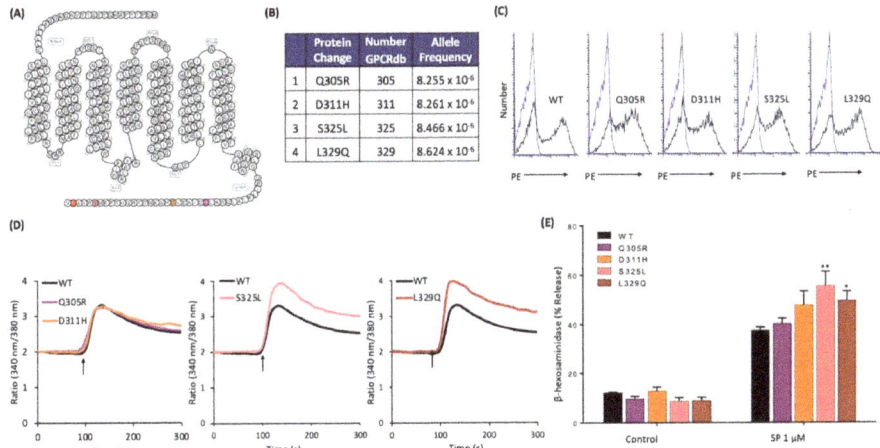

Figure 6. Effects of naturally occurring MRGPRX2 variants within the receptor's carboxyl-terminus (Q305R, D311H, S325L, and L329Q) on SP-induced responses in transiently transfected RBL-2H3 cells. (**A**) Snake diagram of secondary structure of MRGPRX2. Each circle represents amino acid residue with one letter code. Solid purple, orange, pink, and red backgrounds denote the naturally occurring missense variants Q305R, D311H, S325L, and L329Q, respectively; (**B**) amino acid change for each MRGPRX2 variant with allele frequency; (**C**) cell surface expression of WT-MRGPRX2 and its variants was determined by flow cytometry using PE-anti MRGPRX2 antibody. Representative histograms for WT/variant (black line) and control untransfected cells (blue line) are shown; (**D**) cells expressing WT-MRGPRX2 and its variants were loaded with Fura-2 and intracellular Ca^{2+} mobilization in response to SP (1 µM) was determined. Data shown are representative of three independent experiments; (**E**) cells were exposed to buffer (control) or SP (1 µM) for 30 min, and β-hexosaminidase release was determined. All data points are the mean ± SEM of at least three experiments performed in triplicate. Statistical significance was determined by a nonparametric *t*-test. * $p \leq 0.05$ and ** $p \leq 0.01$.

3. Discussion

Unique features of MRGPRX2 that differentiate it from other class A GPCRs are that it is expressed predominantly in one subtype of MCs and responds to a variety of cationic ligands, including SP [18,41–43]. Structure-based computational modeling and site directed mutagenesis approach have been used to show that negatively charged residues Glu164 (E164) in TM4 (4x60) and Asp184 (D184) in TM5 (5x36) are important for binding opioids and SP [34–36]. We recently showed that missense variants in the MRGPRX2's ligand-binding pocket (G165E and D184H) fail to respond to a variety of cationic ligands including SP, human β-defensin-3, and icatibant (bradykinin B2 receptor antagonist) for receptor activation [36]. In the present study, we utilized information derived from the comparison of crystal structures of a number of class A GPCRs, as well as naturally occurring missense variants in MRGPRX2's predicted G protein coupling domains and potential phosphorylation sites to identify a number of gain and loss of function variants. These findings have important implications for SP/MRGPRX2-mediated conditions such as neurogenic inflammation, pain, atopic dermatitis, and chronic idiopathic urticaria [12,13,18,19].

In the inactive state of class, A GPCRs, the residue at 6x37 is in contact with a conserved hydrophobic residue at position 3x46 [22]. Upon receptor activation, this interaction is rearranged so that residue at 3x46 breaks contact with residue 637 and forms a new contact with a tyrosine residue, Tyr7x53, within the highly conserved NPXXY motif of TM7 [21,22,26]. This rearrangement results in the activation of G proteins. Accordingly, Ala substitution of each of these residues (3x46, 6x37, and 7x53) of the vasopressin V2 receptor results in its uncoupling from Gαs and Gαq [22]. We showed that MRGPRX2 coupled to both Gαi and Gαq families of G proteins for Ca^{2+} mobilization and degranulation in response to SP. Thus, PTx (a Gαi-specific inhibitor) in combination with YM-254890 compound (a Gαq-specific inhibitor) completely inhibited SP-induced MC activation. By contrast, using either PTx or YM-254890 alone was unable to abolish Ca^{2+} and degranulation responses to SP. Of note, many GPCRs have been shown to display distinct intracellular signaling and cellular responses depend on agonist concentrations [44]. It is possible that low-dose SP induces MRGPRX2 to preferentially couple to either Gαi or Gαq, whereas a high concentration of SP mediates MRGPRX2 conformational change to couple to both G proteins. The data presented herein suggest that similar to other class A GPCRs, residues 3x46, 6x37, and 7x53 in MRGPRX2 contribute to coupling to Gαi and Gαq families of G proteins and that naturally occurring missense variants within or near some of these highly conserved residues may contribute to loss of function phenotype for MC activation by SP. One interesting finding of the present study was that while V123A (3x46) mutation resulted in partial inhibition of SP-induced degranulation, the missense variant V123F (3x46) failed to respond to SP for Ca^{2+} mobilization or degranulation. These findings suggest that the presence of a bulky Phe group in the missense variant V123F less effectively breaks the interaction of 3x46 with 6x37 or blocks the formation of new contact Tyr residue at 7x53. Another interesting finding was that while cells expressing I225A mutation (6x37) were resistant to SP-induced Ca^{2+} mobilization and degranulation, a missense mutation T224A responded normally to SP. However, a missense V282M mutation three amino acids way from the Tyr7x53 in the conserved NPXXY motif resulted in complete loss of function phenotype for SP-induced MC degranulation. This finding likely emphasizes the importance of this region of MRGPRX2 for coupling to G proteins.

Additionally, we identified four missense MRGPRX2 variants at the predicted G protein coupling regions within its ICL2. Crystallography and cryogenic electron microscopy studies of GPCR-heterotrimeric G protein complexes have provided evidence that this ICL interacts with Gα subunit to promote GDP dissociation and subsequent GTP binding, resulting in activation of G proteins [27,40]. Mutations of ICL2 in $β_2$ adrenergic receptor have been shown to impair G protein coupling [45]. Here, we found that cells expressing R138C and R141C variants in this region displayed loss of function phenotype in response to SP. By contrast, other MRGPRX2 variants (Y137H and R140C) had no effect on SP-induced MC activation. Intriguingly, this region has also been identified as a cholesterol recognition amino acid consensus (CRAC) motif of MRGPRX2. Cholesterol-rich microdomains (lipid rafts) are membrane microdomains enriched in cholesterol and glycerophospholipids that mediate organization and function of many membrane receptors and biomolecules including GPCRs [46]. The orientation and organization of membrane proteins present in the lipid raft allow greater efficiency and specificity of signal transduction by facilitating protein–protein interactions and preventing crosstalk between competing pathways [46]. Given that MRGPRX2 contains the CRAC motif, it is possible that lipid rafts also contribute to MRGPRX2 activation and G protein coupling. Positively charged Arg residue of MRGPRX2 (R138 and R141) might be necessary to interact with negatively-charged hydroxyl group of cholesterol for proper MRGPRX2 functioning. Substitution of this amino acid with neutral amino acid Cys may disrupt the interaction with lipid raft domains, resulting in loss of function phenotype. The interaction between MRGPRX2 and lipid rafts will be the subject of further investigation to delineate the role of lipid rafts in MRGPRX2 signaling.

While GPCR signaling is essential for regulating physiological function of cells, overstimulation can be deleterious and contributes to pathologic conditions. Thus, following their activation, GPCRs undergo desensitization via phosphorylation of Ser/Thr residues at their carboxyl-terminus [26,31]. Binding of β-arrestin to phosphorylated GPCRs has been implicated in receptor desensitization, endocytosis, and internalization [26,30,31]. It also initiates a distinct downstream signaling pathway known as β-arrestin-mediated activation [26,30,31]. Here, we showed that mutation of all possible phosphorylation sites of MRGPRX2 (ΔST-MRGPRX2) leads to significantly higher SP-induced MC activation. We further examined the effects of naturally occurring missense MRGPRX2 mutations within the carboxyl-terminus. Of these, we identified one missense variant in which a potential phosphorylation site is mutated, S325L. Interestingly, cells expressing this variant exhibited gain of function phenotype for MC degranulation in response to SP. These findings are consistent with previous studies in β$_2$ adrenergic receptor that demonstrated the importance of distal phosphorylation residues for high-affinity β-arrestin binding and receptor desensitization [47]. Distinct GPCR phosphorylation sites have been proposed to be targeted by different GPCR kinases and establish a specific barcode that imparts distinct conformations to the recruited β-arrestin, thus regulating different functional activities, such as desensitization, internalization, and downstream signaling [47]. It is possible that the S325 of MRGPRX2 is responsible for receptor desensitization, thus mutation in this position leads to enhanced SP-induced responses due to impaired desensitization.

In addition, the carboxyl-terminus of MRGPRX2 contains a class I PDZ (PSD-95/Dlg/Zo1) recognition motif S/T-X-φ (where "φ" indicates hydrophobic amino acid and "X" indicates any amino acid). PDZ proteins have been implicated in regulating receptor desensitization, internalization, and signaling for several GPCRs such as β$_2$ adrenergic receptor, parathyroid hormone receptor, and opioid receptors [48]. For example, the PDZ protein, Na$^+$/H$^+$ exchanger regulatory factor 1 (NHERF1) has been shown to regulate type 1 parathyroid hormone receptor signaling by anchoring the receptor to the plasma membrane, thus restricting its desensitization and internalization [49]. Our lab previously demonstrated that these proteins also promote C3a-induced degranulation in human MCs [50]. Given that MRGPRX2 possesses a class I PDZ motif, it is possible that PDZ proteins such as NHERF1 contributes to the regulation of MRGPRX2. It is also possible that missense mutations in the receptor's PDZ motif may enhance the interaction with PDZ proteins, resulting in gain of function phenotype. Altogether, our findings herein indicate the significance of carboxyl-terminal residues for MRGPRX2 regulation and activation. The MRGPRX2 mutations at its carboxyl-terminus may lead to gain of function phenotype for SP-induced MC degranulation due to impaired receptor desensitization, enhanced interaction with PDZ proteins, or both.

Taken together, the data presented herein have identified mutations in MRGPRX2 at the regions involved in the receptor activation pathway. Missense MRGPRX2 mutations in the G protein-coupling regions in TMs and ICL2 fail to activate MC in response to SP, presumably due to impaired G protein coupling. By contrast, MRGPRX2 variants at the carboxyl-terminus, which is responsible for receptor phosphorylation and desensitization, lead to higher responses for MC activation. Thus, individuals with loss of function MRGPRX2 mutation, V123F, R138C, R141C, or V282M may display resistance to developing neurogenic inflammation and chronic inflammatory diseases. By contrast, individuals who harbor the gain of function variant, S325L or L329Q, may be more susceptible to develop these conditions.

4. Materials and Methods

4.1. Materials

All cell culture reagents were obtained from Invitrogen (Gaithersburg, MD, USA). Amaxa transfection kit (Kit V) was obtained from Lonza (Gaithersburg, MD, USA). Q5 Site-Directed Mutagenesis Kit was from New England BioLabs (Ipswich, MA). Substance P (SP) was from AnaSpec (Fremont, CA, USA). Pertussis toxin (PTx) was from List Biological Laboratories (Campbell, CA, USA). YM-254890 was from Wako Chemicals (Richmond, VA, USA) and p-nitrophenyl-N-acetyl-β-D-glucosamine (PNAG) was from Sigma-Aldrich (St. Louis, MO, USA). Fura-2 acetoxymethyl ester was from Abcam (Cambridge, MA, USA). PE-conjugated anti-MRGPRX2 antibody was from BioLegend (San Diego, CA, USA). MRGPRX2 plasmid encoding hemagglutinin (HA)-tagged human MRGPRX2 in pReceiver-M06 vector was obtained from GeneCopoeia (Rockville, MD, USA).

4.2. Cell Culture

Rat basophilic leukemia (RBL-2H3) cells were maintained as monolayer cultures in Dulbecco's modified Eagle's medium (DMEM) supplemented with 10% fetal bovine serum (FBS), L-glutamine (2 mM), penicillin (100 IU/mL), and streptomycin (100 µg/mL) at 37 °C with 5% CO_2 [51]. RBL-2H3 cells stably expressing MRGPRX2 (RBL-MRGPRX2) were maintained similarly in the presence of G-418 (1 mg/mL) [39].

4.3. Construction of MRGPRX2 Variants

Q5 site-directed mutagenesis kit (New England BioLabs, Ipswich, MA, USA) was used to generate MRGPRX2 variants in HA-tagged plasmid. To confirm the correct nucleotide sequences, each mutant was verified by DNA sequencing prior to transfection. The forward and reverse primers used for each variant are listed below.

V123A: Forward: 5'-CTGAGCACCGCCAGCACCGAG-3'
Reverse: 5'-CATGCTCAGGCCTGCAAG-3';
V123F: Forward: 5'-GCTGAGCACCTTCAGCACCGA-3'
Reverse: 5'-ATGCTCAGGCCTGCAAGG-3';
Y137H: Forward: 5'-GCCCATCTGGCATCGCTGCCG-3'
Reverse: 5'-CACAGGACGGACAGGCAG-3';
R138C: Forward: 5'-CATCTGGTATTGCTGCCGCCG-3'
Reverse: 5'-GGCCACAGGACGGACAGG-3';
R140C: Forward: 5'-GTATCGCTGCtGCCGCCCCAG-3'
Reverse: 5'-CAGATGGGCCACAGGACGG-3';
R141C: Forward: 5'-TCGCTGCCGCTGCCCCAGACA-3'
Reverse: 5'-TACCAGATGGGCCACAGGACGG-3';
T224A: Forward: 5'-GCTGTACCTGGCCATCCTGCT-3'
Reverse: 5'-CTGGTCAGTGGCAGACCC-3;
I225A: Forward: 5'-GTACCTGACCGCCCTGCTCACAGTGC-3'
Reverse: 5'-AGCCTGGTCAGTGGCAGA-3';
Y279A: Forward: 5'-CCCCATCATTGCCTTCTTCGTGG-3'
Reverse: 5'-TTGGCACTGCTGTTAAGAG-3';
V282M: Forward: 5'-TTACTTCTTCATGGGCTCTTTTAGG-3'
Reverse: 5'-ATGATGGGGTTGGCACTG-3';
Q305R: Forward: 5'-AGGGCTCTGCGGGACATTGCT-3'
Reverse: 5'-CTGGAGAGCCAGCTTGAG-3';
D311H: Forward: 5'-TGCTGAGGTGCATCACAGTGAAG-3'
Reverse: 5'-ATGTCCTGCAGAGCCCTC-3';
S325L: Forward: 5'-CCGGAGATGTTGAGAAGCAGTCTG-3'
Reverse: 5'-GGTGCCCTGACGGAAGCA-3';
L329Q: Forward: 5'-AGAAGCAGTCAGGTGTAGCTCGAG-3'
Reverse: 5'-CGACATCTCCGGGGTGCC-3'

MRGPRX2 phosphorylation-deficient mutant (Ser/Thr residues mutated to Ala; ∆ST-MRGPRX2) was generated by PCR. Construct was verified by DNA sequencing prior to transfection. The forward and reverse primers used are listed below.

∆ST-MRGPRX2: Forward: 5'-ACATCCGCGGACCATGTACCCTTACGACGTCCCAGACTACGCTGATCCAACCACCCCGGCCTGGGGAACAGAA-3'
Reverse: 5'-ACATCTCGAGCTACACCAGAGCGGCTCTCGCCATCTCCGGGGCGCCCTGACGGAAGCATCCTTCAGCGTGATC-3'

4.4. Generation of Cells Transiently Expressing MRGPRX2 and its Variants

RBL-2H3 cells transiently expressing MRGPRX2 or its missense variants were generated as described previously [36]. Briefly, cells (2×10^6) were transfected with 2 µg of HA-tagged plasmid using the Amaxa Nucleofector Device and Amaxa Kit V according to the manufacturer's protocol. Cells were used within 16–20 h after transfection.

To detect cell surface MRGPRX2 and its variants' expression, transfected RBL-2H3 cells (0.5×10^6) were incubated with PE-conjugated anti-MRGPRX2 antibody for 30 min at 4 °C in the dark, washed in FACS buffer (PBS containing 2% FCS and 0.02% sodium azide), and fixed in 1.5% paraformaldehyde. Cells were acquired using a BD LSR II flow cytometer (San Jose, CA, USA). Results were analyzed using WinList software, version 8.

4.5. Degranulation Assay

The degranulation was measured by β-hexosaminidase release as described previously [51]. Briefly, transfected RBL-2H3 cells (5×10^4 cells per well) were seeded into a 96-well, white, clear-bottom cell culture plate and incubated overnight in a 37 °C incubator with 5% CO_2. To determine the inhibitory effects of PTx and YM-254890 on MC degranulation, cells were pretreated with PTx (100 ng/mL, 16 h) and/or YM-254890 (10 μM, 5 min) prior to stimulation with SP. Cells were then washed twice and suspended in a total volume of 50 μL HEPES buffer containing 0.1% bovine serum albumin (BSA). Experimental groups were stimulated with SP for 30 min at 37 °C. Cells without treatment were designated as controls. To determine the total β-hexosaminidase release, unstimulated cells were lysed in 50 μL of 0.1% Triton X-100. Aliquots (20 μL) of supernatants or cell lysates were incubated with 20 μL of 1 mM p-nitrophenyl-*N*-acetyl-β-*D*-glucosamine (PNAG) for 1 h at 37 °C. The reaction was stopped by adding 250 μL of stop buffer (0.1 M Na_2CO_3/0.1 M $NaHCO_3$). The β-hexosaminidase release was assessed by measuring absorbance at 405 nm using Versamax microplate spectrophotometer (Molecular Devices, San Jose, CA, USA).

4.6. Calcium Mobilization Assay

Transfected RBL-2H3 cells (2×10^6) were loaded with 1 μM Fura-2 acetoxymethyl ester for 30 min at 37 °C, followed by de-esterification in HEPES-buffered saline for additional 15 min at room temperature. Cells were washed, resuspended in 1.5 mL of HEPES-buffered saline containing 0.1% BSA, and then stimulated with SP. In some experiments, cells were treated with PTx (100 ng/mL, 16 h) and/or YM-254890 (10 μM, 5 min), and then stimulated with SP. Ca^{2+} mobilization was determined using a Hitachi F-2700 Fluorescence Spectrophotometer with dual excitation wavelength of 340 and 380 nm, and an emission wavelength of 510 nm.

4.7. Statistical Analysis

Data shown are mean ± standard error of the mean (SEM) values derived from at least three independent experiments. GraphPad Prism scientific software version 6.07 was used for statistical analysis. Statistical significance was determined using a nonparametric *t*-test and two-way ANOVA due to non-normal distribution data. Differences were considered as statistically significant at a value of * $p \leq 0.05$, ** $p \leq 0.01$, *** $p \leq 0.001$, and **** $p \leq 0.0001$.

Author Contributions: Conceptualization, H.A.; investigation, C.C.N.A., S.R., I.A., and A.G.; resources, H.A.; writing—original draft preparation, C.C.N.A. and S.R.; writing—review and editing, H.A.; supervision, H.A.; project administration, H.A.; funding acquisition, H.A.

Funding: This work was supported by National Institutes of Health Grant R01-AI124182 to H.A.

Acknowledgments: We thank the FACS core facilities of the School of Dental Medicine, University of Pennsylvania, for flow cytometry data acquisition and analysis. We also thank Hariharan Subramanian for generating MRGPRX2 phosphorylation-deficient mutant (ΔST-MRGPRX2).

Conflicts of Interest: The authors declare no conflict of interest.

Abbreviations

MC	Mast cell
SP	Substance P
NK-1R	Neurokinin-1 receptor
MRGPRX2	Mas-related G protein-coupled receptor-X2
GPCR	G protein-coupled receptor
TM	Transmembrane
ICL	Intracellular loop
PTx	Pertussis toxin
RBL-2H3	Rat basophilic leukemia-2H3 cells
RBL-MRGPRX2	RBL-2H3 cells stably expressing MRGPRX2
GPCRdb	GPCR database
WT	Wild-type
PE	Phycoerythrin
CRAC	Cholesterol recognition amino acid consensus
NHERF	Na^+/H^+ exchanger regulatory factor

References

1. Theoharides, T.C.; Alysandratos, K.D.; Angelidou, A.; Delivanis, D.A.; Sismanopoulos, N.; Zhang, B.; Asadi, S.; Vasiadi, M.; Weng, Z.; Miniati, A.; et al. Mast Cells and Inflammation. *Biochim. Biophys. Acta* **2012**, *1822*, 21–33. [CrossRef] [PubMed]
2. Choi, H.W.; Suwanpradid, J.; Kim, I.H.; Staats, H.F.; Haniffa, M.; MacLeod, A.S.; Abraham, S.N. Perivascular Dendritic Cells Elicit Anaphylaxis by Relaying Allergens to Mast Cells Via Microvesicles. *Science* **2018**, *362*. [CrossRef] [PubMed]
3. Karhausen, J.; Abraham, S.N. How Mast Cells make Decisions. *J. Clin. Invest.* **2016**, *126*, 3735–3738. [CrossRef] [PubMed]
4. Kleij, H.P.; Bienenstock, J. Significance of Conversation between Mast Cells and Nerves. *Allergy Asthma Clin. Immunol.* **2005**, *1*, 65–80. [CrossRef] [PubMed]
5. Forsythe, P. Mast Cells in Neuroimmune Interactions. *Trends Neurosci.* **2019**, *42*, 43–55. [CrossRef]
6. Gupta, K.; Harvima, I.T. Mast Cell-Neural Interactions Contribute to Pain and Itch. *Immunol. Rev.* **2018**, *282*, 168–187. [CrossRef]
7. Shim, W.S.; Oh, U. Histamine-Induced Itch and its Relationship with Pain. *Mol. Pain* **2008**, *4*, 2–29. [CrossRef]
8. Kulka, M.; Sheen, C.H.; Tancowny, B.P.; Grammer, L.C.; Schleimer, R.P. Neuropeptides Activate Human Mast Cell Degranulation and Chemokine Production. *Immunology* **2008**, *123*, 398–410. [CrossRef]
9. Mashaghi, A.; Marmalidou, A.; Tehrani, M.; Grace, P.M.; Pothoulakis, C.; Dana, R. Neuropeptide Substance P and the Immune Response. *Cell Mol. Life Sci.* **2016**, *73*, 4249–4264. [CrossRef]
10. Ren, K.; Dubner, R. Interactions between the Immune and Nervous Systems in Pain. *Nat. Med.* **2010**, *16*, 1267–1276. [CrossRef]
11. Sagi, V.; Mittal, A.; Gupta, M.; Gupta, K. Immune Cell Neural Interactions and their Contributions to Sickle Cell Disease. *Neurosci. Lett.* **2019**, *699*, 167–171. [CrossRef]
12. Serhan, N.; Basso, L.; Sibilano, R.; Petitfils, C.; Meixiong, J.; Bonnart, C.; Reber, L.L.; Marichal, T.; Starkl, P.; Cenac, N.; et al. House Dust Mites Activate Nociceptor-Mast Cell Clusters to Drive Type 2 Skin Inflammation. *Nat. Immunol.* **2019**. [CrossRef] [PubMed]
13. Fujisawa, D.; Kashiwakura, J.; Kita, H.; Kikukawa, Y.; Fujitani, Y.; Sasaki-Sakamoto, T.; Kuroda, K.; Nunomura, S.; Hayama, K.; Terui, T.; et al. Expression of Mas-Related Gene X2 on Mast Cells is Upregulated in the Skin of Patients with Severe Chronic Urticaria. *J. Allergy Clin. Immunol.* **2014**, *134*, 62–633.e9. [CrossRef] [PubMed]
14. Garcia-Recio, S.; Gascon, P. Biological and Pharmacological Aspects of the NK1-Receptor. *Biomed. Res. Int.* **2015**, *2015*, 495704.
15. Borsook, D.; Upadhyay, J.; Klimas, M.; Schwarz, A.J.; Coimbra, A.; Baumgartner, R.; George, E.; Potter, W.Z.; Large, T.; Bleakman, D.; et al. Decision-Making using fMRI in Clinical Drug Development: Revisiting NK-1 Receptor Antagonists for Pain. *Drug Discov. Today* **2012**, *17*, 964–973. [CrossRef] [PubMed]

16. Tatemoto, K.; Nozaki, Y.; Tsuda, R.; Konno, S.; Tomura, K.; Furuno, M.; Ogasawara, H.; Edamura, K.; Takagi, H.; Iwamura, H.; et al. Immunoglobulin E-Independent Activation of Mast Cell is Mediated by Mrg Receptors. *Biochem. Biophys. Res. Commun.* **2006**, *349*, 1322–1328.
17. McNeil, B.D.; Pundir, P.; Meeker, S.; Han, L.; Undem, B.J.; Kulka, M.; Dong, X. Identification of a Mast-Cell-Specific Receptor Crucial for Pseudo-Allergic Drug Reactions. *Nature* **2015**, *519*, 237–241. [CrossRef]
18. Green, D.P.; Limjunyawong, N.; Gour, N.; Pundir, P.; Dong, X. A Mast-Cell-Specific Receptor Mediates Neurogenic Inflammation and Pain. *Neuron* **2019**, *101*, 41–420.e3. [CrossRef]
19. Navratilova, E.; Porreca, F. Substance P and Inflammatory Pain: Getting it Wrong and Right Simultaneously. *Neuron* **2019**, *101*, 353–355. [CrossRef]
20. Katritch, V.; Cherezov, V.; Stevens, R.C. Diversity and Modularity of G Protein-Coupled Receptor Structures. *Trends Pharmacol. Sci.* **2012**, *33*, 17–27. [CrossRef]
21. Venkatakrishnan, A.J.; Deupi, X.; Lebon, G.; Tate, C.G.; Schertler, G.F.; Babu, M.M. Molecular Signatures of G-Protein-Coupled Receptors. *Nature* **2013**, *494*, 185–194. [CrossRef] [PubMed]
22. Venkatakrishnan, A.J.; Deupi, X.; Lebon, G.; Heydenreich, F.M.; Flock, T.; Miljus, T.; Balaji, S.; Bouvier, M.; Veprintsev, D.B.; Tate, C.G.; et al. Diverse Activation Pathways in Class A GPCRs Converge Near the G-Protein-Coupling Region. *Nature* **2016**, *536*, 484–487. [CrossRef] [PubMed]
23. Isberg, V.; de Graaf, C.; Bortolato, A.; Cherezov, V.; Katritch, V.; Marshall, F.H.; Mordalski, S.; Pin, J.P.; Stevens, R.C.; Vriend, G.; et al. Generic GPCR Residue Numbers-Aligning Topology Maps while Minding the Gaps. *Trends Pharmacol. Sci.* **2015**, *36*, 22–31. [CrossRef] [PubMed]
24. Munk, C.; Isberg, V.; Mordalski, S.; Harpsoe, K.; Rataj, K.; Hauser, A.S.; Kolb, P.; Bojarski, A.J.; Vriend, G.; Gloriam, D.E. GPCRdb: The G Protein-Coupled Receptor Database-an Introduction. *Br. J. Pharmacol.* **2016**, *173*, 2195–2207. [CrossRef]
25. Wootten, D.; Christopoulos, A.; Marti-Solano, M.; Babu, M.M.; Sexton, P.M. Mechanisms of Signalling and Biased Agonism in G Protein-Coupled Receptors. *Nat. Rev. Mol. Cell Biol.* **2018**, *19*, 638–653.
26. Hilger, D.; Masureel, M.; Kobilka, B.K. Structure and Dynamics of GPCR Signaling Complexes. *Nat. Struct. Mol. Biol.* **2018**, *25*, 4–12. [CrossRef]
27. Rasmussen, S.G.; DeVree, B.T.; Zou, Y.; Kruse, A.C.; Chung, K.Y.; Kobilka, T.S.; Thian, F.S.; Chae, P.S.; Pardon, E.; Calinski, D.; et al. Crystal Structure of the Beta2 Adrenergic Receptor-Gs Protein Complex. *Nature* **2011**, *477*, 549–555. [CrossRef]
28. Gupta, K.; Subramanian, H.; Klos, A.; Ali, H. Phosphorylation of C3a Receptor at Multiple Sites Mediates Desensitization, Beta-Arrestin-2 Recruitment and Inhibition of NF-kappaB Activity in Mast Cells. *PLoS ONE* **2012**, *7*, e46369. [CrossRef]
29. Guo, Q.; Subramanian, H.; Gupta, K.; Ali, H. Regulation of C3a Receptor Signaling in Human Mast Cells by G Protein Coupled Receptor Kinases. *PLoS ONE* **2011**, *6*, e22559. [CrossRef]
30. Cahill, T.J., 3rd; Thomsen, A.R.; Tarrasch, J.T.; Plouffe, B.; Nguyen, A.H.; Yang, F.; Huang, L.Y.; Kahsai, A.W.; Bassoni, D.L.; Gavino, B.J.; et al. Distinct Conformations of GPCR-Beta-Arrestin Complexes Mediate Desensitization, Signaling, and Endocytosis. *Proc. Natl. Acad. Sci. USA* **2017**, *114*, 2562–2567. [CrossRef]
31. Gurevich, V.V.; Gurevich, E.V. GPCR Signaling Regulation: The Role of GRKs and Arrestins. *Front. Pharmacol.* **2019**, *10*, 125. [CrossRef] [PubMed]
32. Roy, S.; Ganguly, A.; Haque, M.; Ali, H. Angiogenic Host Defense Peptide AG-30/5C and Bradykinin B2 Receptor Antagonist Icatibant are G Protein Biased Agonists for MRGPRX2 in Mast Cells. *J. Immunol.* **2019**, *202*, 1229–1238. [CrossRef] [PubMed]
33. Subramanian, H.; Gupta, K.; Guo, Q.; Price, R.; Ali, H. Mas-Related Gene X2 (MrgX2) is a Novel G Protein-Coupled Receptor for the Antimicrobial Peptide LL-37 in Human Mast Cells: Resistance to Receptor Phosphorylation, Desensitization, and Internalization. *J. Biol. Chem.* **2011**, *286*, 44739–44749. [CrossRef] [PubMed]
34. Lansu, K.; Karpiak, J.; Liu, J.; Huang, X.P.; McCorvy, J.D.; Kroeze, W.K.; Che, T.; Nagase, H.; Carroll, F.I.; Jin, J.; et al. In Silico Design of Novel Probes for the Atypical Opioid Receptor MRGPRX2. *Nat. Chem. Biol.* **2017**, *13*, 529–536. [CrossRef] [PubMed]
35. Reddy, V.B.; Graham, T.A.; Azimi, E.; Lerner, E.A. A Single Amino Acid in MRGPRX2 Necessary for Binding and Activation by Pruritogens. *J. Allergy Clin. Immunol.* **2017**, *140*, 1726–1728. [CrossRef]

36. Alkanfari, I.; Gupta, K.; Jahan, T.; Ali, H. Naturally Occurring Missense MRGPRX2 Variants Display Loss of Function Phenotype for Mast Cell Degranulation in Response to Substance P, Hemokinin-1, Human Beta-Defensin-3, and Icatibant. *J. Immunol.* **2018**, *201*, 343–349. [CrossRef]
37. Subramanian, H.; Gupta, K.; Lee, D.; Bayir, A.K.; Ahn, H.; Ali, H. Beta-Defensins Activate Human Mast Cells Via Mas-Related Gene X2. *J. Immunol.* **2013**, *191*, 345–352. [CrossRef]
38. Takasaki, J.; Saito, T.; Taniguchi, M.; Kawasaki, T.; Moritani, Y.; Hayashi, K.; Kobori, M. A Novel Galphaq/11-Selective Inhibitor. *J. Biol. Chem.* **2004**, *279*, 47438–47445. [CrossRef]
39. Gupta, K.; Subramanian, H.; Ali, H. Modulation of Host Defense Peptide-Mediated Human Mast Cell Activation by LPS. *Innate Immun.* **2016**, *22*, 21–30. [CrossRef]
40. Zhang, Y.; Sun, B.; Feng, D.; Hu, H.; Chu, M.; Qu, Q.; Tarrasch, J.T.; Li, S.; Sun Kobilka, T.; Kobilka, B.K.; et al. Cryo-EM Structure of the Activated GLP-1 Receptor in Complex with a G Protein. *Nature* **2017**, *546*, 248–253. [CrossRef]
41. Meixiong, J.; Anderson, M.; Limjunyawong, N.; Sabbagh, M.F.; Hu, E.; Mack, M.R.; Oetjen, L.K.; Wang, F.; Kim, B.S.; Dong, X. Activation of Mast-Cell-Expressed Mas-Related G-Protein-Coupled Receptors Drives Non-Histaminergic Itch. *Immunity* **2019**, *50*, 116–1171.e5. [CrossRef]
42. Pundir, P.; Liu, R.; Vasavda, C.; Serhan, N.; Limjunyawong, N.; Yee, R.; Zhan, Y.; Dong, X.; Wu, X.; Zhang, Y.; et al. A Connective Tissue Mast-Cell-Specific Receptor Detects Bacterial Quorum-Sensing Molecules and Mediates Antibacterial Immunity. *Cell. Host Microbe.* **2019**, *26*, 11–122.e8. [CrossRef] [PubMed]
43. Subramanian, H.; Gupta, K.; Ali, H. Roles of Mas-Related G Protein-Coupled Receptor X2 on Mast Cell-Mediated Host Defense, Pseudoallergic Drug Reactions, and Chronic Inflammatory Diseases. *J. Allergy Clin. Immunol.* **2016**, *138*, 700–710. [CrossRef] [PubMed]
44. Civciristov, S.; Ellisdon, A.M.; Suderman, R.; Pon, C.K.; Evans, B.A.; Kleifeld, O.; Charlton, S.J.; Hlavacek, W.S.; Canals, M.; Halls, M.L. Preassembled GPCR Signaling Complexes Mediate Distinct Cellular Responses to Ultralow Ligand Concentrations. *Sci. Signal.* **2018**, *11*. [CrossRef] [PubMed]
45. Moro, O.; Lameh, J.; Hogger, P.; Sadee, W. Hydrophobic Amino Acid in the I2 Loop Plays a Key Role in Receptor-G Protein Coupling. *J. Biol. Chem.* **1993**, *268*, 22273–22276. [PubMed]
46. Villar, V.A.; Cuevas, S.; Zheng, X.; Jose, P.A. Localization and Signaling of GPCRs in Lipid Rafts. *Methods Cell Biol.* **2016**, *132*, 3–23.
47. Nobles, K.N.; Xiao, K.; Ahn, S.; Shukla, A.K.; Lam, C.M.; Rajagopal, S.; Strachan, R.T.; Huang, T.Y.; Bressler, E.A.; Hara, M.R.; et al. Distinct Phosphorylation Sites on the Beta(2)-Adrenergic Receptor Establish a Barcode that Encodes Differential Functions of Beta-Arrestin. *Sci. Signal.* **2011**, *4*, ra51. [CrossRef]
48. Ardura, J.A.; Friedman, P.A. Regulation of G Protein-Coupled Receptor Function by Na+/H+ Exchange Regulatory Factors. *Pharmacol. Rev.* **2011**, *63*, 882–900. [CrossRef]
49. Wang, B.; Yang, Y.; Abou-Samra, A.B.; Friedman, P.A. NHERF1 Regulates Parathyroid Hormone Receptor Desensitization: Interference with Beta-Arrestin Binding. *Mol. Pharmacol.* **2009**, *75*, 1189–1197. [CrossRef]
50. Subramanian, H.; Gupta, K.; Ali, H. Roles for NHERF1 and NHERF2 on the Regulation of C3a Receptor Signaling in Human Mast Cells. *PLoS ONE* **2012**, *7*, e51355. [CrossRef]
51. Ali, H.; Richardson, R.M.; Tomhave, E.D.; DuBose, R.A.; Haribabu, B.; Snyderman, R. Regulation of Stably Transfected Platelet Activating Factor Receptor in RBL-2H3 Cells. Role of Multiple G Proteins and Receptor Phosphorylation. *J. Biol. Chem.* **1994**, *269*, 24557–24563. [PubMed]

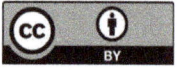

© 2019 by the authors. Licensee MDPI, Basel, Switzerland. This article is an open access article distributed under the terms and conditions of the Creative Commons Attribution (CC BY) license (http://creativecommons.org/licenses/by/4.0/).

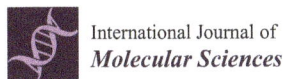

Article

Co-Stimulation of Purinergic P2X4 and Prostanoid EP3 Receptors Triggers Synergistic Degranulation in Murine Mast Cells

Kazuki Yoshida [1], Makoto Tajima [1], Tomoki Nagano [1], Kosuke Obayashi [1], Masaaki Ito [1], Kimiko Yamamoto [2] and Isao Matsuoka [1,*]

1. Laboratory of Pharmacology, Faculty of Pharmacy, Takasaki University of Health and Welfare, Takasaki-shi, Gunma 370-0033, Japan; yoshida-k@takasaki-u.ac.jp (K.Y.); 1321057@takasaki-u.ac.jp (M.T.); 1321067@takasaki-u.ac.jp (T.N.); 0821024@takasaki-u.ac.jp (K.O.); mito@takasaki-u.ac.jp (M.I.)
2. Department of Biomedical Engineering, Graduate School of Medicine, The University of Tokyo, Tokyo 113-0033, Japan; k-yamamoto@umin.ac.jp
* Correspondence: isao@takasaki-u.ac.jp; Tel.: +81-27-352-1180

Received: 4 October 2019; Accepted: 16 October 2019; Published: 17 October 2019

Abstract: Mast cells (MCs) recognize antigens (Ag) via IgE-bound high affinity IgE receptors (FcεRI) and trigger type I allergic reactions. FcεRI-mediated MC activation is regulated by various G protein-coupled receptor (GPCR) agonists. We recently reported that ionotropic P2X4 receptor (P2X4R) stimulation enhanced FcεRI-mediated degranulation. Since MCs are involved in Ag-independent hypersensitivity, we investigated whether co-stimulation with ATP and GPCR agonists in the absence of Ag affects MC degranulation. Prostaglandin E_2 (PGE_2) induced synergistic degranulation when bone marrow-derived MCs (BMMCs) were co-stimulated with ATP, while pharmacological analyses revealed that the effects of PGE_2 and ATP were mediated by EP3 and P2X4R, respectively. Consistently, this response was absent in BMMCs prepared from P2X4R-deficient mice. The effects of ATP and PGE_2 were reduced by PI3 kinase inhibitors but were insensitive to tyrosine kinase inhibitors which suppressed the enhanced degranulation induced by Ag and ATP. MC-dependent PGE_2-triggered vascular hyperpermeability was abrogated in a P2X4R-deficient mouse ear edema model. Collectively, our results suggest that P2X4R signaling enhances EP3R-mediated MC activation via a different mechanism to that involved in enhancing Ag-induced responses. Moreover, the cooperative effects of the common inflammatory mediators ATP and PGE_2 on MCs may be involved in Ag-independent hypersensitivity *in vivo*.

Keywords: extracellular ATP; P2X4 receptor; prostaglandin E_2; EP3 receptor; bone marrow-derived mast cell; mast cell degranulation; Ca^{2+} influx; PI3 kinase

---

1. Introduction

Mast cells (MC) are widely distributed in the body and abundant in tissues that contact with the external environment, such as the intestine, respiratory tract, and skin [1]. MCs are replete with secretory granules containing a variety of preformed mediators, such as histamine, cytokines, and proteases, that they release in response to various harmful pathogens or invading external substances [2]. This process is thought to initiate immunoregulatory reactions by providing a microenvironment that recruits and activates other immunocompetent cells; however, such reactions are sometimes inappropriately enhanced under certain conditions, causing hypersensitivity and allergic inflammation [3]. The most well-known MC activation pathway involves high affinity IgE receptors (FcεRI), which enable MCs to form a barrier against pathogen invasion [4]. When antigens (Ag) cross-link the IgE-FcεRI complex, many signaling molecules are phosphorylated by the protein tyrosine kinase Lyn and subsequently recruited Syk, activating multiple pathways involving processes such as degranulation, cytokine production, and lipid mediator production [5]. MCs are known to express various immunoregulatory receptors, including toll-like receptors, stem cell factor (SCF) receptors, and G-protein-coupled receptors (GPCR), whose stimulation has been reported to promote IgE-dependent MC degranulation [6]. For instance, it has been shown that PGE$_2$, which is known to mediate inflammation [7], and adenosine, which accumulates extracellularly under ischemic conditions [8], enhance Ag-mediated MC degranulation [9–11]. The effects of PGE$_2$ and adenosine are mediated by the EP3 receptor (EP3R) and A$_3$ receptor (A$_3$R), respectively, and are commonly transmitted via the pertussis toxin (PTX)-sensitive Gi protein, suggesting a similar underlying mechanism. Indeed, several studies have demonstrated that enhancing Ag-induced MC degranulation by co-stimulation with Gi-coupled receptor agonists requires the activation of phosphoinositide 3-kinase (PI3K) γ, a PI3K subclass regulated by the Gi protein βγ subunit [10,11]. These enhanced responses are thought to be involved in exacerbating allergic reactions.

In addition to Gi-coupled receptor agonists, we recently reported that extracellular ATP also enhances the Ag-induced degranulation response in bone marrow-derived MCs (BMMCs) by activating the P2X4 receptor (P2X4R), a ligand-gated ion channel [12]. Unlike Gi-coupled receptor agonists, P2X4R stimulation does not induce the PI3K signaling pathway, but enhances the Ag-induced tyrosine phosphorylation of signaling molecules including Syk and phospholipase C (PLC) γ [13]. Based on these results, we hypothesized that stimulation of MCs with ATP and Gi-coupled receptor agonists may cause MC degranulation in an IgE-independent manner. Indeed, we previously showed that co-stimulating BMMCs with ATP and adenosine induced synergistic degranulation via A$_3$R [12].

With respect to IgE-independent MC activation, MCs express several pattern recognition-receptors, such as toll-like receptor 2 and 4, which are stimulated by micro-organism specific molecular motif, triggering the innate immune responses [14]. In this category, extracellular ATP is also considered to act as a danger signal, because living cells contain high concentrations of ATP and release it to extracellular space under adverse conditions, like tissue damage, necrosis, and pyroptosis [15]. The accumulation of ATP is detected by surrounding cells through a wide variety of receptors; not only G protein-coupled receptors (P2Y$_{1,2,4,6,11,12,13,14}$), but also ionotropic receptors (P2X1-7). Upon stimulation through different mechanism, MC is known to be capable of producing a wide variety of inflammatory and anti-inflammatory cytokines, no less than other immune cells such as macrophages and lymphocytes [16]. Indeed, MCs have quite recently been implicated in the pathogenesis of systemic lupus erythematosus [17] and neurofibromatosis [18]. In such inflammatory diseases, MC activation cannot be explained only by the IgE-dependent mechanism. Since, extracellular ATP is suggested to be released from cells via mechanical stress such as itching-induced scratching behavior [19,20], MCs must be exposed to ATP and various humoral factors in the inflammatory environment.

This study therefore investigated whether combining ATP with GPCR agonists affected MC degranulation, finding that co-stimulation with ATP and PGE$_2$ induced synergistic MC degranulation by activating P2X4 and EP3R, respectively, via a novel mechanism that is different to the Ag-induced response.

2. Results

2.1. Effects of ATP and GPCR Agonist co-Stimulation on BMMC Degranulation

We first examined the effect of ATP and GPCR agonist co-stimulation on the degranulation of BMMCs. We tested the GPCR agonists sphingosine-1-phosphate (S1P) (1 µM), PGE$_2$ (1 µM), histamine (100 µM), C5a (10 nM), PGD$_2$ (1 µM), UDP-glucose (100 µM), and compound 48/80 (10 µM), all of which constantly increased the intracellular Ca^{2+} concentration ([Ca^{2+}]i) of Fura-2 loaded BMMCs, albeit to varying degrees (data not shown). Although these GPCR agonists had no effect on BMMC degranulation when tested alone, PGE$_2$ markedly induced degranulation when concurrently stimulated with 100 µM ATP (Figure 1A). Time course experiments revealed that co-stimulation with ATP and

PGE$_2$ induced degranulation rapidly, with the response initiated within 2 min and reaching the maximum steady state in 5 min (Figure 1B). Different PGE$_2$ concentrations only induced BMMC degranulation in a concentration-dependent manner in the presence of 100 μM ATP, with PGE$_1$ inducing similar effects (Figure 1C). Moreover, the effects of ATP on degranulation in the presence of PGE$_2$ were concentration-dependent (Figure 1D). On the basis of these results, we examined the effects of co-stimulation with 100 μM ATP and 1 μM PGE$_2$ for 5 min in the following experiments.

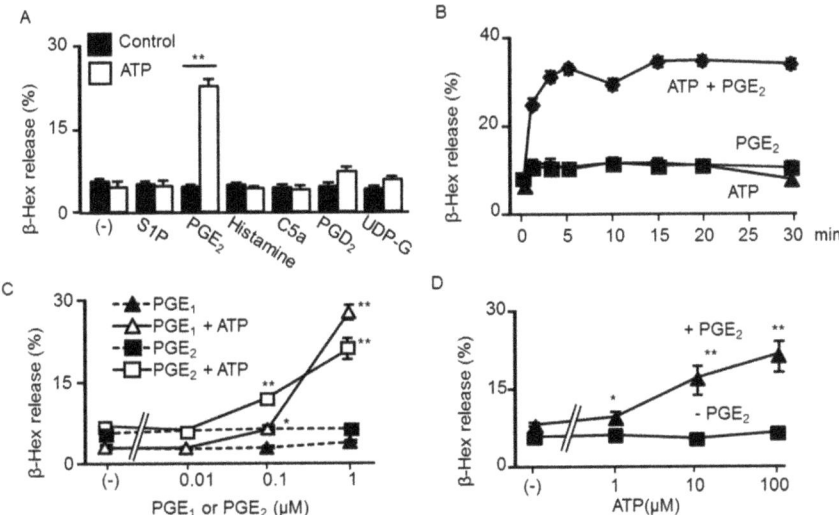

Figure 1. Synergistic effects of ATP and prostaglandin (PG)E$_2$ on mast cell (MC) degranulation. (**A**) Bone marrow-derived MCs (BMMCs) were stimulated with sphingosine-1-phosphate (S1P) (1 μM), PGE$_2$ (1 μM), histamine (100 μM), C5a (10 nM), PGD$_2$ (1 μM), and UDP-glucose (100 μM) with or without ATP (100 μM) (n = 3, mean ± SEM). ** p < 0.01 indicates a significant difference from the control. (**B**) BMMCs were stimulated for 1–30 min with ATP (100 μM, ▲) and PGE$_2$ (1 μM, ■) alone or simultaneously (♦; n = 3, mean ± SEM). (**C**) BMMCs were stimulated with different concentrations (0.01–1 μM) of PGE$_1$ (△, ▲) and PGE$_2$ (□, ■) with (△, □) or without (▲, ■) ATP (100 μM) (n = 3, mean ± SEM). * p < 0.05 and ** p < 0.01 indicate significant differences compared to ATP alone. (**D**) BMMCs were stimulated with different concentrations of ATP (1–100 μM) with (▲) or without (■) PGE$_2$ (1 μM) (n = 3, mean ± SEM). * p < 0.05 and ** p < 0.01 indicate significant differences compared to PGE$_2$ alone.

2.2. Involvement of Gi-Coupled EP3R in Synergistic Degranulation Induced by PGE$_2$ and ATP

The biological effects of PGE$_2$ are known to be mediated by four different EP receptors. Quantitative reverse transcription-polymerase chain reaction (qRT-PCR) revealed that the BMMCs used in this study expressed EP1, EP3, and EP4 receptor mRNAs, while pharmacological experiments with selective EPR antagonists revealed that only the EP3 antagonist ONO-AE3-208 inhibited the degranulation induced by PGE$_2$ and ATP (Figure 2A). Consistently, only the ONO-AE-248 agonist against EP3R, a Gi-coupled receptor, induced degranulation in the presence of ATP (Figure 2B). Moreover, the degranulation induced by PGE$_2$ and ATP was abolished by pretreating the BMMCs with 50 ng/mL of PTX (Figure 2C).

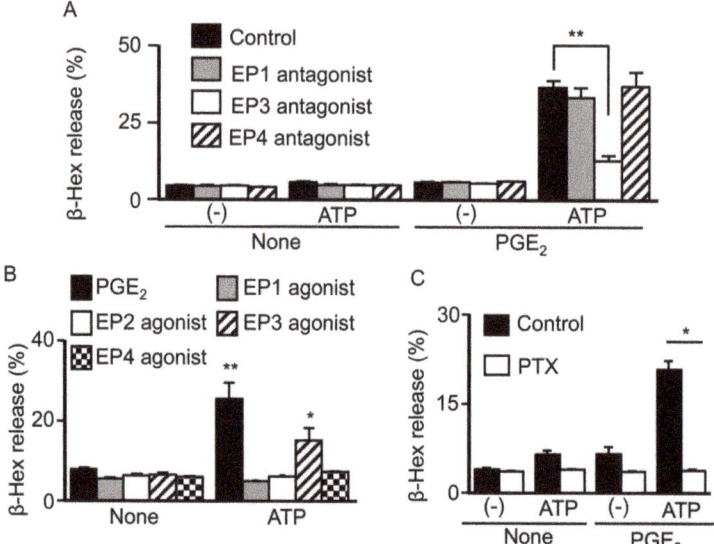

Figure 2. Involvement of EP3 receptor activation in the synergistic effect of prostaglandin (PG)E$_2$ and ATP on mast cell (MC) degranulation. (**A**) Bone marrow-derived MCs were preincubated with a vehicle, ONO-8713 (EP1 antagonist), ONO-AE3-240 (EP3 antagonist), and ONO-AE3-208 (EP4 antagonist) at 1 µM for 5 min and then stimulated with vehicle (-) or ATP (100 µM) with or without PGE$_2$ (1 µM) for 5 min. Data are shown as the mean ± SEM ($n = 3$). * $p < 0.05$ indicates a significant difference from the control. (**B**) BMMCs were stimulated with PGE$_2$, ONO-DI-004 (EP1 agonist), ONO-AE1-259 (EP2 agonist), ONO-AE-248 (EP3 agonist), or ONO-AE1-329 (EP4 agonist) at 1 µM with or without ATP (100 µM). Data are shown as the mean ± SEM ($n = 3$). * $p < 0.05$ and ** $p < 0.01$ indicate significant differences from the response without ATP (none). (**C**) BMMCs were treated with or without pertussis toxin (PTX, 50 ng/mL) overnight and stimulated with ATP (100 µM) with or without PGE$_2$ (1 µM) for 5 min. Data are shown as the mean ± SEM ($n = 3$). * $p < 0.05$ indicates a significant difference from the control.

2.3. Involvement of Ionotropic P2X4R in the Effect of ATP and PGE$_2$ on Degranulation

We next attempted to identify the P2 receptor subtype that mediates the effect of ATP on degranulation with PGE$_2$. We previously reported that under our experimental conditions, BMMCs express ionotropic P2X1, 4, and 7, which are all stimulated by ATP, and G protein-coupled P2Y$_{1, 2,}$ and $_{14}$ receptors, which are stimulated by ADP, UTP, and UDP-glucose, respectively [21]. Since UDP-glucose had little effect (Figure 1A), we examined the effects of ADP and UTP on degranulation with PGE$_2$. As shown in Figure 3A, ADP and UTP had weak effects on degranulation with PGE$_2$ compared to ATP. Consistently, the effect of ATP on degranulation with PGE$_2$ was not affected by the P2Y$_1$ antagonist MRS2179 or P2Y$_2$ antagonist AR-C118925 (Figure 3B). Among the P2X receptor antagonists, degranulation induced by ATP and PGE$_2$ was inhibited by the P2X4 antagonist 5-BDBD, but not the P2X1 antagonist NF449 or P2X7 antagonist AZ10606120 (Figure 3C,D). Furthermore, the effect of ATP on degranulation with PGE$_2$ was enhanced by the P2X4R positive allosteric modulator ivermectin (Figure 3D) but totally absent in BMMCs prepared from P2X4R-deficient mice (Figure 3E).

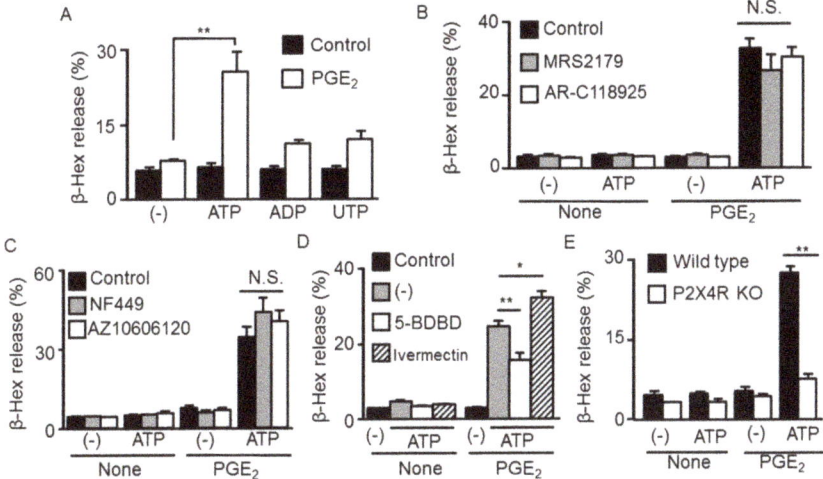

Figure 3. Involvement of P2X4 receptor (P2X4R) activation in the synergistic effect of prostaglandin (PG) E_2 and ATP on mast cell (MC) degranulation. (**A**) Bone marrow-derived MCs (BMMCs) were stimulated concurrently with PGE_2 (1 μM) and a vehicle, ATP, ADP, or UTP (100 μM) for 5 min. (**B**) BMMCs were preincubated with a vehicle, the $P2Y_1$ antagonist MRS2179 (10 μM), or the $P2Y_2$ antagonist AR-C118925 (10 μM) for 5 min and then stimulated with ATP (100 μM) with or without PGE_2 (1 μM) for 5 min. (**C**) BMMCs were preincubated with a vehicle, the P2X1 antagonist NF449 (10 μM), or the P2X7 antagonist AZ10606120 (1 μM) for 3 min and then stimulated with ATP (100 μM) with or without PGE_2 (1 μM) for 5 min. (**D**) BMMCs were preincubated with a vehicle, the P2X4 antagonist 5-BDBD (10 μM), or the P2X4R positive allosteric modulator ivermectin (10 μg/mL) for 5 min and then stimulated with ATP (100 μM) with or without PGE_2 (1 μM) for 5 min. (**E**) BMMCs prepared from wild type and P2X4R-deficient mice (P2X4R KO) were stimulated with ATP (100 μM) with or without PGE_2 (1 μM) for 5 min. Data are shown as the mean ± SEM (n = 3). N.S. no significant difference, * $p < 0.05$ and ** $p < 0.01$ indicate significant differences.

2.4. Mechanism underlying the Synergistic Degranulation Induced by ATP and PGE_2

We recently reported that stimulating P2X4R enhanced Ag-induced degranulation and increased Src tyrosine kinase signaling pathways, such as Syk and phospholipase $C\gamma$ (MS submitted). Therefore, we examined effects of the Src family tyrosine kinase inhibitor PP2 and the Syk inhibitor R406 on degranulation induced by ATP and PGE_2. As shown in Figure 4A,B, although both PP2 and R406 effectively inhibited the degranulation induced by co-stimulation with ATP and Ag, they had little effect on that induced by ATP and PGE_2. It has been reported that MC degranulation induced by PGE_2 is mediated by PI3K [10]. Consistent with the previous report, MC degranulation induced by co-stimulation with ATP and PGE_2 was inhibited by the non-selective PI3 kinase inhibitor LY294002 but not the structurally similar negative control LY303511 (Figure 4C). The response was also inhibited by AS605240, a specific PI3Kγ inhibitor that is activated by G protein $\beta\gamma$ subunits (Figure 4D), whereas the Akt inhibitor triciribine had no effect on the degranulation induced by ATP and PGE_2 (Figure 4E). These results suggest that P2X4R stimulation enhanced EP3R-mediated signaling in a PI3K-dependent but Akt-independent manner.

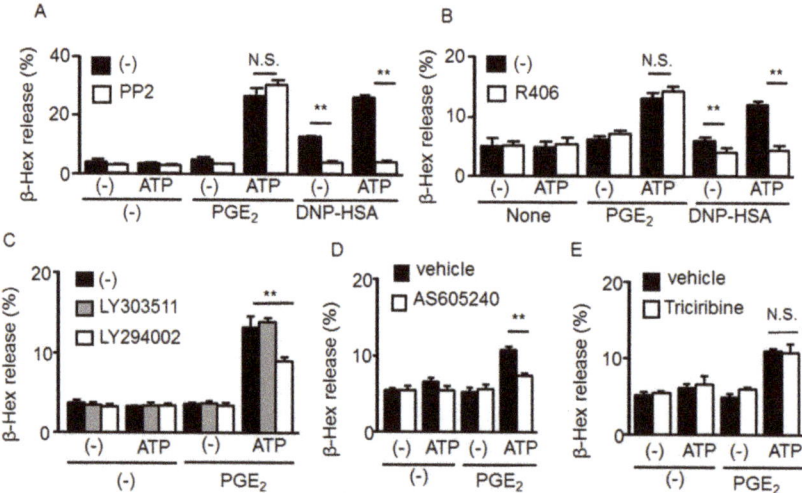

Figure 4. Effect of tyrosine kinase and phosphoinositide 3-kinase (PI3K)/Akt signaling pathway inhibitors on mast cell (MC) degranulation induced by co-stimulation with ATP and prostaglandin (PG)E$_2$. (**A**) Bone marrow-derived MCs (BMMCs) were preincubated with a vehicle or the Src tyrosine kinase inhibitor PP2 (1 µM) for 5 min and then stimulated with ATP (100 µM) with or without PGE$_2$ (1 µM) or 2,4-dinitrophenyl human serum albumin (DNP-HSA, 10 ng/mL). (**B**) BMMCs were preincubated with a vehicle or the Syk inhibitor R406 (2 µM) for 5 min and then stimulated with ATP (100 µM) with or without PGE$_2$ (1 µM) ($n = 3$). (**C**) BMMCs were preincubated with a vehicle, the PI3K inhibitor LY294002 (10 µM), or the control compound LY303511 (10 µM) for 5 min and then stimulated with ATP (0.1 mM) with or without PGE$_2$ (1 µM) ($n = 3$). (**D**) BMMCs were preincubated with a vehicle or the PI3Kγ inhibitor AS605240 (1 µM) for 5 min and then stimulated with ATP (100 µM) with or without PGE$_2$ (1 µM) ($n = 3$). (**E**) BMMCs were preincubated with a vehicle or the Akt inhibitor triciribin (10 µM) for 5 min, and then stimulated with ATP (100 µM) with or without PGE$_2$ (1 µM) ($n = 3$). Data are shown as the mean ± SEM. N.S. no significant difference, ** $p < 0.01$ indicates a significant difference.

2.5. Effects of Co-Stimulating BMMCs with ATP and PGE$_2$ on ERK1/2, Akt, and Syk Phosphorylation

As shown previously, ATP enhanced Ag-induced Syk phosphorylation (Figure 5A) in BMMCs; however, neither PGE$_2$ nor co-stimulation with PGE$_2$ and ATP affected Syk phosphorylation (Figure 5A). In contrast, stimulation with PGE$_2$ and ATP alone induced ERK1/2 and Akt phosphorylation in a time-dependent manner. Furthermore, Syk phosphorylation in response to ATP and Ag was greater than the response to either alone, whereas the Akt and ERK1/2 phosphorylation induced by co-stimulation with ATP and PGE$_2$ was slightly lower (Figure 5B).

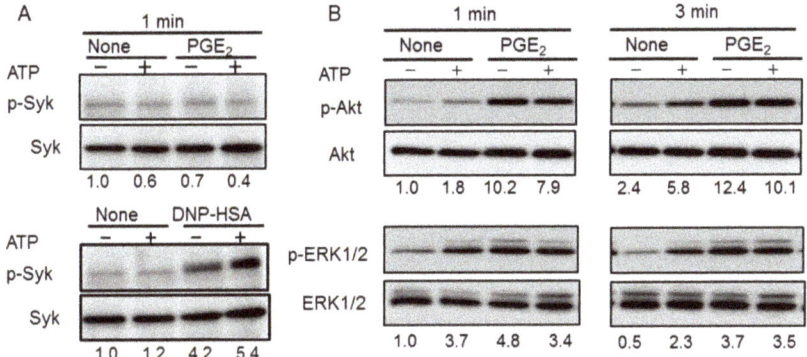

Figure 5. Effect of co-stimulation with ATP and prostaglandin (PG)E_2 on Syk, extracellular signal-regulated kinase (ERK)1/2, and Akt phosphorylation in bone marrow-derived mast cells (BMMCs). (**A**) BMMCs were stimulated with ATP (100 µM) with or without PGE_2 (1 µM, upper) or 2,4-dinitrophenyl human serum albumin (DNP-HAS,10 ng/mL, lower) for 1 min. Cell lysates were subjected to western blot analysis for phospho-Syk and total-Syk. (**B**) BMMCs were stimulated with ATP (100 µM) with or without PGE_2 (1 µM) for 1 (left) or 3 (right) min. Cell lysates were subjected to western blot analysis for phospho-Akt and total Akt (upper) or phospho-ERK 1/2 and total-ERK 1/2 (lower). The numbers below each image indicate normalized relative phosphorylated protein intensity; the results for no stimulation are set to one. Blots are representative of three independent experiments.

2.6. Effects of Co-Stimulating BMMCs with ATP and PGE_2 on $[Ca^{2+}]i$

In Fura-2-loaded BMMCs, ATP stimulation induced a rapid increase in $[Ca^{2+}]i$ which decreased to a sustained steady state, whereas PGE_2 induced a similar $[Ca^{2+}]i$ increase, but to a weaker extent than that induced by ATP. Co-stimulation with ATP and PGE_2 resulted in a sustained increase in $[Ca^{2+}]i$ that was greater than the additive responses elicited by ATP or PGE_2 alone, but was not evident in BMMCs obtained from P2X4-deficient mice (Figure 6A,B), and was inhibited by the PI3Kγ inhibitor AS605240 (Figure 6C,D).

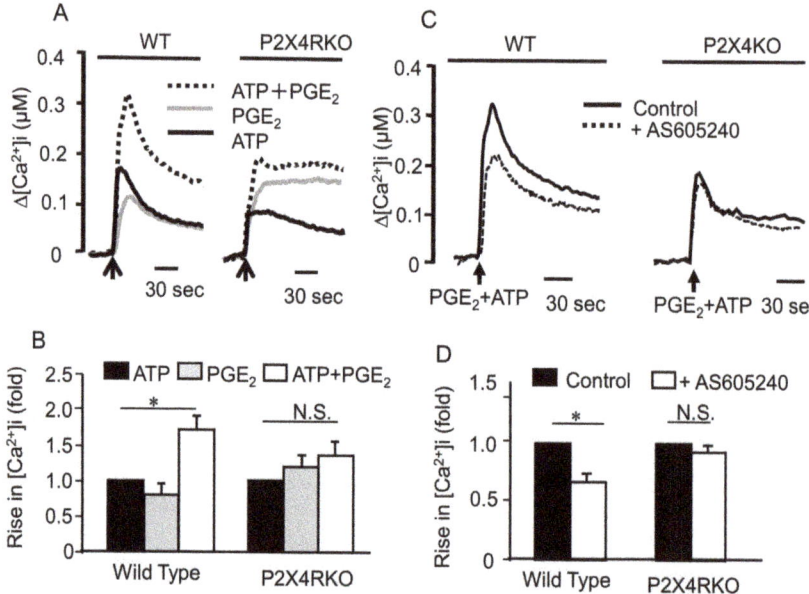

Figure 6. Effects of co-stimulating bone marrow-derived mast cells (BMMCs) with ATP and prostaglandin (PG)E$_2$ on intracellular Ca^{2+} concentration ([Ca^{2+}]i) levels. (**A**) BMMCs prepared from widg type (WT) or P2X4 receptor deficient (P2X4RKO) mice were loaded with Fura-2 acetoxymethyl ester and changes in [Ca^{2+}]i were monitored after stimulating with ATP (black line), PGE$_2$ (gray line), or ATP plus PGE$_2$ (dotted line) at the time indicated by the arrow. The Ca^{2+} data are representative of four independent experiments. (**B**)Summary of the data obtained in A. Results are indicated as fold of ATP-induced response (WT; 205 ± 38 nM, n = 4, P2X4RKO; 115 ± 16 nM, n = 4). Data are shown as the mean ± SEM (n = 4). N.S.; no significant difference, * p < 0.05 indicates a significant difference. (**C**) BMMCs prepared from WT or P2X4RKO were preincubated with or without the PI3Kγ inhibitor AS605240 (1 µM) for 5 min and then stimulated with ATP (100 µM) plus PGE$_2$ (1 µM). The superimposed [Ca^{2+}]i changes are representative of at least four different BMMC preparations obtained from different animals. (**D**) Summary of the data obtained in C. Results are indicated as fold of control response (WT; 342 ± 45 nM, n = 3, P2X4RKO; 158 ± 29 nM, n = 4). Data are shown as the mean ± SEM (n = 3–4). N.S.; no significant difference, * p < 0.05 indicates a significant difference.

2.7. Role of P2X4R Signaling in PGE$_2$-Induced Skin MC Activation in Vivo

Administering PGE$_2$ to mouse ears reportedly induces edema due to increased extravasation via the EP3R-mediated activation of resident MCs [22]; therefore, we examined whether P2X4R contributed toward this response. Intradermally injecting PGE$_2$ into the auricle of wild type mice caused significant Evans blue leakage compared to solvent-injected auricles (Figure 7); however, these effects were absent in MC-deficient Kit$^{Wsh/Wsh}$ mice, confirming that MCs are involved in the PGE$_2$-induced effects. Moreover, the effect of PGE$_2$ on dye leakage was significantly abrogated in P2X4R-deficient mice (Figure 7).

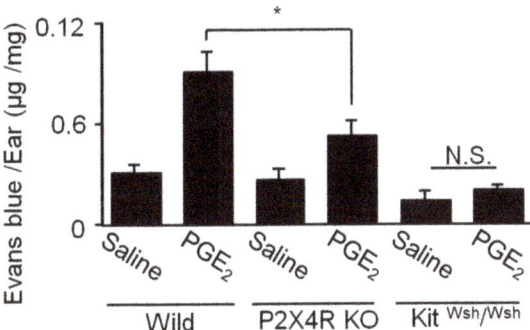

Figure 7. Comparison of prostaglandin (PG) E_2-induced hyperpermeability in wild type, P2X4 receptor-deficient (P2X4RKO), and mast cell-deficient Kit $^{Wsh/Wsh}$ mice. PGE_2 (1.5 nmol) was intradermally injected into the ear and vascular permeability measured 30 min later. Data are shown as the mean ± SEM (n = 5–6). N.S. no significant difference, * $p < 0.05$ indicates a significant difference.

3. Discussion

Previously, we reported that Ag-induced MC degranulation was enhanced by extracellular ATP [12]. Although various GPCR agonists have been shown to enhance Ag-induced degranulation, particularly those acting on Gi-coupled receptors [9,11], we found that the ATP-induced response was mediated by the ionotropic P2X4R [12]. This study examined whether P2X4R stimulation affected IgE-independent MC activation in combination with the GPCR agonists S1P, compound 48/80, UDP-glucose, C5a, histamine, PGD_2, and PGE_2, which reportedly activate MCs via the $S1P_2$, MRGPRB2, $P2Y_{14}$, C5a, H_3, DP2, and EP3 receptors, respectively [6]. In this study, these agonists had little effect on MC degranulation alone, with only PGE_2 causing a strong degranulation response when co-stimulated with ATP. Since ATP is known to promote PG production in various tissues [23,24], this finding may help understand the physiological functions of MCs.

The biological effects of PGE_2 are mediated by four different receptor subtypes, EP1, EP2, EP3, and EP4Rs [25]. EP3R has been well characterized as the site of action via which PGE_2 stimulates MC degranulation alone or in the presence of Ag [9,10,22]. In this study, pharmacological investigation using receptor subtype selective agonists and antagonists indicated that the costimulatory effects of PGE_2 and ATP on degranulation were also mediated by EP3R. In particular, the effect of PGE_2 was inhibited by the selective EP3 antagonist ONO-AE3-208 and mimicked by the selective EP3 agonist ONO-AE-2248. Furthermore, our observation that the effect of PGE_2 was abolished by the PTX-mediated inactivation of Gi-dependent signals is consistent with the fact that EP3R is the only Gi-coupled EP receptor subtype [25]. With respect to ATP receptors, we previously demonstrated that BMMCs express mRNA for the P2X1, P2X4, P2X7, $P2Y_1$, $P2Y_2$ and $P2Y_{14}$ receptors [12]. Several results obtained in this study clearly suggest that the effect of ATP was mediated by P2X4R, similar to enhanced Ag-induced degranulation [12]. First, combining PGE2 with the $P2Y_1$ agonist ADP, $P2Y_2$ agonist UTP, and $P2Y_{14}$ agonist UDP-glucose did not mimic the effect of ATP on degranulation. In addition, the effect of ATP and PGE_2 was affected by neither the $P2Y_1$ antagonist MRS2179 nor the $P2Y_2$ antagonist AR-C118925, indicating that G protein-coupled P2Y receptors are not involved in ATP and PGE_2-induced degranulation. Moreover, degranulation induced by ATP and PGE_2 was inhibited by the P2X4 antagonist 5-BDBD but not the P2X1 antagonist NF449 or P2X7 antagonist AZ10606120, and was enhanced by the P2X4R positive allosteric modulator ivermectin [26]. Finally, the degranulation induced by ATP and PGE_2 was impaired in BMMCs prepared from P2X4R-deficient mice, suggesting that co-activation of Gi-coupled EP3R and ionotropic P2X4R induces MC degranulation.

Previously, we demonstrated that P2X4R stimulation promotes Ag-induced tyrosine phosphorylation signaling, providing a possible mechanism for synergistic MC degranulation in response to Ag and ATP [13]. However, this mechanism was not involved in the effect of ATP and PGE$_2$ on MC degranulation, since the response to ATP and PGE$_2$ was insensitive to the tyrosine kinase inhibitor PP2 or Syk inhibitor R406, both of which inhibited the synergistic degranulation induced by Ag and ATP. Furthermore, ATP, PGE$_2$, and their combination failed to induce Syk phosphorylation. It has been demonstrated that stimulating EP3R with PGE$_2$ in BMMCs induces Gβγ-mediated PLCγ and PI3Kγ activation, increased phosphorylation of Akt (a kinase downstream of PI3K), and functionally promotes Ca^{2+} influx [9,11]. In this study, degranulation induced by ATP and PGE$_2$ was inhibited by the non-selective PI3K inhibitor LY294002 and PI3Kγ selective inhibitor AS605240; however, ATP did not enhance PGE$_2$-induced Akt phosphorylation but rather decreased it slightly. Although ATP itself slightly stimulates Akt phosphorylation, this effect is unchanged in P2X4R KO mice [13], suggesting that ATP-induced Akt phosphorylation is mediated by a receptor other than P2X4R and that P2X4R stimulation does not affect Gβγ-mediated PI3Kγ activation. These results suggest that PI3Kγ activation is necessary for ATP and PGE$_2$-induced degranulation but that the downstream mechanism differs to that described for the combination of Ag and PGE$_2$ [9,11].

In the Ca^{2+} assay, we observed an enhanced [Ca^{2+}]i response to ATP and PGE$_2$ that was abrogated in BMMCs obtained from P2X4R KO mice and partly suppressed by inhibiting PI3Kγ with AC605240. Assuming that Ca^{2+} influx through P2X4R is crucial for degranulation in response to ATP and PGE$_2$, two potential mechanisms could be inferred. First, since it has been reported that P2X4R channel activity is enhanced by membrane PI(3,4,5)P3 accumulation [27], EP3R-mediated PI3Kγ activation may cause PI(3,4,5)P3 accumulation which in turn promotes P2X4R-mediated Ca^{2+} influx. Second, MCs have been reported to possess functional G protein-coupled inwardly-rectifying K$^+$ channel (GIRK), a Gβγ-gated K$^+$ channels [28]; therefore, EP3R activation may open these channels, hyperpolarizing the membrane and increasing in driving force of Ca^{2+} influx [29] through the P2X4 receptor. Similar methods of regulation have been demonstrated in Ag-induced MC activation, where Ca^{2+}-activated K$^+$ channels play a critical role in facilitating Ca^{2+} influx via store-operated Ca^{2+} channels [30]. Further research using electrophysiological analysis is required to explore the precise mechanism of crosstalk between EP3 and P2X4R signaling.

Local PGE$_2$ administration has been reported to enhance vascular permeability by directly activating MCs via EP3R activation [22]. In this study, a similar effect of PGE$_2$ was reproduced in WT mice but not MC-deficient Kit $^{Wsh/Wsh}$ mice, while the PGE$_2$-induced increase in vascular permeability was shown to be significantly attenuated in P2X4R-deficient mice. These results indicate that ATP positively controls the responsiveness of MCs to PGE$_2$ via P2X4R *in vivo*. Since both ATP and PGE$_2$ are extracellular mediators that accumulate in damaged or inflamed tissues, the response described here may help to understand the role of MCs in Ag-independent hypersensitivity [14].

Recent accumulating evidence suggest that P2X4R signal is involved in several inflammatory diseases, including neuropathic pain induced by nerve injury [31], joint inflammation in rheumatoid arthritis [32], rejection to transplanted tissue [33], and allergic airway inflammation [34]. The present study focused on the MC degranulation response, an early event in MC activation. As mentioned earlier, MCs can produce wide variety of cytokines [16], which affect chronic responses related to inflammatory diseases. It is therefore important to examine whether P2X4R signaling would affect the MC cytokine production.

In summary, this study demonstrated that co-stimulating MCs with ATP and PGE$_2$ synergistically induces degranulation via ionotropic P2X4R and Gi-coupled EP3R, respectively (Figure 8). Moreover, this reaction is independent of the tyrosine kinase cascade, which plays a major role in the Ag-induced response, and is likely to involve enhanced Ca^{2+} influx in a manner dependent on EP3R-mediated PI3K activation. Previously, we reported that ATP also promotes Ag-induced allergic reactions via P2X4R activation; therefore, P2X4R signaling is suggested to act as an enhancer for both Ag-dependent and -independent MC activation. Taken together, targeting the ionotropic P2X4R may be a novel strategy for controlling allergic reactions.

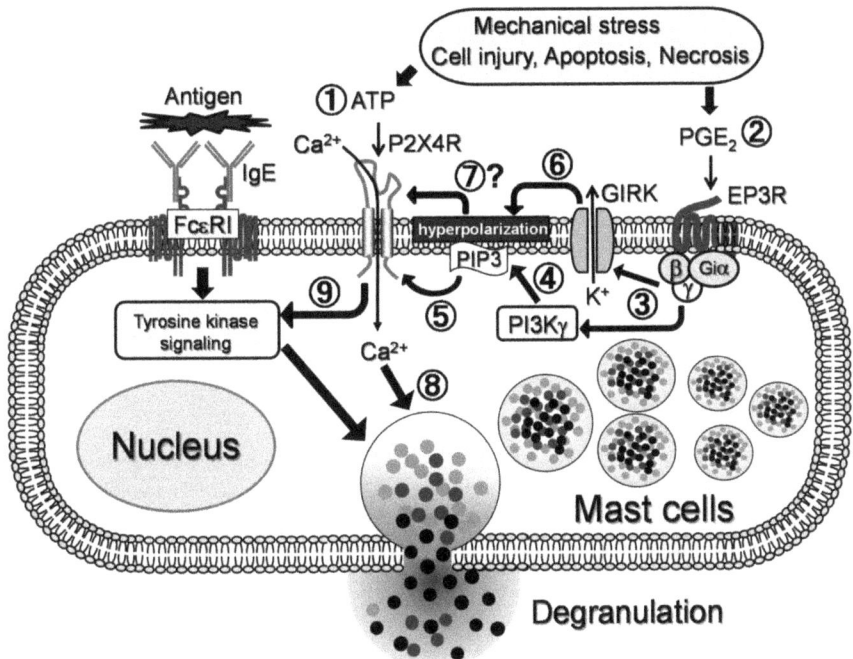

Figure 8. Proposed mechanism of interaction between P2X4 receptor (P2X4R) and EP3 receptor (EP3R) signals for the synergistic degranulation in mast cells(MCs). Extracellular ATP released from damaged cells stimulates MC P2X4R ①, leading to Ca^{2+} influx. Such conditions are accompanied by an inflammation with increased production of prostaglandin (PG)E_2. In MCs, PGE_2 stimulates Gi-coupled EP3R ②, leading to activation of phosphoinositide 3-kinase (PI3K)γ and G protein-coupled inwardly-rectifying K^+ channel (GIRK) via βγ-complex of the G protein ③. Activation of PI3Kγ increases phosphoinositide-3,4,5-trisphosphate (PIP3) levels in plasma membrane ④, thereby promoting P2X4R channel activity ⑤. GIRK activation may cause hyperpolarization of the membrane potential ⑥, which would increase the driving force of Ca^{2+} inflow through P2X4R ⑦. These interactions between P2X4R and EP3R signals lead to the observed synergy in MC degranulation ⑧. P2X4R signal also promotes IgE-dependent tyrosine kinase-mediated signals to induce facilitated degranulation, as described previously ⑨ [12].

4. Materials and Methods

4.1. Materials

UTP, ATP, ADP, PGE_1, PGE_2, 2,4-dinitrophenyl human serum albumin (DNP-HSA), anti-DNP IgE (clone SPE-7), *p*-nitrophenyl *N*-acetyl-β-d-glucosaminide, and the GenElute Mammalian Total RNA miniprep kit were obtained from Sigma-Aldrich (Tokyo, Japan). Allophycocyanin (APC)-conjugated rat anti-mouse c-Kit antibodies (clone 2B8) were obtained from BD Pharmingen (Tokyo, Japan). Phycoerythrin (PE)-conjugated mouse anti-mouse FcεRIα antibodies (clone MAR-1) were obtained from eBioscience (San Diego, CA, USA). Recombinant mouse interleukin (IL)-3 and recombinant mouse SCF were obtained from Peprotech (London, UK). MRS2179, AR-C118925, NF449, AZ10606120, 5-BDBD, Ivermectin, PP2, LY303511, LY294002, Triciribine, and AS605240 were obtained from Tocris Bioscience (Bristol, UK). R406 was obtained from Cayman Chemical (Michigan, USA). Fura-2-acetoxymethylester (AM) and PTX were obtained from Wako (Osaka, Japan). Anti-phospho-Syk, anti-Syk, anti-phospho-ERK1/2, anti-ERK1/2, anti-phospho-Akt, and anti-Akt antibodies were obtained from Cell Signaling Technology (Danvers, MA, USA). ONO-DI-004 (selective EP1 agonist),

ONO-AE1-259-01 (selective EP2 agonist), ONO-AE-248 (selective EP3 agonist), and ONO-AE1-329 (selective EP4 agonist) were obtained from ONO Pharmaceuticals (Osaka, Japan). All other chemicals were of reagent-grade or the highest quality available.

4.2. Animals

P2X4R-deficient mice were generated by Dr. Yamamoto (University of Tokyo), as described previously [35]. C57BL/6 and Kit$^{Wsh/Wsh}$ mice were purchased from SLC Japan (Hamamatsu, Japan) and RIKEN (Ibaraki, Japan), respectively. All mice were maintained under specific pathogen-free conditions at the animal facility of Takasaki University of Health and Welfare. All experiments were performed in accordance with the regulations of the Animal Research Committee of Takasaki University of Health and Welfare.(Approval number: 1813, 1 April, 2018)

4.3. Cell Culture

BMMCs were established using bone marrow from C57BL/6 mice, as described previously [36]. Briefly, bone marrow cells were collected from the femur and cultured in RPMI1640 medium containing 10% fetal bovine serum, 100 units/mL penicillin, 100 μg/mL streptomycin, and 10 ng/mL recombinant IL-3. After 2 weeks, the cells were cultured with 10 ng/mL of recombinant SCF for 4–6 weeks. After these treatments, almost all (>95%) cells displayed an MC phenotype, as indicated by CD117 (c-Kit) and FcεRI expression measured using a FACSCant II flow cytometer (BD Biosciences, Tokyo, Japan).

4.4. Degranulation Assay

Degranulation was evaluated by measuring β-hexosaminidase release, as described previously [36]. BMMCs were sensitized with 50 ng/mL anti-DNP IgE overnight in RPMI 1640 growth medium. Cells were washed twice with phosphate buffered saline (PBS), suspended in Krebs-Ringer-HEPES (KRH) buffer (130 mM NaCl, 4.7 mM KCl, 4.0 mM NaHCO$_3$, 1.2 mM KH$_2$PO$_4$, 1.2 mM MgSO$_4$, 1.8 mM CaCl$_2$, 11.5 mM glucose) and 10 mM HEPES (pH 7.4) containing 0.1% bovine serum albumin (BSA), and then stimulated under various conditions for 5 min at 37 °C. Reactions were terminated by placing the cells on ice and centrifuging them. Supernatants were collected and the cell pellets were lysed in 1 % Triton X-100. The supernatant and cell lysate were incubated with an equal volume of 1 mM p-nitrophenyl N-acetyl-β-D-glucosaminide dissolved in citrate buffer (pH 4.5) in a 96-well plate at 37 °C for 30 min. Na$_2$CO$_3$/NaHCO$_3$ buffer (pH 10.4) was then added and the absorbance was measured at 405/655 nm.

4.5. [Ca^{2+}]i Measurement

Cells were collected and washed twice with KRH containing 0.1 % BSA, suspended in KRH-BSA buffer, and treated with 1 μM Fura-2 AM at 37 °C for 20 min. The Fura-2-loaded cells were washed twice with KRH-BSA buffer and adjusted to 1–2 × 10^5 cells/mL. Changes in Fura-2 fluorescence were measured as described previously [36].

4.6. Western Blot

Cells were collected, washed with PBS, and resuspended in KRH. The reaction was performed in KRH buffer and terminated by adding 4× sample buffer. The lysate was separated by 10% sodium dodecyl sulfate polyacrylamide gel electrophoresis (SDS-PAGE) and transferred to Immobilon-P polyvinylidene fluoride (PVDF) membranes. The PVDF membranes were blocked with 5% BSA-TBST for 1 h at room temperature, exposed to primary antibodies overnight at 4 °C, and secondary antibodies for 2 h at room temperature. Antibodies were diluted as follows: anti-phospho-Syk (1:1000), anti-syk (1:1000), anti-phospho-ERK1/2 (1:1000), anti-ERK1/2 (1:1000), anti-phospho-Akt (1:1000), anti-Akt (1:1000), and horseradish peroxidase (HRP)-linked anti-rabbit IgG (1:10000). The entire western blots were shown in Supplementary Materials.

4.7. Quantitative RT-PCR (qRT-PCR)

Total RNA was isolated using the GenElute Mammalian Total RNA miniprep kit. First-strand cDNA was synthesized using Moloney Murine Leukemia Virus reverse transcriptase with a 6-mer random primer. qRT-PCR was performed using an SYBR green kit, as described previously [37].

4.8. PGE_2-Induced Skin Edema

Mice were anesthetized with isoflurane, injected intravenously with 200 µL 0.5% Evans blue diluted in PBS, and injected intradermally in the right ear with PGE_2 (1.5 nmol) in 20 µL saline and in the left ear with a vehicle of 0.1% ethanol in saline. After 30 min, the mice were sacrificed and their ears collected and weighed. Evans blue dye was extracted from the ears with 1 mL formamide at 55 °C for 24 h and absorbance measured at 620 nm. Data are expressed as µg of Evans blue per mg of ear.

4.9. Statistics

All experiments were repeated at least three times, yielding similar results. Data represent the mean ± standard error of the mean (SEM). Statistical analyses were performed using the Student's *t*-test for two sample comparisons and one-way analysis of variance (ANOVA) with Dunnett's two-tailed test for multiple comparisons. *p* values < 0.05 were considered statistically significant.

Supplementary Materials: The following are available online at http://www.mdpi.com/1422-0067/20/20/5157/s1.

Author Contributions: Conceptualization, K.Y. (Kazuki Yoshida), M.I. and I.M.; Methodology, K.Y. (Kazuki Yoshida), M.I. and I.M.; Formal analysis, K.Y. (Kazuki Yoshida); Investigation, K.Y. (Kazuki Yoshida), M.T., T.N. and K.O.; Resources, K.Y. (Kimiko Yamamoto); Data curation, K.Y. (Kazuki Yoshida); Writing—Original draft preparation, K.Y. (Kazuki Yoshida); Writing—Review and editing, I.M.

Funding: This research was funded by JSPS KAKENHI, grant numbers 18K14925 to K.Y and 19K07328 to I.M., and by the The Japan Science Society, Sasakawa Scientific Research Grant to K.Y.

Conflicts of Interest: The authors declare no conflict of interest.

Abbreviations

$[Ca^{2+}]i$	Intracellular Ca^{2+} concentration
A_3R	A_3 receptor
Ag	Antigen
APC	Allophycocyanin
BMMCs	Bone marrow-derived mast cells
DNP-HSA	2,4-dinitrophenyl human serum albumin
EP3R	EP3 receptor
FcεRI	High affinity IgE receptors
GPCR	G-protein-coupled receptors
IL	Interleukin
KRH	Krebs-Ringer-HEPES
MC	Mast cell
P2X4R	P2X4 receptor
PE	Phycoerythrin
PG	Prostaglandin
PI3K	Phosphoinositide 3-kinase
PLC	Phospholipase C
PTX	Pertussis toxin
PVDF	Immobilon-P polyvinylidene fluoride
qRT-PCR	Quantitative reverse transcription-polymerase chain reaction
S1P	Sphingosine-1-phosphate
SDS-PAGE	Sodium dodecyl sulfate polyacrylamide gel electrophoresis

References

1. Metcalfe, D.D.; Baram, D.; Mekori, Y. Mast cells. *Pharmacol. Rev.* **1997**, *77*, 1033–1079. [CrossRef] [PubMed]
2. Da Silva, E.Z.M.; Jamur, M.C.; Oliver, C. Mast cell function: A new vision of an old cell. *J. Histochem. Cytochem.* **2014**, *62*, 698–738. [CrossRef] [PubMed]
3. Metcalfe, D.D.; Peavy, R.D.; Gilfillan, A.M. Mechanisms of mast cell signaling in anaphylaxis. *J. Allergy Clin. Immunol.* **2009**, *124*, 639–646. [CrossRef] [PubMed]
4. Metzger, H. The receptor with high affinity for IgE. *Immunol. Rev.* **1992**, *125*, 37–48. [CrossRef]
5. Gilfillan, A.M.; Tkaczyk, C. Integrated signalling pathways for mast-cell activation. *Nat. Rev. Immunol.* **2006**, *6*, 218–230. [CrossRef]
6. Kuehn, H.S.; Gilfillan, A.M. G protein-coupled receptors and the modification of FcεRI-mediated mast cell activation. *Immunol. Lett.* **2007**, *113*, 59–69. [CrossRef]
7. Moncada, S.; Ferreira, S.; Vane, J. Prostaglandins, aspirin-like drugs and the oedema of inflammation. *Nature* **1973**, *246*, 217–219. [CrossRef]
8. Borea, P.A.; Gessi, S.; Merighi, S.; Varani, K. Adenosine as a multi-signalling guardian angel in human diseases: When, where and how does it exert its protective Effects? *Trends Pharmacol. Sci.* **2016**, *37*, 419–434. [CrossRef]
9. Kuehn, H.S.; Beaven, M.A.; Ma, H.-T.; Kim, M.-S.; Metcalfe, D.D.; Gilfillan, A.M. Synergistic activation of phospholipases Cγ and Cβ: A novel mechanism for PI3K-independent enhancement of FcεRI-induced mast cell mediator release. *Cell. Signal.* **2008**, *20*, 625–636. [CrossRef]
10. Kuehn, H.S.; Jung, M.-Y.; Beaven, M.A.; Metcalfe, D.D.; Gilfillan, A.M. Prostaglandin E 2 activates and utilizes mTORC2 as a central signaling locus for the regulation of mast cell chemotaxis and mediator release. *J. Biol. Chem.* **2011**, *286*, 391–402. [CrossRef]
11. Laffargue, M.; Calvez, R.; Finan, P.; Trifilieff, A.; Barbier, M.; Altruda, F.; Hirsch, E.; Wymann, M.P. Phosphoinositide 3-kinase γ is an essential amplifier of mast cell function. *Immunity* **2002**, *16*, 441–451. [CrossRef]
12. Yoshida, K.; Ito, M.; Matsuoka, I. Divergent regulatory roles of extracellular ATP in the degranulation response of mouse bone marrow-derived mast cells. *Int. Immunopharmacol.* **2017**, *43*, 99–107. [CrossRef] [PubMed]
13. Yoshida, K.; Ito, M.; Yamamoto, K.; Koizumi, S.; Tanaka, S.; Furuta, K.; Matsuoka, I. Extracellular ATP augments antigen-induced murine mast cell degranulation and allergic responses via P2X4 receptor activation. *J. Immunol.* **2019**. submitted for publication.
14. Redegeld, F.A.; Yu, Y.; Kumari, S.; Charles, N.; Blank, U. Non-IgE mediated mast cell activation. *Immunol. Rev.* **2018**, *282*, 87–113. [CrossRef] [PubMed]
15. Fitz, J.G. Regulation of cellular ATP release. *Trans. Am. Clin. Climatol. Assoc.* **2007**, *118*, 199–208.
16. Gallenga, C.; Pandolfi, F.; Caraffa, A.; Ronconi, G.; Toniato, E.; Martinotti, S.; Conti, P. Interleukin-1 family cytokines and mast cells: activation and inhibition. *J. Biol. Regul. Homeost. Agents* **2019**, *33*, 1–6.
17. Caraffa, A.; Gallenga, C.E.; Kritas, S.K.; Ronconi, G.; Conti, P. Impact of mast cells in systemic lupus erythematosus: can inflammation be inhibited? *J. Biol. Regul. Homeost. Agents* **2019**, *33*, 669–673.
18. Antonopulos, D.; Tsilioni, I.; Balatsos, N.A.A.; Gourgoulianis, K.I.; Theoharides, T.C. The mast cell—Neurofibromatosis connection. *J. Biol. Regul. Homeost. Agents* **2019**, *33*, 657–659.
19. Lazarowski, E.R. Vesicular and conductive mechanisms of nucleotide release. *Purinergic. Signal* **2012**, *8*, 359–373. [CrossRef]
20. Dosch, M.; Gerber, J.; Jebbawi, F.; Beldi, G. Mechanisms of ATP Release by inflammatory cells. *Int. J. Mol. Sci.* **2018**, *19*, 1222. [CrossRef]
21. Burnstock, G. Purinergic signalling: Therapeutic developments. *Front. Pharmacol.* **2017**, *8*, 661. [CrossRef] [PubMed]
22. Morimoto, K.; Shirata, N.; Taketomi, Y.; Tsuchiya, S.; Segi-Nishida, E.; Inazumi, T.; Kabashima, K.; Tanaka, S.; Murakami, M.; Narumiya, S.; et al. Prostaglandin E_2–EP3 signaling induces inflammatory swelling by mast cell activation. *J. Immunol.* **2014**, *192*, 1130–1137. [CrossRef] [PubMed]
23. Needleman, P.; Minkes, M.S.; Douglas, J.R. Stimulation of prostaglandin biosynthesis by adenine nucleotides: Profile of prostaglandin release by perfused organs. *Circ. Res.* **1974**, *34*, 455–460. [CrossRef] [PubMed]

24. Loredo, G.A.; Benton, H.P. ATP and UTP activate calcium-mobilizing P2U-like receptors and act synergistically with interleukin-1 to stimulate prostaglandin E_2 release from human rheumatoid synovial cells. *Arthritis Rheum.* **1998**, *41*, 246–255. [CrossRef]
25. Sugimoto, Y.; Narumiya, S. Prostaglandin E receptors. *J. Biol. Chem.* **2007**, *282*, 11613–11617. [CrossRef]
26. Khakh, B.S.; Proctor, W.R.; Dunwiddie, T.V.; Labarca, C.; Lester, H.A. Allosteric control of gating and kinetics at P2X 4 receptor channels. *J. Neurosci.* **1999**, *19*, 7289–7299. [CrossRef]
27. Bernier, L.-P.; Ase, A.R.; Chevallier, S.; Blais, D.; Zhao, Q.; Boue-Grabot, E.; Logothetis, D.; Seguela, P. Phosphoinositides regulate P2X4 ATP-gated channels through direct interactions. *J. Neurosci.* **2008**, *28*, 12938–12945. [CrossRef]
28. Qian, Y.X.; McCloskey, M.A. Activation of mast cell K^+ channels through multiple G protein-linked receptors. *Proc. Natl. Acad. Sci. USA* **1993**, *90*, 7844–7848. [CrossRef]
29. Ashmole, I.; Bradding, P. Ion channels regulating mast cell biology. *Clin. Exp. Allergy* **2013**, *43*, 491–502. [CrossRef]
30. Shumilina, E.; Lam, R.S.; Wölbing, F.; Matzner, N.; Zemtsova, I.M.; Sobiesiak, M.; Mahmud, H.; Sausbier, U.; Biedermann, T.; Ruth, P.; et al. Blunted IgE-mediated activation of mast cells in mice lacking the Ca^{2+}-Activated K^+ channel K Ca 3.1. *J. Immunol.* **2008**, *180*, 8040–8047. [CrossRef]
31. Tsuda, M.; Shigemoto-Mogami, Y.; Koizumi, S.; Mizokoshi, A.; Kohsaka, S.; Salter, M.W.; Inoue, K. P2X4 receptors induced in spinal microglia gate tactile allodynia after nerve injury. *Nature* **2003**, *424*, 778–783. [CrossRef] [PubMed]
32. Li, F.; Guo, N.; Ma, Y.; Ning, B.; Wang, Y.; Kou, L. Inhibition of P2X4 suppresses joint inflammation and damage in collagen-induced arthritis. *Inflammation* **2014**, *37*, 146–153. [CrossRef] [PubMed]
33. Ledderose, C.; Fakhari, M.; Lederer, J.A.; Robson, S.C.; Visner, G.A.; Junger, W.G.; Liu, K.; Kondo, Y.; Slubowski, C.J.; Dertnig, T.; et al. Purinergic P2X4 receptors and mitochondrial ATP production regulate T cell migration. *J. Clin. Invest.* **2018**, *128*, 3583–3594. [CrossRef] [PubMed]
34. Zech, A.; Wiesler, B.; Ayata, C.K.; Schlaich, T.; Dürk, T.; Hoßfeld, M.; Ehrat, N.; Cicko, S.; Idzko, M.; Zech, A.; et al. P2rx4 deficiency in mice alleviates allergen-induced airway inflammation. *Oncotarget* **2016**, *7*, 80288–80297. [CrossRef] [PubMed]
35. Yamamoto, K.; Sokabe, T.; Matsumoto, T.; Yoshimura, K.; Shibata, M.; Ohura, N.; Fukuda, T.; Sato, T.; Sekine, K.; Kato, S.; et al. Impaired flow-dependent control of vascular tone and remodeling in P2X4-deficient mice. *Nat. Med.* **2006**, *12*, 133–137. [CrossRef]
36. Yoshida, K.; Ito, M.; Matsuoka, I. P2X7 receptor antagonist activity of the anti-allergic agent oxatomide. *Eur. J. Pharmacol.* **2015**, *767*, 41–51. [CrossRef]
37. Ito, M.; Matsuoka, I. Inhibition of $P2Y_6$ receptor-mediated phospholipase C activation and Ca^{2+} signalling by prostaglandin E_2 in J774 murine macrophages. *Eur. J. Pharmacol.* **2015**, *749*, 124–132. [CrossRef]

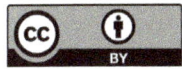

© 2019 by the authors. Licensee MDPI, Basel, Switzerland. This article is an open access article distributed under the terms and conditions of the Creative Commons Attribution (CC BY) license (http://creativecommons.org/licenses/by/4.0/).

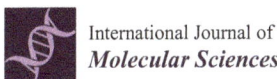

Article

Repeated Vaginal Exposures to the Common Cosmetic and Household Preservative Methylisothiazolinone Induce Persistent, Mast Cell-Dependent Genital Pain in ND4 Mice

Erica Arriaga-Gomez [1,†], Jaclyn Kline [1,†], Elizabeth Emanuel [1], Nefeli Neamonitaki [1], Tenzin Yangdon [1], Hayley Zacheis [1], Dogukan Pasha [1], Jinyoung Lim [2], Susan Bush [3], Beebie Boo [1], Hanna Mengistu [1], Ruby Kinnamon [1], Robin Shields-Cutler [1], Elizabeth Wattenberg [4] and Devavani Chatterjea [1,*]

1. Biology Department, Macalester College, Saint Paul, MN 55105, USA; arriagagomez.erica@gmail.com (E.A.-G.); jaclynmlkline@gmail.com (J.K.); elizabethe819@gmail.com (E.E.); nefnea@gmail.com (N.N.); tyangdon@macalester.edu (T.Y.); hzacheis@macalester.edu (H.Z.); dpasha@macalester.edu (D.P.); beebieboo@gmail.com (B.B.); hmengist@umn.edu (H.M.); rkinnamo@macalester.edu (R.K.); rshield2@macalester.edu (R.S.-C.)
2. Mathematics, Statistics & Computer Science Department, Macalester College, Saint Paul, MN 55105, USA; jlim2@macalester.edu
3. Biology Department, Trinity College, Hartford, CT 06106, USA; susan.bush@trincoll.edu
4. Division of Environmental Health Sciences, University of Minnesota School of Public Health, Minneapolis, MN 55455, USA; watte004@umn.edu
* Correspondence: chatterjead@macalester.edu; Tel.: +1-(651)-696-6621
† These authors contributed equally to this work.

Received: 12 September 2019; Accepted: 24 October 2019; Published: 28 October 2019

Abstract: A history of allergies doubles the risk of vulvodynia—a chronic pain condition of unknown etiology often accompanied by increases in numbers of vulvar mast cells. We previously established the biological plausibility of this relationship in mouse models where repeated exposures to the allergens oxazolone or dinitrofluorobenzene on the labiar skin or inside the vaginal canal of ND4 Swiss Webster outbred mice led to persistent tactile sensitivity and local increases in mast cells. In these models, depletion of mast cells alleviated pain. While exposure to cleaning chemicals has been connected to elevated vulvodynia risk, no single agent has been linked to adverse outcomes. We sensitized female mice to methylisothiazolinone (MI)—a biocide preservative ubiquitous in cosmetics and cleaners—dissolved in saline on their flanks, and subsequently challenged them with MI or saline for ten consecutive days in the vaginal canal. MI-challenged mice developed persistent tactile sensitivity, increased vaginal mast cells and eosinophils, and had higher serum Immunoglobulin E. Therapeutic and preventive intra-vaginal administration of Δ^9-tetrahydrocannabinol reduced mast cell accumulation and tactile sensitivity. MI is known to cause skin and airway irritation in humans, and here we provide the first pre-clinical evidence that repeated MI exposures can also provoke allergy-driven genital pain.

Keywords: mast cells; allergy; vulvar pain; methylisothiazolinone; Δ-9 tetrahydrocannabinol

1. Introduction

Debilitating, unexplained provoked localized vulvar pain or vulvodynia affects a significant proportion (~8%) of women [1,2] and is epidemiologically linked to a history of both seasonal and contact allergies [3]. Vulvar biopsies from diagnosed patients show increases in mast cells and nerves [4–6]. To recapitulate and dissect the pathobiology of allergy-driven tactile sensitivity and to inform novel therapies, we established mouse models of allergy-driven genital pain [7–9]. We have shown that contact hypersensitivity to the commonly used laboratory haptens oxazolone (Ox) on the labiar skin or dinitrofluorobenzene (DNFB) on the labiar skin or vaginal canal induces persistent tactile genital pain and increased accumulation of mast cells in the labiar tissues of outbred, female ND4 mice well beyond the resolution of visible inflammation. Chemical depletion of labiar mast cells reduced Ox-driven painful responses [8] and therapeutic topical administration of Δ-9-tetrahydrocannabinol (THC) in the vaginal canal alleviated DNFB-induced pain and reduced numbers of accumulated mast cells in the affected tissue [9]. Here, we examined the potential of a common household chemical, 2-methyl-4-isothiazolin-3-one/methylisothiazolinone (MI), to induce contact hypersensitivity reactions and consequent allergy-driven genital pain in ND4 female outbred mice. MI is a biocide preservative present in soaps, shampoos, vaginal washes, household cleaners, and paints [10,11]. Recent evidence suggests that a significant portion of people exposed to MI developed the capacity for an allergic response [11,12], showed exacerbated inflammatory responses [13], and experienced tissue injury in the skin or lungs [12,14] after exposure. Allergic responses to MI have also been linked to vulvar dermatitis [15,16], but no connections between such dermatoses and the later development of vulvar pain have been made in the published clinical literature. Recently, Reed and colleagues identified exposures to household and workplace chemicals as a possible risk factor for the development of vulvodynia [17]. Our previously published mouse models demonstrated the biological plausibility of the epidemiological link between chemical exposures and the development of genital pain. However, a specific link between vulvodynia and a known environmental chemical does not yet exist. We suggest that MI is a plausible candidate for an environmental irritant/allergen, and that exposure to MI might drive allergy-provoked pain. Here, we repeatedly applied MI dissolved in saline (a surrogate for water-based cleansers that typically contain MI as a preservative) topically within the vaginal canals of mice and characterized consequent allergic inflammation, accumulation of mast cells, and ano-genital sensitivity to pressure. We also assessed the effects of therapeutic and preventive administration of topical THC treatments in the vaginal canal on mast cell abundance and painful sensitivity.

2. Results

2.1. Meta-Analysis of Patch-Testing Studies Reveals Widespread Sensitization to MI in Populations Tested in Europe and North America

MI has been in use as a biocide preservative for many decades by itself and, earlier, in conjunction with methylchloroisothiazolinone (MCI), and adverse allergic reactions to these chemicals were reported as early as the 1980s [18,19] in both clinical and pre-clinical studies [20,21]. MCI was considered a strong sensitizer and subsequently discontinued; MI, which was previously used at a lower concentration in the MI/MCI mixture, was used at a higher concentration by itself, and safe limits for MI in cosmetic preparations were set at 100 ppm [22]. However, reports of allergic outcomes as well as sensitization of populations exposed to the purported safe doses of MI via household and industrial contexts have continued to rise. We conducted a meta-analysis of studies that reported MI-sensitivity via patch testing to evaluate the epidemiological trends of allergic sensitivity to MI. Of the 163 epidemiological studies, between 1995 and 2019, reported on PubMed.gov, most were conducted in Europe, along with a few North American investigations (Figure 1A). One article without MI parts per million (ppm) tested was excluded from plotting [23]. Sample sizes varied between fewer than 100 and more than 10,000 human subjects and concentrations of MI used varied between 500 and 2000 ppm. By 2012, studies reporting 5–10% of participants being MI-sensitive were more prevalent, while the majority of studies reporting 1% of participants sensitized to MI were published prior to 2012 (Figure 1B). In 2013, the American Contact Dermatitis Society named MI the Allergen of the Year [24]. Sensitivity to MI is clear and present in populations within North America and Europe, and adverse health outcomes related to MI are on the rise. Given that exposure to household cleaning products is a risk factor for developing vulvodynia [17], we found it important to investigate whether repeated exposure to MI provoked persistent pain in laboratory mice.

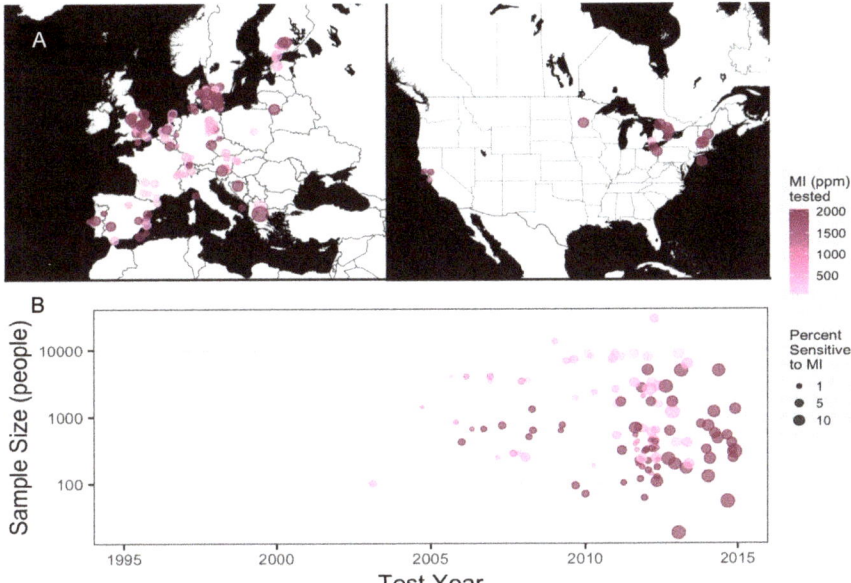

Figure 1. Population level sensitization to methylisothiazolinone (MI) in Europe and North America. (**A**) Location of epidemiological studies conducted in Europe (left) and North America (right); all points plotted at the approximate latitude and longitude of the original study with random noise added for easier visualization. (**B**) Sample size reported by epidemiological studies in Europe and North America using MI patch tests. Point placement corresponds with the year each study ended. Sample size may include multi-year studies if yearly data were not available. Color gradient indicates the highest concentration of MI in parts per million (ppm) tested in each study and the size of the point represents the proportion of the population that tested sensitive to MI. Studies in which MI ppm were not reported are excluded from the plot. The size of each point represents the percent of participants that were found to be sensitized to MI ($n = 151$ studies).

2.2. Repeated Exposures to MI in the Vaginal Canal Induce Painful Ano-Genital Responses to Touch and Aberrant Mast Cell Accumulation in the Affected Tissues

Using standard conventions of species scaling practices, we used 10,000 ppm (1% w/v in saline; 100 times the safe human dose [22] of 100 ppm, i.e., ppm) as a sensitizing dose and a lower 0.5% dose for subsequent challenges of MI dissolved in saline in our experiments using 6–8-week-old outbred ND4 female mice. These doses are similar to those used for dermal sensitization and challenge using MI in CBA [25] mice, as well as dermal and airway sensitization and challenge with MI in C57BL/6 and BALB/C mouse strains [26]. To our knowledge, we are the first to use MI in ND4 mice and, therefore, we first confirmed that these sensitization and challenge doses caused detectable and significant ear-swelling responses in flank-sensitized ND4 mice after three topical challenges on the ear (Figure S1).

Next, we sensitized mice with 1% and 0.5% MI dissolved in saline on their shaved flanks before administering 10 daily challenges of 0.5% MI or saline in their vaginal canals (Figure 2A). We assessed changes in tissue mast cells after 10 intra-vaginal challenges with 0.5% MI or saline and found that one day after 10 MI challenges, there were 1.75 times as many mast cells in the vaginal canal tissue of sensitized female ND4 Swiss mice compared with vehicle-challenged controls, although this increase was no longer detectable by 21 days (Figure 3A–G). This was accompanied by a significant increase in serum IgE levels in MI-challenged mice one day after the cessation of challenges (Figure 3H); circulating IgE is important for mast cell expansion and survival [27,28]. Furthermore, we observed that sensitized female ND4 Swiss mice were more sensitive to touch, as measured with an electronic Von Frey meter, with a 60% decrease in withdrawal threshold one day after 10 exposures to MI in the vaginal canal (Figure 3I). Shaved and sensitized mice that were treated with 0.9% saline were significantly less sensitive than their MI-treated counterparts and did not display a similar decrease from baseline. MI-challenged mice remained significantly more sensitive than saline-treated controls for up to 14 days (Figure 3I). These observations of early mast cell accumulation, elevated serum IgE, and consequent painful sensitivity in response to MI exposures are congruent with similar outcomes we have previously described in mice exposed to commonly used laboratory haptens Ox and DNFB [7–9], and suggest that this ubiquitous household preservative can induce allergy-provoked pain.

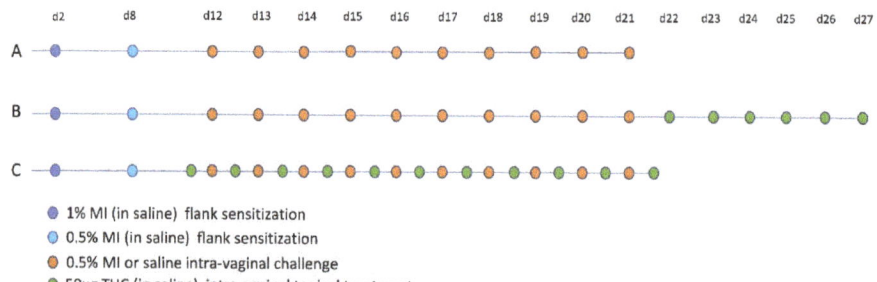

Figure 2. Sensitization, challenge, and treatment timelines. Schedule of MI in saline flank sensitizations and challenges (**A–C**). (**B**) Therapeutic intra-vaginal Δ-9-tetrahydrocannabinol (THC) treatment timeline. (**C**) Preventative intra-vaginal THC treatments.

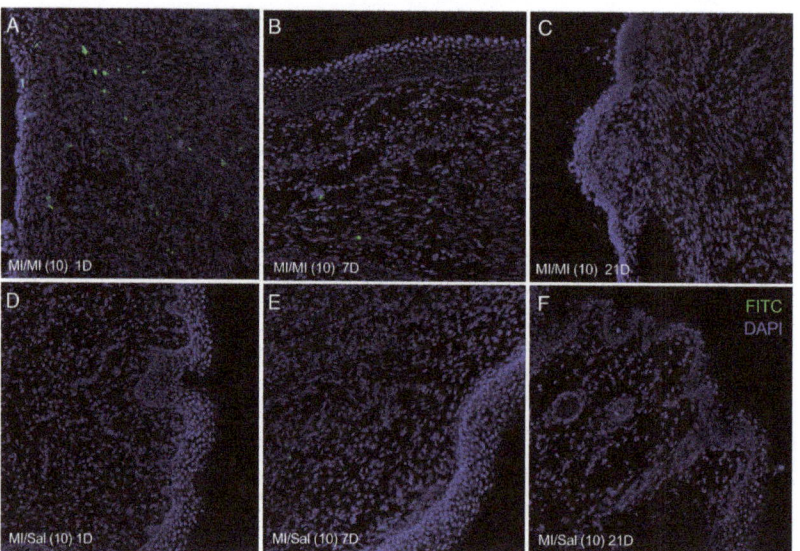

Figure 3. *Cont.*

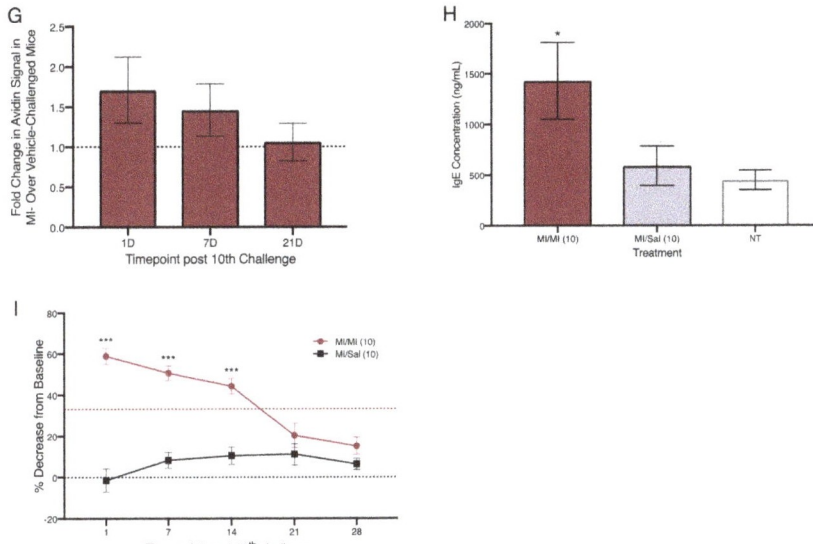

Figure 3. Increased mast cell density in the vaginal canal and elevated tactile ano-genital sensitivity after 10 intra-vaginal MI challenges in previously sensitized ND4 female mice. Representative confocal images of vaginal canal tissue from MI sensitized mice challenged with MI (**A–C**) or saline **D–F**) at 1, 7, and 21 days after the 10th MI challenge, respectively. Mast cells stained with FITC-conjugated avidin (green) and nuclei counterstained with DAPI (blue); 200× magnification. (**G**) Density of avidin$^+$ mast cells in 12 μm vaginal canal cryo-sections from sensitized mice challenged with MI or saline. Results reported as fold change in avidin signal in MI- over saline-treated mice. Dotted line denotes no change. Data pooled from 5–6 mice. (**H**) Serum IgE content in mice treated with MI or saline in the vaginal canal 1 day after the last MI/saline challenge. NT bar denotes serum IgE levels in naïve age-matched, untreated mice. Significance with respect to vehicle control group * = $p < 0.05$; 4–6 mice/treatment group. (**I**) Tactile sensitivity in MI and saline challenged mice, reported as mean ± SEM of the percent decrease from baseline in the withdrawal threshold for each treatment group; $n = 17$–18 mice/treatment group. Red dotted line = 33% hyperalgesia threshold. Significance with respect to vehicle control group *** $p < 0.001$.

2.3. Repeated Exposures to MI in the Vaginal Canal Induce Inflammatory Changes in the Vaginal Mucosa and in the Spinal Cord of Mice

In our previous experiments, we found that repeated intra-vaginal exposures to the hapten DNFB induced increased levels of *interleukin (IL)-6* and *interferon-γ (IFN-γ)* transcripts in the vaginal canal [9]. Here, we found that one day after the 10th MI challenge, average relative transcript abundance of mRNAs encoding *IFN-γ* and *IL-6* in the vaginal canal tissue of MI-treated ND4 Swiss mice increased twofold over vehicle-challenged mice (Figure 4A). However, at seven days following 10 MI challenges, the amount of *IFN-γ* and *IL-6* transcripts was comparable to vehicle-challenged controls (Figure 4A).

As painful responses to touch persisted for more than two weeks after the cessation of MI exposures in the vaginal canal, we next looked for changes in levels of immunomodulatory factors in the spinal cord of MI-treated versus control mice. IL-1 and IL-6 signaling in the spinal cord are associated with low grade chronic inflammation [29], and intra-thecal injection of anti-IL-6 antibodies has been shown to alleviate pathological pain [30]. We evaluated the relative transcript abundance of *IL-1β* and *IL-6* in the spinal cord of both MI-treated and control mice one and seven days after the 10th challenge. The levels of *IL-1β* were increased by 1.5-fold in the spinal cord one day after 10 challenges, but this increase was resolved by seven days after cessation of challenges (Figure 4B). *IL-6* transcripts were slightly elevated by 0.75-fold to 2-fold in the spinal cord of MI-treated mice at one day after 10 challenges, but the increase was also no longer detected at seven days.

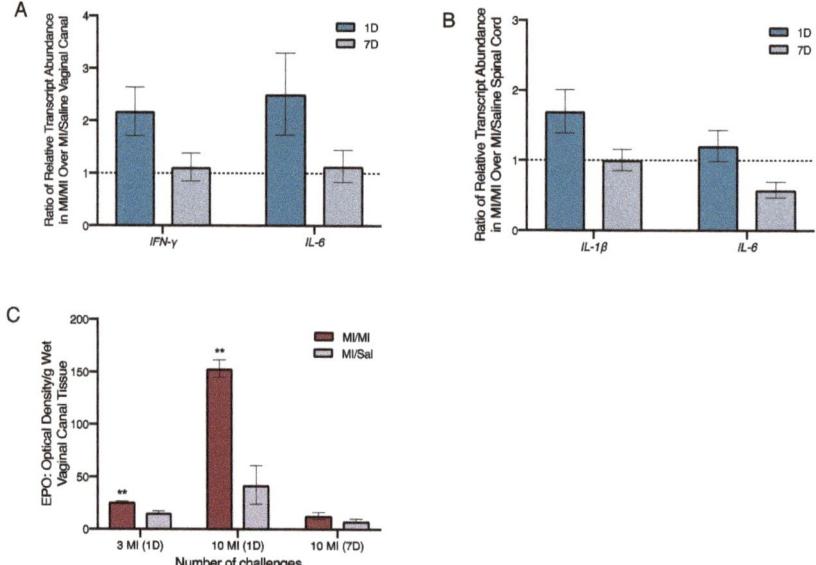

Figure 4. Inflammatory changes in the vaginal canal and spinal cord, and increased eosinophil activity after 10 intra-vaginal MI challenges in previously sensitized ND4 female mice. Relative transcript abundance of *interferon-γ (IFN-γ)* and *interleukin (IL)-6* transcripts in the vaginal canal tissue (**A**) and *IL-1β* and *IL-6* in spinal cord tissue (**B**) of MI challenged mice one and seven days after 10 challenges, normalized to *β2-microglobulin* mRNA levels; 5–6 mice/treatment group. Black dotted line denotes no change in the relative abundance of transcripts. (**C**) Tissue eosinophil peroxidase levels measured by optical density (OD)/g of wet tissue, in the vaginal canal of mice one day after the 3rd and 10th MI challenge; 3–5 mice/treatment group. Significance with respect to vehicle control group ** $p < 0.01$. EPO, eosinophil peroxidase.

Given the increase in eosinophils accompanying pain-inducing allergic exposures to hapten oxazolone we observed earlier [7], we measured the levels of eosinophil peroxidase (EPO; a tissue marker for activated eosinophils) in the vaginal canal after 10 exposures to MI. One day after both 3 and 10 MI challenges, the levels of EPO were significantly higher in MI-treated vaginal canals than in vaginal canals exposed to saline. One day after 10 challenges, mice had around three times higher levels of EPO in MI-treated vaginal canal tissue than controls (Figure 4C). Seven days after the 10th challenge, eosinophil activity in the tissue was no longer increased as compared with saline controls. Mice that were multiply exposed to oxazolone showed neutrophil influx into the painful, allergic tissue [7]. Here, we saw a slight, but not significant increase in myeloperoxidase activity, indicating neutrophil influx into MI-challenged tissue after 1–3 administrations of MI in the vaginal canals of sensitized mice; however, by one day after the 10th administration of MI, we could see no differences in myeloperoxidase activity between saline-challenged and MI-challenged mice (Figure S2).

2.4. Therapeutic Administration of THC in the Vaginal Canal after 10 MI Exposures Reduces Both Mast Cell Numbers as Well as Painful Sensitivity to Touch

Intra-vaginal therapeutic application of THC alleviated DNFB-provoked allergy-driven genital pain in our previous studies [9]. To assess any effects of therapeutic THC treatment following induction of MI-provoked mast cell increase and heightened tactile sensitivity, we administered 50 μg of THC intra-vaginally in 20 µl saline for six consecutive days in the vaginal canal beginning one day after the tenth MI challenge (Figure 2B). One day after six THC treatments, mast cell numbers decreased by 45% compared with mice that received no THC (Figure 5A–C). Seven days after THC treatment, mast cells were slightly decreased by 7% of those observed in untreated MI-challenged mice. By 21 days after the last THC treatment, mast cell numbers for both the no treatment (NT) and THC treatment groups were indistinguishable from one another (Figure 5B); this coincided with the resolution of mast cells to baseline levels after 10 MI challenges (Figure 3A–G). We evaluated tactile sensitivity in mice treated with therapeutic THC and found that, one day following cessation of THC treatment, tactile sensitivity was significantly reduced compared with untreated mice, with THC-treated mice displaying a ~20% decrease from baseline and mice not treated with THC displaying a 45% decrease (Figure 5D). By seven days after the last THC treatment, the sensitivity thresholds for mice treated with THC were at the same levels as mice that did not receive THC.

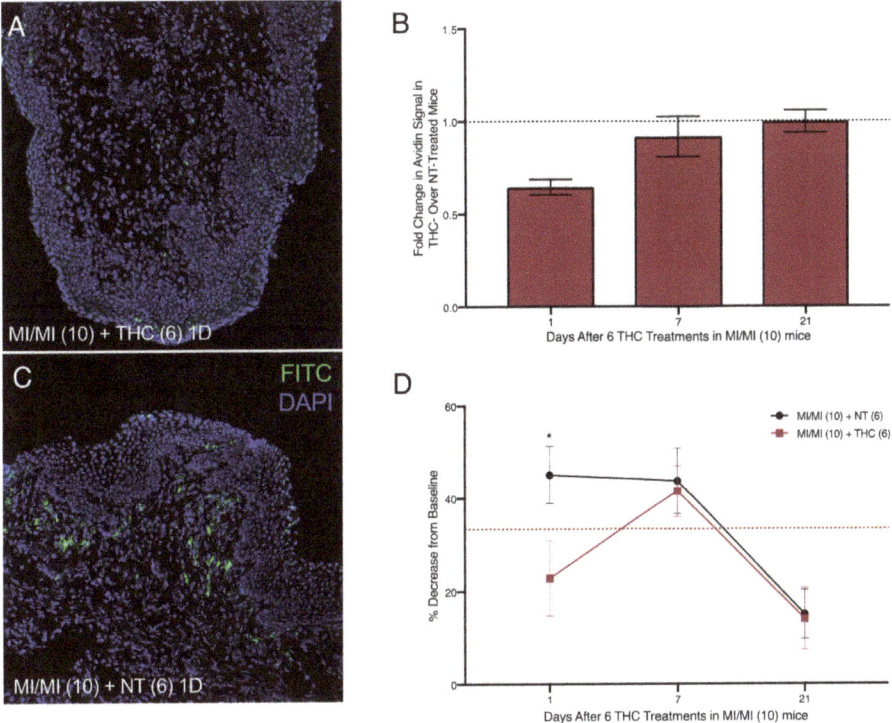

Figure 5. Reduced vaginal mast cell density and ano-genital sensitivity following six intra-vaginal therapeutic THC treatments after 10 vaginal MI challenges in previously sensitized ND4 female mice. (**A,C**) Representative confocal images of vaginal canal tissue from mice that were sensitized and challenged with MI and subsequently treated with THC (**A**) or untreated, that is, NT (**C**), at one day after the last treatment, respectively. Mast cells stained with FITC-conjugated avidin (green) and nuclei counterstained with DAPI (blue); 200× magnification. (**B**) Mast cell density displayed as fold change in avidin signal in THC-treated over NT mice at 1, 7, and 10 days after the 6th THC treatment; 6–7 mice/treatment group. Black dotted line denotes no change in MC abundance. (**D**) Anogenital tactile sensitivity of MI challenged mice treated with NT (black) or therapeutic THC (red) 1, 7, and 10 days after the 6th THC treatment; $n = 8–9$ mice/treatment group. Results displayed as mean ± SEM. Significance with respect to control group * $p < 0.05$.

2.5. Preventive Administration of THC in the Vaginal Canal before and during 10 MI Exposures Reduces Both Mast Cell Numbers as Well as Painful Sensitivity to Touch

We next treated MI-challenged mice with THC before and during exposures to MI to evaluate the potential preventive effects of THC in MI-driven allergy-induced pain. We applied THC inside the vaginal canal 12 h before each MI challenge as well as once 12 h after the 10th challenge (Figure 2C). One day after the cessation of MI challenges, and 12 h after the last THC treatment, mast cell numbers in the THC-treated vaginal canal tissue showed a ~0.6-fold decrease in comparison with non-THC treated mice exposed to MI in the vaginal canal daily for 10 days (Figure 6A,C,D). This comparative decrease persisted at seven days after the last MI challenge; with avidin signal intensity of THC treated MI-challenged mice decreased by ~50% (Figure 6B,C,E). At 21 days after the 10th MI challenge, mast cell numbers between THC-treated and control MI-challenged mice were similar, reflecting the decrease in mast cell density seen at 21 days after 10 MI challenges. Importantly, preventive THC treatment resulted in a significant, persistent reduction in mean tactile sensitivity at one and seven days after cessation of treatment, compared with NT controls (Figure 6F). We observed decreases from the baseline of only 30% and 25% in mice treated preventively with THC at one and seven days after the cessation of MI challenges, respectively, compared with mice not treated with THC, who displayed a 55% decrease from the baseline at one day and a 50% decrease at seven days.

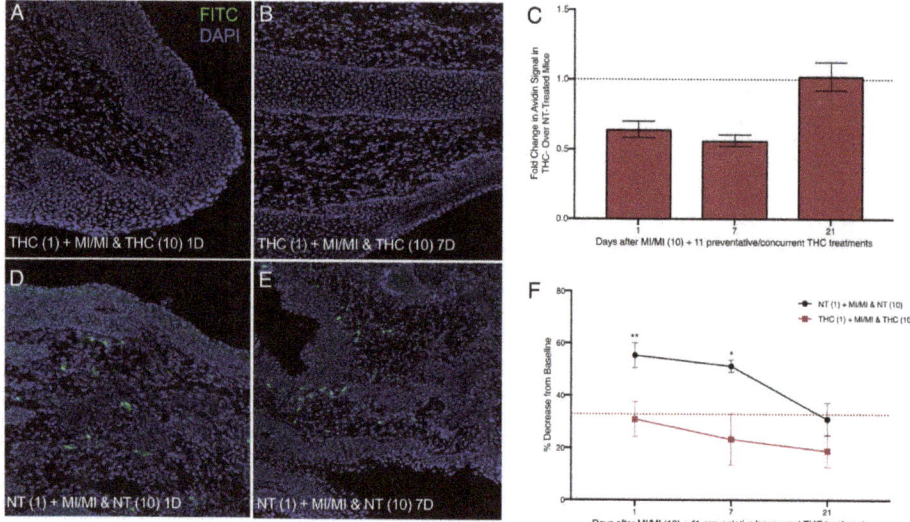

Figure 6. Reduced vaginal mast cell density and ano-genital sensitivity following intra-vaginal preventive THC treatments before and during 10 vaginal MI challenges in previously sensitized ND4 female mice. (**A,B,D,E**) Representative images of vaginal canal tissue from THC-treated (**A,B**) and NT (**D,E**) MI-challenged mice one and seven days after the 10th MI challenge. Mast cells stained with FITC-conjugated avidin (green) and nuclei counterstained with DAPI (blue); 200× magnification. (**C**) Mast cell density displayed as fold change in avidin$^+$ signal intensity of the THC-treated over NT mice; n = 3–7 mice/treatment group. (**F**) Ano-genital tactile sensitivity of preventive THC-treated and NT mice at 1, 7, and 21 days after the 10th MI challenge; 8–9 mice/treatment group. Red dotted line denotes 33% hyperalgesia threshold. Results displayed as mean ± SEM. Significance with respect to control group * $p < 0.05$ and ** $p < 0.01$.

3. Discussion

Our collective understanding of risk factors, etiologies, and effective interventions for vulvodynia continues to evolve. Histories of seasonal and contact allergies [3], recurrent urinogenital infections [31], and chronic psychological stress [32,33] have all been positively associated with individual- and population-level vulvodynia risk. In our previously published work, we have demonstrated the biological plausibility of contact allergy reactions in labiar skin [7,8] and vaginal canal [9] tissues, driving subsequent persistent painful sensitivity to touch in the ano-genital ridge of ND4 female mice. We used hapten irritants, oxazolone and DNFB, commonly used in the laboratory, to study contact hypersensitivity in mice and found a common pattern in the pathogenesis of allergy-driven pain. Multiple exposures to haptens led to abnormal tissue mast cell accumulation and tactile pain. Mast cell depletion, either via intra-labiar secretagogue compound 48/80 [8] or intra-vaginal topical THC [9], led to a temporary alleviation of painful symptoms.

A recent study by Reed et al. [17] suggests that environmental exposure to household and work-related toxins may amplify vulvodynia risk. Accordingly, we demonstrate here that the biocide preservative MI triggers allergy-driven, mast cell-dependent pain responses in a mouse model of vulvodynia. MI is widely used in cosmetics and cleaners, and has been the target of recent scrutiny as a population-level sensitizing allergen [12] and a risk factor for skin and airway injury [12,14]. Our meta-analysis of patch-testing studies (Figure 1) demonstrates significant recent clinical and epidemiological attention paid to MI toxicity in Europe. In 2014, the European Commission's Scientific Committee on Consumer Safety regulated MI out of leave-on cosmetic products and lowered the safe limit of MI in rinse-off cosmetics from 100 ppm to 15 ppm [34]. In contrast, MI is still widely used at 100 ppm in cosmetics in the United States [24].

A limited number of mouse studies of MI toxicity in the past have used sensitizing doses of 1–2% MI followed by 0.5% MI used for elicitation [25,26]. We found that 10 intra-vaginal exposures to 0.5% MI in previously sensitized ND4 female mice caused painful ano-genital sensitivity and vaginal mast cell expansion at one and seven days after cessation of MI challenges, accompanied by increased local transcription of IFN-γ and IL-6 genes and higher levels of circulating IgE. As avidin binds to proteoglycans present in granules, we acknowledge that it is possible that some of the avidin staining we see in the vaginal canal after 10 consecutive MI challenges might be coming from eosinophils or possibly neutrophils present in the tissue. However, as we show in Figure S2 and Figure 4, eosinophils and neutrophils (as measured by tissue peroxidase activity) are no longer increased in the vaginal canal tissue by the time 10 MI challenges have been administered. These outcomes of MI exposure are similar to what we have observed with labiar and vaginal exposures to common laboratory haptens [7–9]. Mast cells are present in murine [35] and human [36] vaginal canal and are known to participate in local inflammatory responses to parasites [37], bacteria [38], and yeast [39]. Mast cell increases have been reported in subsets of vulvodynia patients [5,6], but not in others [40]. Foster and colleagues have described increased levels of inflammatory cytokines in vulvar tissue [41,42], while Reed et al. have reported not finding such differences in the population they studied [43]. However, taken together, multiple lines of evidence suggest that dysregulated inflammation is a part of the pathobiology of vulvodynia.

Pathological inflammation in allergic diseases has been linked, in part, to the bacterial dysbiosis and disruption of the commensal microflora of the gut, lungs, and skin [44]. Altered gut microbiomes have been reported in fibromyalgia patients experiencing chronic widespread pain [45] and associated with visceral abdominal pain [46]. In a pilot study of the effects of MI on the mouse vaginal microbiota, we found that repeated exposures to MI as well as saline vehicle initially disrupt the vaginal microbiota in our mouse model (Figure S3). However, beta diversity analyses suggest that only MI challenges continue to disrupt the microbiota, while saline-treated control mice return toward baseline stability (Figure S3A). This difference in compositional stability between MI and saline treatments is greatest at days 16–17 post-sensitization (Figure S3B). We are currently conducting further experiments to monitor changes in both vaginal and gut microbiota after MI exposures and to investigate resulting dysregulated inflammation in the vaginal canal. Disruptions of this ecosystem have been linked to increased susceptibility to several diseases including bacterial vaginosis [47,48], chlamydia [49], and endometriosis [50], and thus are of interest to the larger pathological implications of this work. In our pilot studies, we see that after three exposures, MI-treated mice also had detectably higher levels of IL-1 and CXCL-2 in vaginal lysates and continued to have higher expression of the genes encoding these cytokines up to a week after MI challenges ended (Figure S3C,D), suggesting continued heightened inflammation in the vaginal canal. The dynamics of the vaginal microbiome in health and disease [51] are relatively understudied and may be a fruitful direction to pursue in understanding the inflammatory correlates of vulvodynia. Given the role of spinal IL-6 in chronic inflammation and pathological pain [30], we tested inflammatory gene expression in the sacral spinal cord of MI-challenged mice and found slight increases in both *IL-6* and *IL-1β* transcripts one day after 10 challenges (Figure 4). IL-1β, released by spinal microglia, has been implicated in inflammatory pain that lasts beyond the presence of the noxious environmental stimulus that triggered it in the first place [52]; this is similar to hapten allergen-driven pain that persists well after antigen challenge in our past and current mouse studies. Systemic increases in nerve growth factor (NGF) have been reported in the serum of some vulvodynia patients [45], and central sensitization of the nervous system reported in others [53]. As such, cellular and molecular mechanisms underlying central sensitization and its contributions to vulvar pain need to be further elucidated to determine whether novel biomarkers and/or targeted therapies can be developed to help at least a subset of the population in need. Although a history of allergies is known to amplify vulvodynia risk, eosinophil levels and activity have not, to our knowledge, been studied in vulvodynia patients. Eosinophils are critical mediators of allergic responses as well as long-term esophageal and airway remodeling [54]. We see MI-driven early increases in eosinophil activity (Figure 3); while specific roles of eosinophils in pain pathologies remain to be characterized, eosinophilia accompanies many painful chronic conditions, including endometriosis [55]. Eosinophils may be another important cellular player to consider in the pathogenesis of vulvar pain.

Vulvodynia is a multifactorial condition and likely has different, potentially overlapping etiologies. Our pre-clinical findings and those from clinical studies affirm that identifying inflammatory biomarkers and cellular mechanisms of action for different etiologies is warranted and may lead to novel effective, targeted therapies. We have observed before [8,9], and see here again, that in tissue allergy-driven persistent pain, mast cell depletion can help relieve tactile sensitivity. Six daily doses of intra-vaginal administration of 50 μg THC after multiple MI exposures alleviates painful responses temporarily for up to seven days, along with a concomitant ~50% reduction in tissue mast cells (Figure 5). Additionally, if pre-sensitized mice are treated daily with THC beginning 12 h before the first MI challenge until 12 h after the last MI challenge, they do not develop painful ano-genital tactile sensitivity (Figure 6). Our results suggest that mast cells may play a role in the cannabinoid-mediated pain reduction of allergy-triggered genital pain in our model, although the effects of cannabinoid signaling on mast cell survival are not known. While topical mast cell granule stabilizer cromolyn has not been efficacious in relief of vulvodynia in the clinic [56], to our knowledge, mast cell depletion therapies have not been tested. Similarly, effects of cannabis-based medicines in vulvodynia pain relief have not been investigated and may well warrant a closer look.

The vaginal mucosa, while susceptible to noxious environmental stimuli, is also known to induce tolerance [57], and we have previously seen that 10 labiar exposures to the hapten DNFB produce longer lasting pain compared with 10 vaginal exposures [9]. While our findings here provide critical support for the idea that intra-vaginal MI exposures can provoke local inflammation and genital pain, human populations are exposed to MI through multiple routes, including skin and airways, and to cumulatively higher doses than the likely already unsafe limit of 100 ppm. The ubiquitous use of methylisothiazolinone in a wide range of consumer products raises the concern that repeated exposures to methylisothiazolinone from multiple sites could exceed the 100 ppm limit, and consequently increase the risk of sensitization in the population. To investigate this idea, we are currently conducting studies to determine whether cumulative exposure to methylisothiazolinone from multiple routes of exposure elicits sensitization as effectively as exposure through a single, localized route. From a regulatory perspective, it is also important to understand the biological threshold at which sensitization and pain occur. Accordingly, we are conducting dose-response studies to determine the doses required to elicit sensitization and pain. In the context of increasing scrutiny of MI toxicity in both the scientific [12] and popular [58] literature, our work here draws attention to a hitherto overlooked harmful outcome of MI exposure—its potential to contribute to allergy-driven persistent genital pain. While a potential link between methylisothiazolinone, mast cells, and vulvar pain may provide new tools for prevention and intervention for those living with vulvodynia, increased understanding of mechanistic connections between chemical exposures, allergies, and chronic pain may well be of even broader use and importance.

4. Materials and Methods

4.1. Meta-Analysis of MI Sensitization Studies

A total of 164 studies of MI-sensitization published from 1995 to 2019 were collected from PubMed.gov using "methylisothiazolinone AND (patch test)" as search terms. All articles were parsed with Python using xml.etree.ElementTree API to extract author names, title, publication year, and journal title. For each study in which patch testing was used to determine sensitization, testing locations, percent sensitivity to MI (ppm), and testing year(s) were extracted manually. Graphs were plotted using R. Scatter plots were generated using the gather() function from the tidyr package and ggplot() function from the ggplot2 package [59]; maps were generated with get_stamenmap() and ggmap() functions in the ggmap package [60].

4.2. Animal Usage

Six to twelve-week-old naive female ND4 Swiss mice (Harlan Laboratories, Indianapolis, IN, USA) were housed with a 12 h light/dark cycle and free access to food and water in Macalester College's animal facilities. Mice were euthanized using 100% CO_2 inhalation at predetermined timepoints. This study was performed in accordance with the Guide for the Care and Use of Laboratory Animals of the National Institutes of Health. All experimental protocols were approved by Macalester College's Institutional Animal Care and Use Committee (IACUC B16Su2, approved on 1 July 2016).

4.3. MI Sensitization and Challenge

For MI challenges on ears, mice were anesthetized with isoflurane (Baxter Healthcare Corporation, Deerfield, IL, USA) and their backs were shaved on day 1. Sensitization was performed on the following day with 100 µL of 1% MI in a 4:1 mixture of acetone and olive oil (Sigma-Aldrich, St. Louis, MO, USA). On day 8, mice were sensitized a second time with 100 µL of 0.5% MI. Beginning on day 12, mice were challenged with 20 µL of 0.5% MI on each ear, 10 µL on each side, once every day at the same time for three days.

For vaginal canal challenges, mice were shaved on the flank on day 1 and sensitized on the flank with 100 µL of 1% methylisothiazolinone (MI) (Sigma-Aldrich, St. Louis, MO, USA) dissolved in 0.9% saline on the next day. Four days later, mice were sensitized again on the flank with 100 µL 0.5% MI in 0.9% saline (Figure 2). From day 12 onwards, mice were challenged with 20 µL of either 0.5% MI or vehicle (saline) in the vaginal canal. Mice were challenged daily at the same time for either three (Figure S2) or ten days (Figure 2).

4.4. Ear Edema Measurements

Ear thickness was measured using digital calipers (±0.1 mm; VWR, Radnor, PA, USA) one and two days prior to the start of the experiment to establish the baseline for each mouse. Measurements were repeated 6 and 24 h after the third challenge. The percent difference between the baseline and post-challenge values was calculated for each mouse and then for each experimental group.

4.5. THC Treatments

THC was precipitated from a methanol extract (Sigma-Aldrich, St. Louis, MO, USA) and resuspended in 0.9% saline with a few drops of olive oil (Sigma-Aldrich, St. Louis, MO, USA) to promote emulsification. Then, 50 µg of THC in 20 µL of saline solution was gently pipetted into the vaginal canals of mice. Therapeutic treatments were administered for six consecutive days after the 10th MI challenge (Figure 2B). Preventive treatments were administered daily starting 12 h prior to the first MI challenge and ending 12 h after the 10th MI challenge (Figure 2C).

4.6. Tissue Collection and Storage

Whole blood was collected immediately after euthanasia via heart puncture; cells were removed by centrifugation, serum aliquoted, and stored at −80 °C. Vaginal canal and spinal cord tissues were carefully extracted 1, 7, and 21 days after MI challenges or THC treatment, as indicated in the figures. Vaginal canals were carefully extracted, and the section between the cervix and introitus was used for further analyses. Sacral sections 1 and 2 of the spinal cord were identified as described [61], collected, and flushed with cold 1× phosphate buffered saline (PBS) (MidSci, St. Louis, MO, USA). All tissues extracted for semi-quantitative real-time reverse transcription PCR (sqRT-PCR) were weighed immediately after collection, flash-frozen, and stored at −80 °C. Tissues extracted for immunofluorescent staining were flash-frozen and stored at −80 °C. Tissues extracted for eosinophil peroxidase analyses were weighed after extraction, stored in 0.5% hexadecyl trimethylammonium bromide (HTAB) buffer at a volume 5.6 times the wet tissue mass, flash-frozen, and stored at −80 °C. Vaginal canal tissues used for protein quantification were flash-frozen and stored at −80 °C.

4.7. Tactile Sensitivity

Mechanical sensitivity was measured in a 2 × 2 mm area of the ano-genital ridge of mice with an electronic von Frey Anesthesiometer (IITC Corporation, Woodland Hills, CA, USA). Mice were allowed to acclimate in individual Plexiglass von Frey chambers over a wire mesh grating 15 min prior to any sensitivity measurements. Two baseline measurements were taken one and two days prior to MI sensitization; mice were screened for optimal responsiveness and sorted into experimental groups with comparable average baseline responses, as previously described [7–9]. Three to four experimental measurements were taken at described timepoints after 10 MI challenges and/or THC treatments by an experimenter blinded to the treatment groups. The averages of experimental measurements were calculated for each timepoint and reported as a percent decrease from the baseline. Percent decreases from the baseline of 33% or higher were considered hyperalgesic [7,8,62].

4.8. Immunofluorescent Staining and Microscopy

Flash-frozen vaginal canal samples collected from mice 1, 7, and 21 days after ten challenges were embedded in optimal cutting temperature compound (Sakara Finetek, Torrance, CA, USA) and 12 µm sections were cut using a Leica CM 1860 cryostat. Sections were fixed in 4% paraformaldehyde (Sigma-Alrich, St. Louis, MO, USA; pH 8.5), permeabilized for 30 min with 0.1% Triton (Sigma-Aldrich, St. Louis, MO, USA)/PBS, and blocked for one hour in 5% normal donkey serum/PBS. For mast cell staining, slides were incubated for one hour with Fluorescein Avidin D (Vector Laboratories; Burlingame, CA, USA) (1:1000) to stain polysaccharides in mast cell granules, as described by Kakurai et al. [63] and in our own previous studies [7–9]. For mast cell quantification after MI or saline challenges, all slides were coverslipped with Vectashield + DAPI (Vector Laboratories, Burlingame, CA). Sections were imaged using a Zeiss LSM 800 laser scanning confocal microscope. Composite images of ten optical 1 µm sections projected on the z-axis were analyzed using Zen2.1 software (Carl Zeiss AG, Oberkochen, Germany). Mast cell density was determined by fluorescent pixel intensity measurements, taken in four representative 5000 µm^2 regions of interest from one section. Three sections per slide were quantified for three slides per mouse. For mast cell quantification after THC administration, four representative 5000 µm² regions of interest, as well as one blank region of interest outside of the tissue, were measured for three sections per each slide. The average of the four representative sections was taken, subtracted by the blank region of interest, and then divided by 5000 µm² to give a value of the average fluorescent intensity/µm² for each section quantified. Three sections per slide were quantified per mouse.

4.9. RNA Isolation and Quantification of Gene Expression

Total RNA was extracted from flash-frozen vaginal canal or spinal cord tissues using the Total RNA Mini Kit (Midwest Scientific, St. Louis, MO, USA). RNA was eluted with RT-PCR grade water, and quantified using either a Nanodrop ND-1000 Spectrophotometer (Thermo Fisher Scientific, Wilmington, DE, USA) or NanoPhotometer NP80 (Implen, West Lake Village, CA, USA). mRNA was reverse-transcribed in a 2720 Thermal Cycler (Thermo Fisher Scientific) using Superscript III First-Strand Synthesis System (Thermo Fisher Scientific). Relative transcript abundance was determined by sqRT-PCR using TaqMan Gene Expression Assay Primer/Probe Sets: interleukin-6 (IL-6; Mm00446190_m1), interferon-γ (IFN-γ; Mm01168134_m1), chemokine C–X–C motif ligand (CXCL-2; Mm00436450_m1), interleukin-1 β (IL-1β; Mm00434228_m1), and MasterMix (Life Technologies) in a StepOnePlus Real-Time PCR System (Life Technologies). The results were normalized to the expression of housekeeping gene β-2-microglobulin (β2M; Mm00437764_m1) and then calculated as fold-expression over vehicle controls [64], following methods used in previous studies [7–9].

4.10. Protein Quantification

Protein concentrations in serum and in vaginal canal lysates were determined using enzyme-linked immunosorbent assay (ELISA). IgE concentration was measured using an IgE ELISA kit (Bethyl Laboratories, Montogomery, TX, USA). CXCL2 and IL-1β levels were quantified using cytokine specific ELISA kits (R&D Systems, Minneapolis, MN, USA) from whole cell lysates, as previously described [8,9]. Absorbances for all ELISAs were measured at 450 nm and 570 nm using a PowerWave XZ microplate spectrophotometer (Biotek Instruments, Winooski, VT, USA). The recorded optical density measurements (OD) were then used to determine the protein concentration for each sample from a standard curve. Total protein concentrations in all samples were determined using a Detergent Compatible Assay (Bio-Rad, Hercules, CA, USA) following the manufacturers' directions. Total protein concentrations were used to normalize concentrations of target proteins derived from ELISA assays.

4.11. Quantification of Eosinophil Activity

Vaginal canals stored in hexadecyl trimethylammonium bromide (HTAB) buffer were homogenized into whole cell lysates after adding 0.5% HTAB at a volume of four times larger than the storage buffer. All samples were sonicated, freeze-thawed thrice, re-sonicated for optimal homogenization, and centrifuged to separate cellular debris, after which the resulting supernatant was incubated in a substrate solution containing 0.025% hydrogen peroxide, 16 mmol/L o-phenylenediamine, and PBS in a 96-well plate. After 30 min, absorbances were read at 490 nm. All measured optical densities (OD) were divided by the mass of wet tissue to obtain OD/g of wet tissue.

4.12. Vaginal 16S rRNA-Based Microbiome Profiling and Analysis

To investigate the effect of MI sensitization and challenge on the vaginal microbiota, we collected vaginal microbial biomass by lavage as previously described [8] using 100 µl of sterile PBS before sensitization (day 0), post-sensitization (day 6), and after 3 and 10 daily challenges of MI or saline (experiment days 7 and 14). Lavage samples were frozen immediately at –80 °C until processing. Genomic DNA was extracted by the University of Minnesota Genomics Center, followed by 16S rRNA gene amplification using Nextera library-compatible primers flanking the V3–V4 hypervariable regions in a dual-indexing protocol [65]. Libraries were verified with 16S qPCR and normalized based on molecular copy number, and then sequenced on an Illumina MiSeq with v3 reagents in 2 × 300 paired-end mode.

We used the quality control pipeline SHI7 [66] to stich paired reads, trim adaptors, and a quality filter with a trimming threshold of 32 and a mean quality score of 33. This yielded 1,671,150 reads that were then aligned to a custom database from the NCBI RefSeq 16S rRNA Targeted Loci Project (https://www.ncbi.nlm.nih.gov/refseq/targetedloci/) at 97% identity with the accelerated optimal gapped alignment engine BURST [66], run in CAPITALIST mode. OTUs present in less than 5% of samples, and samples with less than 200 counts, were dropped, leaving 33 samples for downstream analysis, with an average read count of 10,411 per sample. Initial diversity analyses were performed using QIIME2 v.2018.11 (https://qiime2.org/) [67], and further statistical tests and visualizations were performed in R v3.5.0 (R Foundation for Statistical Computing, Vienna, Austria; https://www.R-project.org/), using the packages ggplot2 and splinectomeR [68].

4.13. Statistical Analysis

Data were processed using Excel (Microsoft, Redmond, WA, USA) or FlowJo Software (FlowJo, Ashland, OR, USA) and graphed using PRISM 5.0 (GraphPad, San Diego, CA, USA). One-way analysis of variance (ANOVA), post hoc Tukey honest significant different (HSD) analyses, or unpaired Student's *t*-test were run using JMP software (v. 10, SAS, Cary, NC, USA) to compare treatment groups at designated time points. Statistical significance will be defined as $p < 0.05$, $p < 0.01$, and $p < 0.001$ between the two treatment groups and indicated by *, **, and ***, respectively.

Supplementary Materials: Supplementary materials can be found at http://www.mdpi.com/1422-0067/20/21/5361/s1.

Author Contributions: Conceptualization: D.C., E.A.-G., and E.E.; Data curation: E.A.-G. and D.C.; Formal analysis: E.A.-G., J.K., E.E., H.Z., D.P., N.N., and J.L.; Funding acquisition: D.C.; Investigation: E.A.-G., J.K., E.E., H.Z., D.P., N.N., J.L., H.M., B.B., R.K., and T.Y.; Methodology: D.C., E.A.-G., E.E., S.B., and R.S.-C.; Project administration: D.C.; Resources: D.C.; Supervision: D.C.; Validation: D.C.; Visualization: E.A.-G., E.E., J.K., N.N., H.Z., D.P., R.S.-C., and D.C.; Writing—original draft: D.C., J.K., and E.A.-G.; Writing—review & editing: D.C. and E.W.

Funding: These studies were supported by NIH 1R15AI113620-01A1 to D.C., the Biology Department at Macalester College, and intramural undergraduate summer research stipends from Macalester College.

Acknowledgments: The authors thank Gitanjali Matthes and Megan Vossler for graphic design and artwork, Patty Byrne Pfalz for administrative assistance, Jamie Atkins for animal care, Tijana Martinov for feedback on the manuscript, and past and current members of the Chatterjea lab for their help and support.

Conflicts of Interest: The authors declare no conflict of interest. The funders had no role in the design of the study; in the collection, analyses, or interpretation of data; in the writing of the manuscript, or in the decision to publish the results.

References

1. Reed, B.D.; Harlow, S.D.; Sen, A.; Legocki, L.J.; Edwards, R.M.; Arato, N.; Haefner, H.K. Prevalence and demographic characteristics of vulvodynia in a population-based sample. *Am. J. Obstet. Gynecol.* **2012**, *206*, 170. [CrossRef] [PubMed]
2. Harlow, B.L.; Kunitz, C.G.; Nguyen, R.H.N.; Rydell, S.A.; Turner, R.M.; MacLehose, R.F. Prevalence of symptoms consistent with a diagnosis of vulvodynia: Population-based estimates from 2 geographic regions. *Am. J. Obstet. Gynecol.* **2014**, *210*, 40. [CrossRef] [PubMed]
3. Harlow, B.L.; He, W.; Nguyen, R.H.N. Allergic reactions and risk of vulvodynia. *Ann. Epidemiol.* **2009**, *19*, 771–777. [CrossRef] [PubMed]
4. Weström, L.V.; Willén, R. Vestibular nerve fiber proliferation in vulvar vestibulitis syndrome. *Obstet. Gynecol.* **1998**, *91*, 572–576. [CrossRef] [PubMed]
5. Bornstein, J.; Goldschmid, N.; Sabo, E. Hyperinnervation and mast cell activation may be used as histopathologic diagnostic criteria for vulvar vestibulitis. *Gynecol. Obstet. Invest.* **2004**, *58*, 171–178. [CrossRef]

6. Bornstein, J.; Cohen, Y.; Zarfati, D.; Sela, S.; Ophir, E. Involvement of heparanase in the pathogenesis of localized vulvodynia. *Int. J. Gynecol. Pathol.* **2008**, *27*, 136–141. [CrossRef]
7. Martinov, T.; Glenn-Finer, R.; Burley, S.; Tonc, E.; Balsells, E.; Ashbaugh, A.; Swanson, L.; Daughters, R.S.; Chatterjea, D. Contact hypersensitivity to oxazolone provokes vulvar mechanical hyperalgesia in mice. *PLoS ONE* **2013**, *8*, e78673. [CrossRef]
8. Landry, J.; Martinov, T.; Mengistu, H.; Dhanwada, J.; Benck, C.J.; Kline, J.; Boo, B.; Swanson, L.; Tonc, E.; Daughters, R.; et al. Repeated hapten exposure induces persistent tactile sensitivity in mice modeling localized provoked vulvodynia. *PLoS ONE* **2017**, *12*, e0169672. [CrossRef]
9. Boo, B.; Kamath, R.; Arriaga-Gomez, E.; Landry, J.; Emanuel, E.; Joo, S.; Saldías Montivero, M.; Martinov, T.; Fife, B.T.; Chatterjea, D. Tetrahydrocannabinol Reduces Hapten-Driven Mast Cell Accumulation and Persistent Tactile Sensitivity in Mouse Model of Allergen-Provoked Localized Vulvodynia. *Int. J. Mol. Sci.* **2019**, *20*, 2163. [CrossRef]
10. Schwensen, J.F.; Lundov, M.D.; Bossi, R.; Banerjee, P.; Giménez-Arnau, E.; Lepoittevin, J.P.; Lidén, C.; Uter, W.; Yazar, K.; White, I.R.; et al. Methylisothiazolinone and benzisothiazolinone are widely used in paint: A multicentre study of paints from five European countries. *Contact Dermatitis* **2015**, *72*, 127–138. [CrossRef]
11. Yazar, K.; Lundov, M.D.; Faurschou, A.; Matura, M.; Boman, A.; Johansen, J.D.; Lidén, C. Methylisothiazolinone in rinse-off products causes allergic contact dermatitis: A repeated open-application study. *Br. J. Dermatol.* **2015**, *173*, 115–122. [CrossRef] [PubMed]
12. Lundov, M.D.; Opstrup, M.S.; Johansen, J.D. Methylisothiazolinone contact allergy–growing epidemic. *Contact Derm.* **2013**, *69*, 271–275. [CrossRef] [PubMed]
13. Popple, A.; Williams, J.; Maxwell, G.; Gellatly, N.; Dearman, R.J.; Kimber, I. T lymphocyte dynamics in methylisothiazolinone-allergic patients. *Contact Derm.* **2016**, *75*, 1–13. [CrossRef] [PubMed]
14. Lundov, M.D.; Krongaard, T.; Menné, T.L.; Johansen, J.D. Methylisothiazolinone contact allergy: A review. *Br. J. Dermatol.* **2011**, *165*, 1178–1182. [CrossRef] [PubMed]
15. Vij, A.; Sood, A.; Piliang, M.; Mesinkovska, N.A. Infection or allergy? The multifaceted nature of vulvar dermatoses. *Int. J. Women's Dermatol.* **2015**, *1*, 170–172. [CrossRef] [PubMed]
16. Marfatia, Y.S.; Patel, D.; Menon, D.; Naswa, S. Genital contact allergy: A diagnosis missed. *Indian J. Sex. Transm. Dis. AIDS* **2016**, *37*, 1–6. [CrossRef]
17. Reed, B.D.; McKee, K.S.; Plegue, M.A.; Park, S.K.; Haefner, H.K.; Harlow, S.D. Environmental Exposure History and Vulvodynia Risk: A Population-Based Study. *J. Women's Health* **2019**, *28*, 69–76. [CrossRef]
18. Hannuksela, M. Rapid increase in contact allergy to Kathon CG in Finland. *Contact Derm.* **1986**, *15*, 211–214. [CrossRef]
19. De Groot, A.C.; Weyland, J.W. Kathon CG: A review. *J. Am. Acad. Dermatol.* **1988**, *18*, 350–358. [CrossRef]
20. Bruze, M.; Dahlquist, I.; Fregert, S.; Gruvberger, B.; Persson, K. Contact allergy to the active ingredients of Kathon CG. *Contact Derm.* **1987**, *16*, 183–188. [CrossRef]
21. Fregert, S.; Trulson, L.; Zimerson, E. Contact allergic reactions to diphenylthiourea and phenylisothiocyanate in PVC adhesive tape. *Contact Derm.* **1982**, *8*, 38–42. [CrossRef] [PubMed]
22. Burnett, C.L.; Bergfeld, W.F.; Belsito, D.V.; Klaassen, C.D.; Marks, J.G.; Shank, R.C.; Slaga, T.J.; Snyder, P.W.; Alan Andersen, F. Final report of the safety assessment of methylisothiazolinone. *Int. J. Toxicol.* **2010**, *29*, 187S–213S. [CrossRef] [PubMed]
23. Goldenberg, A.; Lipp, M.; Jacob, S.E. Appropriate Testing of Isothiazolinones in Children. *Pediatr. Dermatol.* **2017**, *34*, 138–143. [CrossRef] [PubMed]
24. Castanedo-Tardana, M.P.; Zug, K.A. Methylisothiazolinone. *Dermatitis* **2013**, *24*, 2–6. [CrossRef] [PubMed]
25. Basketter, D.A.; Angelini, G.; Ingber, A.; Kern, P.S.; Menné, T. Nickel, chromium and cobalt in consumer products: Revisiting safe levels in the new millennium. *Contact Derm.* **2003**, *49*, 1–7. [CrossRef] [PubMed]
26. Devos, F.C.; Pollaris, L.; Van Den Broucke, S.; Seys, S.; Goossens, A.; Nemery, B.; Hoet, P.H.M.; Vanoirbeek, J.A.J. Methylisothiazolinone: Dermal and respiratory immune responses in mice. *Toxicol. Lett.* **2015**, *235*, 179–188. [CrossRef]
27. Mathias, C.B.; Freyschmidt, E.-J.; Caplan, B.; Jones, T.; Poddighe, D.; Xing, W.; Harrison, K.L.; Gurish, M.F.; Oettgen, H.C. IgE influences the number and function of mature mast cells, but not progenitor recruitment in allergic pulmonary inflammation. *J. Immunol.* **2009**, *182*, 2416–2424. [CrossRef]
28. Bax, H.J.; Keeble, A.H.; Gould, H.J. Cytokinergic IgE Action in Mast Cell Activation. *Front. Immunol.* **2012**, *3*, 229. [CrossRef]

29. DiSabato, D.; Quan, N.; Godbout, J.P. Neuroinflammation: The Devil is in the Details. *J. Neurochem.* **2016**, *139*, 136–153. [CrossRef]
30. Zhou, Y.-Q.; Liu, Z.; Liu, Z.-H.; Chen, S.-P.; Li, M.; Shahveranov, A.; Ye, D.-W.; Tian, Y.-K. Interleukin-6: An emerging regulator of pathological pain. *J. Neuroinflamm.* **2016**, *13*, 141. [CrossRef]
31. Nguyen, R.H.; Swanson, D.; Harlow, B.L. Urogenital infections in relation to the occurrence of vulvodynia. *J. Reprod. Med.* **2009**, *54*, 385–392. [PubMed]
32. Khandekar, M.; Brady, S.S.; Rydell, S.A.; Turner, R.M.; Schreiner, P.J.; Harlow, B.L. Early-life Chronic Stressors, Rumination, and the Onset of Vulvodynia. *J. Sex. Med.* **2019**, *16*, 880–890. [CrossRef] [PubMed]
33. Khandekar, M.; Brady, S.S.; Stewart, E.G.; Harlow, B.L. Is chronic stress during childhood associated with adult-onset vulvodynia? *J. Women's Health (Larchmt)* **2014**, *23*, 649–656. [CrossRef] [PubMed]
34. European Commission. Consumers: Commission Improves Safety of Cosmetics. European Commission Press Release Database. 2014. Available online: https://europa.eu/rapid/press-release_IP-14-1051_en.htm (accessed on 13 September 2019).
35. Majeed, S.K. Mast cell distribution in mice. *Arzneimittelforschung* **1994**, *44*, 1170–1173.
36. Shafik, A.; El-Sibai, E.; Shafik, I.; Shafik, A. Immunohistochemical identification of the pacemaker cajal cells in the normal human vagina. *Arch. Gynecol. Obstet.* **2005**, *272*, 13–16. [CrossRef]
37. Han, H.; Park, S.J.; Ahn, H.; Ryu, J.S. Involvement of mast cells in inflammation induced by *Trichomonas vaginalis* via crosstalk with vaginal epithelial cells. *Parasite Immunol.* **2012**, *34*, 8–14. [CrossRef]
38. Gendrin, C.; Vorhagen, J.; Ngo, L.; Whidbey, C.; Boldenow, E.; Santana-Ufret, V.; Clauson, M.; Burnside, K.; Galloway, D.P.; Waldorf, K.A.; et al. Mast cell degranulation by a hemolytic lipid toxin decreased GBS colonization and infection. *Sci. Adv.* **2015**, *1*, e1400225. [CrossRef]
39. Renga, G.; Borghi, M.; Oikonomou, V.; Mosci, P.; Bartoli, A.; Renauld, J.; Romani, L.; Costantini, C. IL-9 Integrates the Host-*Candida* Cross-Talk in Vulvovaginal Candidiasis to Balance Inflammation and Tolerance. *Front. Immuol.* **2018**, *9*. [CrossRef]
40. Papoutsis, D.; Haefner, H.K.; Crum, C.P.; Opipari, A.W.; Reed, B.D. Vestibular mast cell density in vulvodynia: A case-controlled study. *J. Low. Genit. Tract Dis.* **2017**, *20*, 275–279. [CrossRef]
41. Foster, D.C.; Hasday, J.D. Elevated tissue levels of interleukin-1 beta and tumor necrosis factor-alpha in vulvar vestibulitis. *Obstet. Gynecol.* **1997**, *89*, 291–296. [CrossRef]
42. Foster, D.C.; Pierkarz, K.H.; Murant, T.I.; LaPoint, R.; Haidaris, C.G.; Phipps, R.P. Enhanced synthesis of proinflammatory cytokines by vulvar vestibular fibroblasts: Implications for vulvar vestibulitis. *Am. J. Obstet. Gynecol.* **2007**, *196*, 346. [CrossRef] [PubMed]
43. Reed, B.D.; Plegue, M.A.; Sen, A.; Haefner, H.K.; Siddiqui, J.; Remick, D.G. Nerve Growth Factor and Selected Cytokines in Women with and Without Vulvodynia. *J. Low. Genit. Tract Dis.* **2018**, *22*, 139–146. [CrossRef] [PubMed]
44. Pascal, M.; Perez-Gordo, M.; Caballero, T.; Escribese, M.M.; Lopez Longo, M.N.; Luengo, O.; Manso, L.; Matheu, V.; Seoane, E.; Zamorano, M.; et al. Microbiome and Allergic Diseases. *Front. Immunol.* **2018**, *9*. [CrossRef] [PubMed]
45. Minerbi, A.; Gonzalez, E.; Brereton, N.J.B.; Anjarkouchian, A.; Dewar, K.; Fitzcharles, M.-A.; Chevalier, S.; Shir, Y. Altered microbiome composition in individuals with fibromyalgia. *Pain* **2019**. [CrossRef]
46. Chichlowski, M.; Rudolph, C. Visceral Pain and Gastrointestinal Microbiome. *J. Neurogastroenterol. Motil.* **2015**, *21*, 172–181. [CrossRef]
47. Ling, Z.; Kong, J.; Liu, F.; Zhu, H.; Chen, X.; Wang, Y.; Li, L.; Nelson, K.E.; Xia, T.; Xiang, C. Molecular analysis of the diversity of vaginal microbiota associated with bacterial vaginosis. *BMC Genom.* **2010**, *11*, 488. [CrossRef]
48. Fredricks, D.N.; Fiedler, T.L.; Marrazzo, J.M. Molecular identification of bacteria associated with bacterial vaginosis. *N. Engl. J. Med.* **2005**, *3*, 1899–1911. [CrossRef]
49. Ziklo, N.; Vidgen, M.E.; Taing, K.; Huston, W.M.; Timms, P. Dysbiosis of the vaginal microbiota and higher vaginal kynurenine/tryptophan ratio reveals an association with Chlamydia trachomatis genital infections. *Front. Cell. Infect. Microbiol.* **2018**, *8*, 1. [CrossRef]
50. Ata, B.; Yildiz, S.; Turkgeldi, E.; Brocal, V.P.; Dinleyici, E.C.; Moya, A.; Urman, B. The Endobiota Study: Comparison of Vaginal, Cervical and Gut Microbiota Between Women with Stage 3/4 Endometriosis and Healthy Controls. *Sci. Rep.* **2019**, *9*, 2204. [CrossRef]

51. Greenbaum, S.; Greenbaum, G.; Moran-Gilad, J.; Weintraub, A.Y. Ecological dynamics of the vaginal microbiome in relation to health and disease. *Am. J. Obstet. Gynecol.* **2019**, *220*, 324–335. [CrossRef]
52. Latremoliere, A.; Woolf, C.J. Central sensitization: A generator of pain hypersensitivity by central neural plasticity. *J. Pain* **2009**, *10*, 895–926. [CrossRef] [PubMed]
53. Zhang, Z.; Zolnoun, D.A.; Francisco, E.M.; Holden, J.K.; Dennis, R.G.; Tommerdahl, M. Altered central sensitization in subgroups of women with vulvodynia. *Clin. J. Pain* **2011**, *27*, 755–763. [CrossRef] [PubMed]
54. Nhu, Q.M.; Aceves, S.S. Tissue Remodeling in Chronic Eosinophilic Esophageal Inflammation: Parallels in Asthma and Therapeutic Perspectives. *Front. Med. (Lausanne)* **2017**, *4*, 128. [CrossRef] [PubMed]
55. Vallvé-Juanico, J.; Houshdaran, S.; Giudice, L.C. The endometrial immune environment of women with endometriosis. *Hum. Reprod. Update* **2019**, *25*, 565–592. [CrossRef] [PubMed]
56. Nyirjesy, P. Chronic vulvovaginal candidiasis. *Am. Fam. Physician* **2001**, *63*, 697–702. [PubMed]
57. Black, C.A.; Rohan, L.C.; Cost, M.; Watkins, S.C.; Draviam, R.; Alber, S.; Edwards, R.P. Vaginal mucosa serves as an inductive site for tolerance. *J. Immunol.* **2000**, *165*, 5077–5083. [CrossRef] [PubMed]
58. Abrams, R. Growing Scrutiny for an Allergy Trigger Used in Personal Care Products. *The New York Times.* 24 January 2015. Available online: https://www.nytimes.com/2015/01/24/business/allergy-trigger-found-in-many-personal-care-items-comes-under-greater-scrutiny.html (accessed on 3 September 2019).
59. Wickham, H.; Henry, L. Tidyr: Easily Tidy Data with 'spread()' and 'gather()' Functions, R package version 0.6.3, last modified September 1, 2017. Available online: https://CRAN.R-project.org/package=tidyr (accessed on 10 September 2019).
60. Kahle, D.; Wickham, H. ggmap: Spatial Visualization with ggplot2. *R J.* **2013**, *5*, 144–161. [CrossRef]
61. Harrison, M.; O'Brien, A.; Adams, L.; Cowin, G.; Ruitenberg, M.J.; Sengul, G.; Watson, C. Vertebral landmarks for the identification of spinal cord segments in the mouse. *Neuroimage* **2013**, *68*, 22–29. [CrossRef]
62. Farmer, M.A.; Taylor, A.M.; Bailey, A.L.; Tuttle, A.H.; MacIntyre, L.C.; Milagrosa, Z.E.; Crissman, H.P.; Bennett, G.J.; Ribeiro-da-Silva, A.; Binik, Y.M.; et al. Repeated vulvovaginal fungal infections cause persistent pain in a mouse model of vulvodynia. *Sci. Transl. Med.* **2011**, *3*, 101ra91. [CrossRef]
63. Kakurai, M.; Monteforte, R.; Suto, H.; Tsai, M.; Nakae, S.; Galli, S.J. Mast Cell-Derived Tumor Necrosis Factor Can Promote Nerve Fiber Elongation in the Skin during Contact Hypersensitivity in Mice. *Am. J. Pathol.* **2006**, *169*, 1713–1721. [CrossRef]
64. Livak, K.J.; Schmittgen, T.D. Analysis of relative gene expression data using real-time quantitative PCR and the 2(-Delta Delta C(T)) Method. *Methods* **2001**, *25*, 402–408. [CrossRef] [PubMed]
65. Gohl, D.M.; Vangay, P.; Garbe, J.; MacLean, A.; Hauge, A.; Becker, A.; Gould, T.J.; Clayton, J.B.; Johnson, T.J.; Hunter, R.; et al. Systematic improvement of amplicon marker gene methods for increased accuracy in microbiome studies. *Nat. Biotechnol.* **2016**, *34*, 942–949. [CrossRef] [PubMed]
66. Al-Ghalith, G.A.; Hillmann, B.; Ang, K.; Shields-Cutler, R.; Knights, D. SHI7 Is a Self-Learning Pipeline for Multipurpose Short-Read DNA Quality Control. *mSystems* **2018**, *3*, e00202-17. [CrossRef] [PubMed]
67. Bolyen, E.; Rideout, J.R.; Dillon, M.R.; Bokulich, N.A.; Abnet, C.C.; Al-Ghalith, G.A.; Alexander, H.; Alm, E.J.; Arumugam, M.; Asnicar, F.; et al. Reproducible, interactive, scalable and extensible microbiome data science using QIIME 2. *Nat. Biotechnol.* **2019**, *37*, 852–857. [CrossRef]
68. Shields-Cutler, R.R.; Al-Ghalith, G.A.; Yassour, M.; Knights, D. Splinectome R Enables Group Comparisons in Longitudinal Microbiome Studies. *Front. Microbiol.* **2018**, *9*, 785. [CrossRef]

© 2019 by the authors. Licensee MDPI, Basel, Switzerland. This article is an open access article distributed under the terms and conditions of the Creative Commons Attribution (CC BY) license (http://creativecommons.org/licenses/by/4.0/).

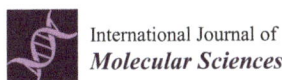

Article

The Putatively Specific Synthetic REV-ERB Agonist SR9009 Inhibits IgE- and IL-33-Mediated Mast Cell Activation Independently of the Circadian Clock

Kayoko Ishimaru [1], Shotaro Nakajima [1,2], Guannan Yu [1], Yuki Nakamura [1] and Atsuhito Nakao [1,3,*]

[1] Department of Immunology, Faculty of Medicine, University of Yamanashi, Yamanashi 409-3821, Japan; ikayoko@yamanashi.ac.jp (K.I.); ipsho555@gmail.com (S.N.); guannan@yamanashi.ac.jp (G.Y.); ynakamura@yamanashi.ac.jp (Y.N.)
[2] Department of Progressive DOHaD Research, School of Medicine, Fukushima Medical University, Fukushima 960-1247, Japan
[3] Atopy Research Center, Juntendo University School of Medicine, Tokyo 113-8421, Japan
* Correspondence: anakao@yamanashi.ac.jp; Tel.: +81-55-273-6752

Received: 4 December 2019; Accepted: 12 December 2019; Published: 14 December 2019

Abstract: The cell-autonomous circadian clock regulates IgE- and IL-33-mediated mast cell activation, both of which are key events in the development of allergic diseases. Accordingly, clock modifiers could be used to treat allergic diseases, as well as many other circadian-related diseases, such as sleep and metabolic disorders. The nuclear receptors REV-ERB-α and -β (REV-ERBs) are crucial components of the circadian clockwork. Efforts to pharmacologically target REV-ERBs using putatively specific synthetic agonists, particularly SR9009, have yielded beneficial effects on sleep and metabolism. Here, we sought to determine whether REV-ERBs are functional in the circadian clockwork in mast cells and, if so, whether SR9009 affects IgE- and IL-33-mediated mast cell activation. Bone marrow-derived mast cells (BMMCs) obtained from wild-type mice expressed REV-ERBs, and SR9009 or other synthetic REV-ERBs agonists affected the mast cell clockwork. SR9009 inhibited IgE- and IL-33-mediated mast cell activation in wild-type BMMCs in association with inhibition of Gab2/PI3K and NF-κB activation. Unexpectedly, these suppressive effects of SR9009 were observed in BMMCs following mutation of the core circadian gene *Clock*. These findings suggest that SR9009 inhibits IgE- and IL-33-mediated mast cell activation independently of the functional circadian clock activity. Thus, SR9009 or other synthetic REV-ERB agonists may have potential for anti-allergic agents.

Keywords: REV-ERBs; mast cells; IgE; IL-33; circadian clock

1. Introduction

The circadian clock controls a large proportion of genes in a cyclic manner, thereby regulating the timing of cellular activities [1,2]. The circadian clock consists of a cell-autonomous transcription–translation feedback loop involving several clock genes. Briefly, the transcription factors BMAL1 (*Arntl*) and CLOCK heterodimerize, bind to E-box motifs throughout the genome, and activate transcription of their own repressors *Period (Per1-3)* and *Cryptochrome (Cry1, 2)*. The PER and CRY proteins form oligomers and enter the nucleus, where they inhibit BMAL1/CLOCK activity. This negative-feedback loop takes ~24 h to be completed, with several post-transcriptional regulation. Accordingly, the circadian clock controls periodic expression of thousands of clock-controlled genes (CCGs) with E-box motifs in their promoter/enhancer regions other than Per and Cry.

Previously, we showed that in mouse mast cells, *Clock* binds to E-box motif in the promoter of β-subunit gene of the high-affinity IgE receptor FcεRIβ or IL-33 receptor ST2 in a circadian manner, contributing to day–night variation in IgE- and IL-33-mediated mast cell activation [3,4]. Because IgE- and IL-33-mediated mast cell activation plays a key role in the development and maintenance of allergic diseases [5,6], synthetic compounds capable of modifying the period, phase, or amplitude of clock gene expression in mast cells may have potential as new anti-allergy drugs [7,8].

The nuclear receptors REV-ERB-α (*Nr1d1*) and REV-ERB-β (*Nr1d2*) (REV-ERBs) function as transcriptional repressors. REV-ERBs regulate the expression of genes involved in the control of circadian rhythm, metabolism, and inflammatory response [9–11]. As components of the circadian clock, REV-ERBs provide a stabilizing loop that regulates the timing and amplitude of Bmal1 [1,2]. Briefly, the BMAL1/CLOCK heterodimer activates transcription of REV-ERBs and, in turn, REV-ERB-α/REV-ERB-β proteins repress *Bmal1* expression by competing bindings of transcriptional activators, RORα and RORγ, to the ROR-response element (RRE) in the *Bmal1* promoter.

Recent studies have shown that pharmacologically targeting of REV-ERBs using putatively specific synthetic agonists, particularly SR9009 [12], has beneficial effects on circadian rhythm disorders, including jet lag, sleep disturbance, metabolic disease, inflammation, and cancer [12–15]. For instance, administration of SR9009 induces wakefulness and reduces rapid-eye-movement (REM) and slow-wave sleep in mice [13]. However, it remains unclear whether mast cells express functional REV-ERBs, and if so, whether synthetic REV-ERB agonists such as SR9009 would have beneficial in these cells.

Hence, in this study, we sought to determine whether mast cells express functional REV-ERBs, and if so, whether SR9009 affects IgE- and IL-33-mediated mast cell activation. Our results revealed that REV-ERBs are functional in mast cells, and that SR9009 inhibits IgE- and IL-33-mediated mast cell activation. Unexpectedly, this inhibition was independent of functional clock activity. These findings suggest that SR9009 or other synthetic REV-ERB agonists may have therapeutic potential against allergic diseases.

2. Results

2.1. Mast Cells Express Functional REV-ERBs

First, we investigated whether REV-ERBs are expressed and functional in mast cells. For this purpose, we examined the kinetics of the mRNA levels of REV-ERB-α and REV-ERB-β as well as two other major clock genes, Per2 and Bmal1, in bone marrow-derived mast cells (BMMCs) from wild-type mice. REV-ERB-α and REV-ERB-β mRNAs were expressed at considerable levels comparable to Per2 and Bmal1 in wild-type BMMCs (Threshold Cycle (Ct value) of each gene in the real-time quantitative PCR experiments were as follows; REV-ERB-α: 32~34, REV-ERB-β: 30~32, Per2: 31~33, Bmal1: 30~32). REV-ERB-α, but not REV-ERB-β, mRNA exhibited oscillations (REB-ERB-α: $p = 4.15 \times 10^{-5}$, REV-ERB-β: $p = 0.26$, one-way ANOVA) with a peak at 18 h following a medium change to synchronize the mast cell clock (Figure 1a). Per2 and Bmal1 mRNA levels exhibited circadian oscillations (Per2: $p = 9.44 \times 10^{-9}$, Bmal1: $p = 9.89 \times 10^{-7}$, One-way ANOVA), as previously reported (Figure 1a) [16]. Because no good anti-REV-ERB-α or -β antibody is available, we were unable to confirm REV-ERB-α and -β expression in BMMCs at the protein level. Consistent with a model in which transcription of REV-ERBs is activated by the BMAL1/CLOCK heterodimer [1,2], BMMCs from Clock-mutated mice [17] expressed significantly much lower levels of REV-ERB-α and REV-ERB-β mRNA expression than BMMCs from wild-type mice (Figure S1).

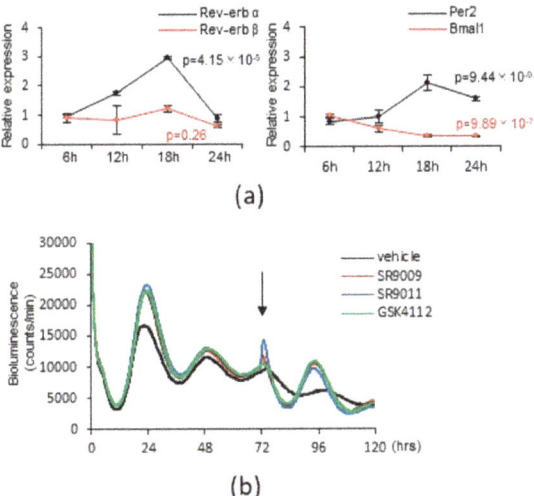

Figure 1. Mast cells express REV-ERBs and synthetic REV-ERB agonists can synchronize the mast cell clockwork. (**a**) Kinetics of the mRNA expression changes of REV-ERB-α, -β, Per2, and Bmal1 at the indicated time points after a medium change in constitutively cultured wild-type BMMCs. The values represent the means ± SD (n = 3) (one-way ANOVA). (**b**) Monitoring of PER2^{LUC} bioluminescence of BMMCs derived from PER2^{LUC} knock-in mice after the medium change for 120 h. Synthetic REV-ERB agonists (10 μM) were added to the culture 72 h after the start of the monitoring (black arrow).

We next examined the effects of SR9009 and other synthetic REV-ERBs agonists SR9011 [12] and GSK4112 [14] on the mast cell clockwork in vitro. We confirmed that treatment of wild-type BMMCs with SR9009, SR9011, or GSK4112 for 24 h at a concentration of 1 or 10 μM did not affect cell viability, as judged by a metabolic assay (NAD(P)H-based: WST-1 assay) (Figure S2a) and expression of Annexin V (Figure S2b); by contrast, a dose of 50 μM exerted cytotoxicity. Therefore, in this study, we used 10 μM, the most commonly used concentration among published studies [12,14,15].

We previously showed that the mast cell clockwork (i.e., the kinetics of PER2 expression) can be evaluated in vitro [3], based on monitoring of bioluminescent emission of BMMCs from Per2^{Luc} knock-in mice, which express PER2 as a luciferase fusion protein [18] (PER2^{LUC} BMMCs). A simple medium change triggers synchronization of the circadian clocks in peripheral cells in vitro [19]. Accordingly, the mast cell clockwork (as reflected by the oscillation of PER2^{LUC}) was observed from 0 to 72 h after a media change, as previously described (Figure 1b) [3]. The PER2^{LUC} oscillation may have been limited to 0–72 h due to a lack of oscillator coupling in dissociated cell cultures without internal zeitgebers ('time givers' in German), leading to damping of the ensemble rhythm at the population level [3]. We found that addition of 10 μM SR9009, SR9011, or GSK4112 72 h after the medium change recovered the mast cell clockwork (i.e., PER2^{LUC} oscillation) for another 48 h (Figure 1b), suggesting that activation of REV-ERBs by these reagents can synchronize the mast cell clockwork at the population level. Collectively, these results suggested that mast cells express functional REV-ERBs, and that SR9009 or other synthetic agonists can affect the mast cell clockwork.

2.2. SR9009 and Other Synthetic Agonists of REV-ERBs Inhibit IgE- and IL-33-Mediated Mast Cell Activation

We next examined the effects of SR9009 and other synthetic REV-ERBs agonists on IgE- and IL-33-mediated activation in mast cells. Pretreatment of wild-type BMMCs for 1 h with 10 μM SR9009, SR9011, or GSK4112 inhibited IgE-mediated degranulation, as judged by β-hexosaminidase release, histamine release, and CD63 expression (Figure 2a, Figure S3). IgE-mediated IL-6 and IL-13 protein expression in wild-type BMMCs was also suppressed by pretreatment with 10 μM SR9009, SR9011, and GSK4112 for 1 h (Figure 2b). Importantly, intraperitoneal administration of SR9009 inhibited passive cutaneous anaphylactic (PCA) reaction, a classical in vivo model of IgE/mast cell-mediated skin allergic response, in wild-type mice (Figure 2c). Similarly, pretreatment of wild-type BMMCs for 1 h with 10 µM SR9009, SR9011, or GSK4112 inhibited IL-33-mediated IL-6 and IL-13 protein expression in wild-type BMMCs (Figure 2d). We also found that pretreatment of wild-type BMMCs for 1 h with 10 µM SR9009, SR9011, or GSK4112 inhibited LPS-mediated IL-6 and IL-13 protein expression in wild-type BMMCs (Figure S4a).

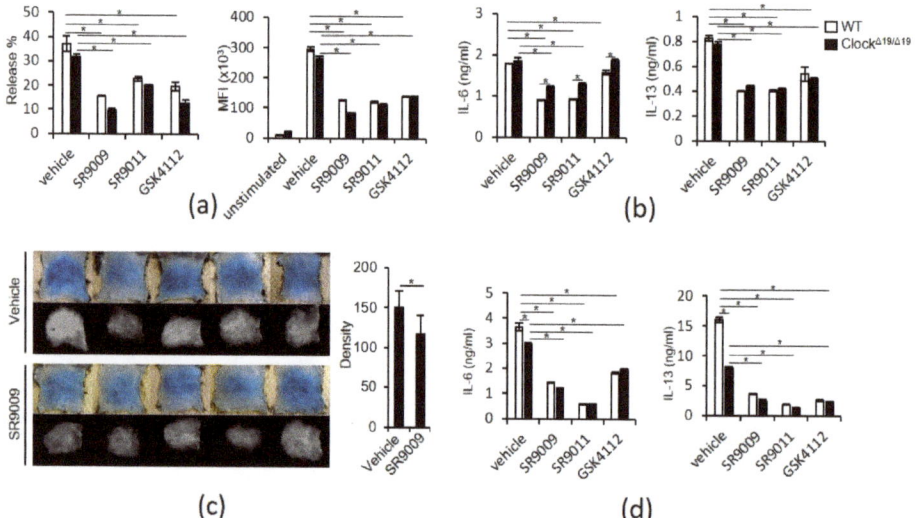

Figure 2. Inhibition of IgE- and IL-33-mediated mast cell activation by synthetic REV-ERB agonists. (**a**) IgE-mediated release of β-hexosaminidase (left) or CD63 upregulation (right) in wild-type and Clock-mutated BMMCs in the presence or absence of 10 µM synthetic REV-ERB agonists ($n = 3$). (**b**) IgE-mediated IL-6 and IL-13 production from wild-type or Clock-mutated BMMCs in the presence or absence of 10 µM synthetic REV-ERB agonists ($n = 4$). (**c**) PCA reactions in wild-type mice i.p. treated with vehicle or 100 mg/kg SR9009. Representative pictures of the skin color reactions (upper left panels) and the digitalized images of the density value evaluations (lower left panels). The quantitative analysis of the data is shown in the right panel. ($n = 5$). (**d**) IL-33-mediated IL-6 and IL-13 production from wild-type or Clock-mutated BMMCs in the presence or absence of 10 µM synthetic REV-ERB agonists ($n = 4$). The values represent the means ± SD (error bars). * $p < 0.05$.

Similar to wild-type BMMCs, 10 µM SR9009, SR9011, and GSK4112 inhibited IgE-mediated degranulation and IgE- and IL-33-mediated IL-6 and IL-13 expression in wild-type fetal skin-derived mast cells (FSMCs), mouse connective tissue-type skin-derived mast cells (Figure S5).

Unexpectedly, these suppressive effects of SR9009, SR9011, and GSK4112 were also observed in BMMCs derived from Clock-mutated mice (Figure 2a–d), suggesting that suppression of IgE- and IL-33-mediated mast cell activation by SR9009 or other synthetic REV-ERB agonists does not require functional circadian clock activity. In addition, we found that IL-33-mediated IL-13 production was significantly lower in Clock-mutated BMMCs than in wild-type BMMCs (Figure 2b,d), suggesting that Clock mutation can affect IL-13 production via IL-33 in mast cells.

2.3. SR9009 Inhibits IgE- and IL-33-Mediated Activation of the Gab2/PI3K and NF-κB Pathways in Mast Cells

To investigate the mechanisms by which SR9009 suppresses IgE- and IL-33-mediated mast cell activation, we examined the drug's effects on IgE- and IL-33–induced intracellular signaling pathways leading to degranulation or cytokine expression such as the Gab2/PI3K pathway and NF-κB and p38 MAPK pathways [5,6,20,21].

The Gab2/PI3K pathway is critical in FcεRI signaling leading to degranulation in mast cells [22]. Briefly, stimulation of FcεRI phosphorylates Gab2 probably by Syk and Src family protein-tyrosine kinases Syk or Lyn. Then, phosphorylated Gab2 binds to the p85 subunit of PI3K and recruits PI3K to its substrate lipids, thereby leading to PLCγ activation and degranulation. Interestingly, SR9009 inhibited IgE-mediated phosphorylation of Gab2 and the p55 subunit of PI3K in wild-type BMMCs (Figure 3a). SR9009 did not affect Gab2 mRNA expression in wild-type BMMCs (Figure S6). In contrast to IgE stimulation, IL-33 did not induce phosphorylaton of Gab2 in wild-type BMMCs.

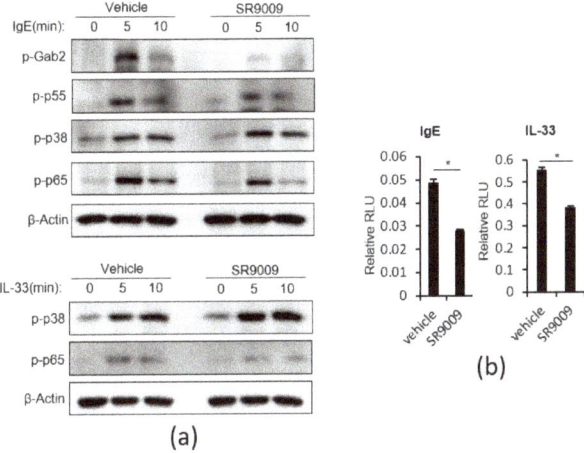

Figure 3. Effects of SR9009 on IgE- and IL-33-mediated intracellular signaling in wild-type BMMCs. (**a**) Western blot analysis of phospho-Gab2, phospho-p55 PI3K, phospho-p38 MAPK, and phospho-p65 in wild-type BMMCs stimulated with IgE or IL-33 for 10 min in the presence or absence of 10 μM SR9009. The level of β-actin is shown at the bottom as a loading control. (**b**) Luciferase assay of NF-κB activity in wild-type BMMCs treated with IgE- or IL-33 in the presence or absence of 10 μM SR9009 ($n = 3$). The values represent the means ± SD. * $p < 0.05$.

Both the NF-κB and p38 MAPK pathways mediate IgE- or IL-33-mediated transcriptonal activation of cytokine gene expression [5,6,20,21]. SR9009 inhibited IgE- and IL-33–induced phosphorylation of p65, a subunit of NF-κB, but did not affect IgE- or IL-33–induced phosphorylation of p38 MAPK in wild-type BMMCs (Figure 3a). In addition, a reporter assay showed that SR9009 suppressed IgE- or IL-33-mediated transcriptional activation of NF-κB in BMMCs (Figure 3b). SR9009 also inhibited LPS-mediated transcriptional activation of NF-κB in BMMCs (Figure S4b). Consistent with these findings, SR9009 inhibited IgE-, IL-33-, and LPS-mediated IL-6 and IL-13 mRNA expression in wild-type BMMCs (Figure S7).

We found that SR9009 did not affect surface expression levels of FcεRI or IL-33 receptor ST2 in wild-type BMMCs (Figure S8). Together, these results suggest that inhibition of the Gab2/PI3K and NF-κB pathways, but not p38 MAPK, contributes to the suppressive effects of SR9009 on IgE- or IL-33-mediated degranulation and cytokine gene expression of mast cells.

2.4. SR9009 May Inhibit IgE- and IL-33-Mediated Mast Cell Activation Independently of REV-ERBs

The inhibitions of mast cell activation by SR9009 appeared to be independent of the functional circadian clock activity (Figure 2). Thus, we asked whether the inhibitory actions of SR9009 depended on its agonistic function. For this purpose, the effects of SR9009 on IgE- or IL-33-mediated mast cell activation were examined when REV-ERBs expression were knocked-down by specific siRNAs in wild-type BMMCs.

Both REV-ERBα and β mRNA expressions were significantly downregulated using the specific siRNAs in wild-type BMMCs by ~80% compared to those in wild-type BMMCs using the control siRNAs (Figure 4a). Unexpectedly, pretreatment of the REV-ERBs knocked-down BMMCs for 1 h with 10 μM SR9009 inhibited IgE-mediated degranulation, as judged by β-hexosaminidase release and CD63 expression (Figure 4b). IgE- and IL-33-mediated IL-13 protein expression was also suppressed by pretreatment with 10 μM SR9009 for 1 h in REV-ERBs knocked-down BMMCs (Figure 4c,d). These results suggest that the inhibitory actions of SR9009 on IgE- and IL-33-mediated mast cell activation may not depend on its agonistic function through REV-ERBs.

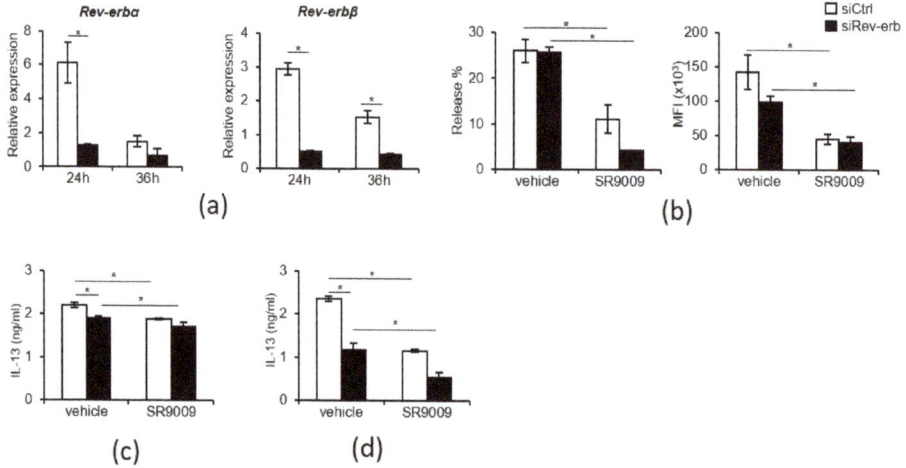

Figure 4. Inhibition of IgE- and IL-33-mediated mast cell activation by SR9009 in REV-ERBs knocked-down BMMCs. (**a**) REV-ERB- α and -β mRNA expression after the specific or control siRNA transfection ($n = 3$). (**b**) IgE-mediated release of β-hexosaminidase (left) or CD63 upregulation (right) in siRNA transfected BMMCs in the presence or absence of 10 μM SR9009 ($n = 3$). (**c**) IgE-mediated IL-13 production from siRNA transfected BMMCs in the presence or absence of 10 μM SR9009 ($n = 3$). (**d**) IL-33-mediated IL-13 production from siRNA transfected BMMCs in the presence or absence of 10 μM SR9009 ($n = 3$). The values represent the means ± SD. *$p < 0.05$.

3. Discussion

Molecular understanding of the circadian clock is opening new therapeutic frontiers for several diseases—including sleep and metabolic disorders, inflammatory diseases, and cancer—through pharmacological targeting of circadian clock components [23]. Given that IgE- and IL-33-mediated mast cell activation is under the control of the circadian clock [3,4] and synthetic REV-ERBs agonists, particularly SR9009, have exhibited many beneficial effects in animal models of circadian-related disorders [12–15], this study sought to determine whether mast cells express functional REV-ERBs and SR9009 affects IgE- and IL-33-mediated mast cell activation. The current results suggest that SR9009 or other synthetic REV-ERB agonists can synchronize the mast cell clockworks and inhibit IgE- and IL-33-mediated mast cell activation.

SR9009 significantly inhibited IgE- and IL-33-mediated mast cell activation (Figure 2). The Gab2/PI3K pathway is critical in FcεRI signaling leading to degranulation in mast cells [22] and the NF-κB pathway mediates IgE- or IL-33-mediated transcriptonal activation of cytokine gene expression [5,6,20,21]. Thus, it is likely that SR9009 and other synthetic REV-ERB agonists inhibited IgE-mediated degranulation and IgE- and IL-33-mediated IL-6 and IL-13 expression through the suppression of the Gab2/PI3K and NF-kB pathways, respectively. Because the Gab2/PI3K pathway play a partial role in IgE-mediated cytokein expression [22], inhibition of this pathway by SR9009 may be also involved in the suppression of IgE-mediated IL-6 and IL-13 expression.

It remains to be determined how SR9009 inhibits the Gab2/PI3K and NF-κB pathways. However, regarding the NF-κB pathway, there were several reports that address the inhibitory mechanisms of SR9009 on the NF-κB pathway, including transcriptional repression of NF-κB–related genes such as IL-6 [24], p65 [25], and induction of FABP4, an intracellular lipid-binding protein [26]. In contrast, it remains totally unclear how SR9009 inhibits IgE-mediated Gab2/PI3K activation in mast cells.

Pretreatment of Clock-mutated BMMCs with SR9009 and other synthetic REV-ERBs agonists for 1 h can suppress IgE- and IL-33-mediated activation, as in wild-type BMMCs (Figure 2). Moreover, given that treatment of wild-type $PER2^{LUC}$ BMMCs with SR9009, SR9011, or GSK4112 did not affect $PER2^{LUC}$ expression 1 h after the addition of the agent (Figure 1b), the suppressive effects of SR9009 or other synthetic REV-ERB agonists may be independent of functional circadian clock activity and PER2 expression in mast cells. The observation that treatment of wild-type BMMCs with SR9009 for 1 h did not affect the expression of FcεRI or ST2 (Figure S8) also support this idea, as expression of FcεRI and ST2 is under the control of mast cell clock activity [3,4].

Surprisingly, SR9009 inhibited IgE- or IL-33-mediated activation in REV-ERBs knocked-down BMMCs (Figure 4). Thus, the inhibitory actions of SR9009 on IgE- and IL-33-mediated mast cell activation may be independent on its agonistic function through REV-ERBs. Most recently, Dierickx et al. reported that SR9009 has REV-ERB-independent effects on cell proliferation and metabolism [27]. They showed that SR9009 can decrease cell viability, rewire cellular metabolism, and alter gene transcription in hepatocytes and embryonic stem cells derived from REV-ERB-α and -β double knockout mice although the mechanisms remain unclear. Thus, SR9009 and possibly other SR9009-related synthetic REV-ERB agonists might inhibit IgE- and IL-33-mediated mast cell activation independently of REV-ERBs. However, it should be noted that REV-ERBs knocked-down BMMCs still express REV-ERB-α and REV-ERB-β mRNAs, albeit at very low levels and SR9009 could exert its function through the residual expression of REV-ERBs.

Clock mutation decreases IL-33-mediated IL-13 production in BMMCs (Figure 2b,d). Kawauchi et al. reported that IL-33-mediated IL-6 and IL-13 production exhibit a time-of-day–dependent variation in synchronized, but not Clock-mutated, BMMCs [4]. Thus, it is likely that Clock may be involved in the circadian regulation of IL-33-mediated IL-13 production, although the mechanisms involved remain to be determined.

In summary, our findings show that activation of REV-ERBs by SR9009 or other synthetic REV-ERBs agonists can inhibit IgE- and IL-33-mediated activation of mast cells in association with suppression of the Gab2/PI3K and NF-κB pathways. Thus, modulation of REV-ERB activity by synthetic REV-ERB agonists may have potential for broad ranges of allergic diseases.

4. Materials and Methods

4.1. Materials

Reagents used in this study were acquired from the indicated suppliers: SR9009 (Merck Millipore, Burlington, MA, USA); SR9011, GSK4112, LPS, and Evans blue (Sigma-Aldrich, St. Louis, MO, USA); recombinant mouse IL-3 (PeproTech, Rocky Hill, NJ, USA); recombinant mouse IL-33 (R & D Systems, Minneapolis, MN, USA); anti-TNP IgE, anti-DNP mouse IgE mAb, anti-mouse CD16/32, PE-conjugated anti-mouse c-kit Ab, and APC-conjugated anti-mouse ST2 Ab (BD Bioscience, San Jose, CA, USA); DNP-BSA (Cosmo Bio, Tokyo, Japan); APC-conjugated anti-mouse CD63 Ab, FITC-conjugated anti-mouse FcεRIα (BioLegend, San Diego, CA, USA); anti-phospho-NF-κB p65 Ab (Ser536; #3033), anti-phospho-p38 MAPK Ab (Thr180/Thy182; #4511), anti-phospho-Gab2 Ab (Tyr452; #3882), anti-phosph-PI3 Kinase p85 (Tyr458)/p55 (Tur199) Ab (#4228), and anti-β-actin Ab (#4970) (Cell Signaling Technology, Danvers, MA, USA).

4.2. Mice

Male 6–8-week-old C57BL/6 mice (Japan SLC, Tokyo, Japan), Per2^{Luciferase} (Per2^{Luc}) knock-in mice (C57BL/6 background) where PERIOD2 (PER2) is expressed as a luciferase fusion protein [18], and C57BL/6 Clock$^{\Delta19/\Delta19}$ mice [17] were kept under 12-hour light / 12-hour dark conditions. Clock$^{\Delta19/\Delta19}$ mice have an A-to-T point mutation in the 5′ splice site of intron 19 and consequently an in-frame deletion of the whole exon 19 (Clock$^{\Delta19/\Delta19}$), resulting in the loss of normal transcriptional activity [17]. All animal experiments were approved by the Institutional Review Board (IRB) of the University of Yamanashi and carried out according to IRB guidelines (ethics committee: Koji Moriishi, Toshiyuki Oda, Hiroaki Nagatomo, Hiroyuki Narita, Jiang Ling, Junichi Miyazaki, Kazuhiro Mori, and Teruhiko Wakayama, approval code: A28-36, 14 August 2019).

4.3. Preparation of Bone Marrow-Derived Mast Cells (BMMCs) and Fetal Skin-Derived Mast Cells (FSMCs)

BMMCs were prepared from femoral bone marrow cell suspensions from male C57BL/6 mice, Per2^{Luc} mice, or Clock$^{\Delta19/\Delta19}$ mice as previously described [3]. Briefly, crude bone marrow cells were cultured in RPMI 1640 supplemented with 10% fetal bovine serum, 2 mM L-glutamine, 10 mM nonessential amino acids, penicillin–streptomycin, 10 mM sodium pyruvate, and 50 μM 2-ME (complete RPMI 1640) in the presence of 10 ng/mL recombinant mouse IL-3 (rmIL-3). Floating cells were refreshed twice per week, and further expanded for 2–4 weeks in fresh complete RPMI 1640 supplied with rmIL-3. Finally, the cells (>90% FcεR1$^+$c-kit$^+$) were used as BMMCs without further purification.

Fetal skin mast cells (FSMCs) were generated from fetal skin of C57BL/6 mice on day 14, as described previously [28]. Briefly, fetal skin was treated with trypsin diluted in medium to form a single cell suspension. Then the cells were cultured in complete medium containing 20 ng/mL rmIL-3 and 20 ng/mL recombinant mouse SCF. After 2 weeks, non-adherent and loosely-adherent cells were collected, and mast cells were collected by Percoll density-gradient centrifugation. Finally, the cells (>90% FcεR1$^+$c-kit$^+$) were used as FSMCs.

4.4. Quantitative Real-Time PCR

Total RNA was isolated from BMMCs using the RNeasy Mini Kit (QIAGEN, Valencia, CA, USA). RNA was quantified on a NanoDrop ND-1000 spectrophotometer (Thermo Fisher Scientific, Waltham, MA, USA). Complementary DNA (cDNA) was synthesized using the ReverTra Ace RT-PCR Kit (TOYOBO, Osaka, Japan). Quantitative real-time PCR (qPCR) was performed on a Step One Plus Fast Real-Time PCR System (Applied Biosystems, Carlsbad, CA, USA) using qPCR Master Mix (Applied Biosystems) with specific primers and probes against mouse *REV-ERB-α*, *IL-13* (Applied Biosystems), *REV-ERB-β*, *IL-6*, and *GAPDH* (IDT; Coralville, IA, USA). qPCR data were normalized against the corresponding levels of *GAPDH* mRNA.

4.5. Measurement of Bioluminescence in BMMCs Generated from Per2^{Luc} Mice

BMMCs generated from Per2^{Luc} knock-in mice were centrifuged at 1500 rpm for 5 min, placed in a 35 mm Petri dish and incubated at 37 °C. As previously described, bioluminescence was monitored for 120 h at 10-min intervals using a dish-type luminometer (Kronos DioAB-2550; ATTO, Tokyo, Japan) [3]. After 72 h of medium change for synchronization, 10 μM REV-ERB agonists were added to the culture.

4.6. Flow Cytometry Analysis

BMMCs were stained with PE-conjugated anti-mouse c-kit, FITC-conjugated anti-mouse FcεRI, APC-conjugated anti-mouse ST2, or APC-conjugated anti-mouse CD63 in the presence of rat anti-mouse CD16/32. After washing with PBS, the stained cells were analyzed on a BD Accuri C6 flow cytometer (BD Biosciences). Flow cytometry data were analyzed using the CellQuest software (BD Biosciences).

4.7. Stimulations of BMMCs or FSMCs

BMMCs or FSMCs were incubated with 1 μg/mL anti-DNP mouse IgE mAb for 1 h at 4 °C and, then, incubated with or without REV-ERB agonists for 1 h at 37 °C. Then, these cells were stimulated with 1 μg/mL of anti-mouse IgE antibody for 1 h at 37 °C (for β-Hexosaminidase or histamine measurement) or for 6 h at 37 °C (for IL-6 or IL-13 measurement). BMMCs or FSMCs were incubated with or without REV-ERB agonists for 1 h at 37 °C and then stimulated with 1 ng/mL IL-33 or 1 μg/mL LPS for 6 h at 37 °C, followed by measurement of IL-6 and IL-13 in the culture supernatants.

4.8. Enzyme-Linked Immunosorbent Assay (ELISA)

Concentrations of IL-6, IL-13, and histamine in supernatants of cell cultures were determined by ELISA. Kits for mouse IL-6 (R & D Systems), mouse histamine (Oxford Biomedical Research, Rochester Hills, MI, USA), mouse IL-13 (eBioscience/Thermo Fisher Scientific) were obtained from the indicated suppliers.

4.9. β-Hexosaminidase Release Assay

BMMCs or FSMCs were incubated with 1 μg/mL anti-DNP mouse IgE mAb for 1 h at 4 °C, and then stimulated with 1 μg/mL of anti-mouse IgE antibody with or without REV-ERB agonists for 1 h at 37 °C. Total release was obtained by adding 1% Triton buffer for 40 min. Supernatants were collected from each well and mixed with *p*-nitrophenyl-*N*-acetyl-β-D-glucosaminide to determine the enzymatic activity of the released β-hexosaminidase. After 90 min at 37 °C, the reaction was stopped by addition of 0.2 M glycine solution, and OD (405 nm) was measured on a spectrophotometer.

4.10. Western Blot Analysis

Ten minutes after various stimulations, BMMCs were lysed in RIPA buffer (25 mM Tris-HCl, pH 7.6, 150 mM NaCl, 1% Triton ×100, 1% sodium deoxycholate, 0.1% SDS) with protease inhibitor cocktail (Merck Millipore, Burlington, MA, USA) and vanadate (FUJIFILM Wako Pure Chemical Corporation, Osaka, Japan). Cell lysate was dissolved in sample buffer containing 50 mM dithiothreitol and bromophenol blue, and then boiled for 5 min. Protein concentrations were measured on a NanoDrop ND-1000. Proteins were subjected to SDS-PAGE and transferred to polyvinylidene fluoride membranes. Blots were immersed in 5% milk blocking solution for 1 h at room temperature (RT), followed by incubation with primary antibody solution overnight at 4 °C. Membranes were washed three times with TBS/T, and then incubated in a secondary antibody solution for 1 h at RT. Immunoreactive proteins were visualized using ECL Prime (GE Healthcare).

4.11. Reporter Assays

Using the Mouse Macrophage Nucleofector kit (VPA-1009; Lonza, Basel, Switzerland), BMMCs were transiently transfected with the pNFκB-Luc reporter plasmid, with pRL-CMV as an internal control. After 24 h, the transfected BMMCs were stimulated with IL-33 (1 ng/mL) or anti-mouse IgE antibody (1 μg/mL) or LPS (1 μg/mL) in the absence or presence of REV-ERBs agonists. Relative NF-κB luciferase activity was normalized against transfection efficiency.

4.12. Cell Viability Assay

After stimulations with synthetic REV-ERB agonists for 24 h, cell viability was monitored using the Cell Counting Kit-8 (Dojindo Laboratory, Kumamoto, Japan) and PE-Annexin V apoptosis detection kit (BD Bioscience, San Jose, CA, USA).

4.13. Passive Cutaneous Anaphylaxis

Mouse anti-TNP IgE (100 ng) was intradermally injected into dorsal skin. After 24 h, 15% Cremophor (vehicle) or SR9009 (100 mg/kg) was intraperitoneally injected. After 1 h, the mice were challenged by intravenous injection with 2.5mg/kg of DNP-BSA in PBS containing 0.2% Evans blue dye. Vascular permeability was visualized 40 min later as blue staining of the injection areas on the inside of the skin. Staining sites were digitized using a high-resolution color camera, and images were saved JPEG files. The images analyzed using ImageJ 1.43 (NIH, Bethesda, MD, USA) as previously described [3]. Briefly, the color-scale images (the upper panels) were converted to HSB (hue/saturation/brightness) stack images, which were then split into hue, saturation, and brightness images. The blue-stained areas were selected from the hue image using the threshold tool, afterwards these images were combined with the saturation image. The density values for the blue-stained areas were measured using the analyze tool.

4.14. siRNAs Experiments

All siRNAs were purchased from Invitrogen (now Thermo Fisher, Waltham, MA, USA). Specific siRNAs against NR1D1 (stealth^{TM} RNAi; Nr1d1MSS211361 [3_RNAI]) or NR1D2 (stealth^{TM} RNAi: Nr1d2MSS221355 [3_RNAI]) were used.

Transfection of wild-type BMMCs were performed with Mouse Macrophage Nucleofector Kit (VPA-1009; Lonza, Basel, Switzerland). BMMCs were suspended in Nucleofector Solution to a final concentration of 2×10^6 cells/100μL. The cells were transfected with 500 nM negative control or 250 nM specific siRNA of NR1D1 and NR1D2, respectively, using the Nucleofector II (Amaxa Biosystems, now Lonza) program Y-001. Subsequently, the transferred cells were placed in a 20% FBS medium and cultured in a 24-well plate. After 24 h, the transfected BMMCs were stimulated with anti-mouse IgE antibody (1μg/mL), IL-33 (1 ng/mL), or LPS (1 μg/mL) in the absence or presence of 10 μM SR9009.

4.15. Statistical Analysis

Statistical analyses were performed using the unpaired Student's *t*-test for two-group comparisons. Multigroup comparisons were analyzed by one-way ANOVA with Tukey–Kramer post hoc test. A value of $p < 0.05$ was considered to be significant.

Supplementary Materials: Supplementary materials can be found at http://www.mdpi.com/1422-0067/20/24/6320/s1.

Author Contributions: K.I. and A.N. conceived and designed the experiments and wrote the manuscript. K.I., S.N., Y.N., and G.Y. performed the experiments. K.I. and S.N. analyzed the data. K.I. and A.N. are the guarantors of this work and, as such, had full access to all the data in the study and take responsibility for the integrity of the data and the accuracy of the data analysis.

Funding: This work was supported in part by grants from the Ministry of Education, Culture, Sports, Science and Technology of Japan (to Kayoko Ishimaru [19K08904] and Atsuhito Nakao [18H02848]).

Acknowledgments: We are grateful to Jian Yao for providing us with experimental materials. We thank Tomoko Tohno and Yukino Fukasawa for helpful secretarial assistance, and Maiko Aihara for technical assistance.

Conflicts of Interest: No potential conflicts of interest relevant to this article were reported.

Abbreviations

MAPK	Mitogen-activated protein kinase
NF-κB	Nuclear factor κB

References

1. Bass, J.; Lazar, M.A. Circadian time signatures of fitness and disease. *Science* **2016**, *354*, 994–999. [CrossRef] [PubMed]
2. Takahashi, J.S. Transcriptional architecture of the mammalian circadian clock. *Nat. Rev. Genet.* **2017**, *18*, 164–179. [CrossRef] [PubMed]
3. Nakamura, Y.; Nakano, N.; Ishimaru, K.; Hara, M.; Ikegami, T.; Tahara, Y.; Katoh, R.; Ogawa, H.; Okumura, K.; Shibata, S.; et al. Circadian regulation of allergic reactions by the mast cell clock in mice. *J. Allergy Clin. Immunol.* **2014**, *133*, 568–575. [CrossRef]

4. Kawauchi, T.; Ishimaru, K.; Nakamura, Y.; Nakano, N.; Hara, M.; Ogawa, H.; Okumura, K.; Shibata, S.; Nakao, A. Clock-dependent temporal regulation of IL-33/ST2-mediated mast cell response. *Allergol. Int.* **2017**, *66*, 472–478. [CrossRef] [PubMed]
5. Galli, S.J.; Tsai, M. IgE and mast cells in allergic diseases. *Nat. Med.* **2012**, *18*, 693–704. [CrossRef]
6. Ohno, T.; Morita, H.; Arae, K.; Matsumoto, K.; Nakae, S. Interleukin-33 in allergy. *Allergy* **2012**, *67*, 1203–1214. [CrossRef]
7. Christ, P.; Sowa, A.S.; Froy, O.; Lorentz, A. The Circadian Clock Drives Mast Cell Functions in Allergic Reactions. *Front Immunol.* **2018**, *9*, 1526. [CrossRef]
8. Nakao, A. Clockwork allergy: How the circadian clock underpins allergic reactions. *J. Allergy Clin. Immunol.* **2018**, *142*, 1021–1031. [CrossRef]
9. Kojetin, D.J.; Burris, T.P. REV-ERB and ROR nuclear receptors as drug targets. *Nat. Rev. Drug Discov.* **2014**, *13*, 197–216. [CrossRef]
10. Woldt, E.; Sebti, Y.; Solt, L.A.; Duhem, C.; Lancel, S.; Eeckhoute, J.; Hesselink, M.K.; Paquet, C.; Delhaye, S.; Shin, Y.; et al. Rev-erb-α modulates skeletal muscle oxidative capacity by regulating mitochondrial biogenesis and autophagy. *Nat. Med.* **2013**, *19*, 1039–1046. [CrossRef]
11. Lam, M.T.; Cho, H.; Lesch, H.P.; Gosselin, D.; Heinz, S.; Tanaka-Oishi, Y.; Benner, C.; Kaikkonen, M.U.; Kim, A.S.; Kosaka, M.; et al. Rev-Erbs repress macrophage gene expression by inhibiting enhancer-directed transcription. *Nature* **2013**, *498*, 511–515. [CrossRef] [PubMed]
12. Solt, L.A.; Wang, Y.; Banerjee, S.; Hughes, T.; Kojetin, D.J.; Lundasen, T.; Shin, Y.; Liu, J.; Cameron, M.D.; Noel, R.; et al. Regulation of circadian behaviour and metabolism by synthetic REV-ERB agonists. *Nature* **2012**, *485*, 62–68. [CrossRef] [PubMed]
13. Banerjee, S.; Wang, Y.; Solt, L.A.; Griffett, K.; Kazantzis, M.; Amador, A.; El-Gendy, B.M.; Huitron-Resendiz, S.; Roberts, A.J.; Shin, Y.; et al. Pharmacological targeting of the mammalian clock regulates sleep architecture and emotional behaviour. *Nat. Commun.* **2014**, *5*, 5759. [CrossRef] [PubMed]
14. Gibbs, J.E.; Blaikley, J.; Beesley, S.; Matthews, L.; Simpson, K.D.; Boyce, S.H.; Farrow, S.N.; Else, K.J.; Singh, D.; Ray, D.W.; et al. The nuclear receptor REV-ERBα mediates circadian regulation of innate immunity through selective regulation of inflammatory cytokines. *Proc. Nat. Acad. Sci. USA* **2012**, *109*, 582–587. [CrossRef] [PubMed]
15. Sulli, G.; Rommel, A.; Wang, X.; Kolar, M.J.; Puca, F.; Saghatelian, A.; Plikus, M.V.; Verma, I.M.; Panda, S. Pharmacological activation of REV-ERBs is lethal in cancer and oncogene-induced senescence. *Nature* **2018**, *553*, 351–355. [CrossRef] [PubMed]
16. Nakamura, Y.; Harama, D.; Shimokawa, N.; Hara, M.; Suzuki, R.; Tahara, Y.; Ishimaru, K.; Katoh, R.; Okumura, K.; Ogawa, H.; et al. Circadian clock gene Period2 regulates a time-of-day-dependent variation in cutaneous anaphylactic reaction. *J. Allergy Clin. Immun.* **2011**, *127*, 1038–1045. [CrossRef]
17. Vitaterna, M.H.; King, D.P.; Chang, A.M.; Kornhauser, J.M.; Lowrey, P.L.; McDonald, J.D.; Dove, W.F.; Pinto, L.H.; Turek, F.W.; Takahashi, J.S. Mutagenesis and mapping of a mouse gene, Clock, essential for circadian behavior. *Science* **1994**, *264*, 719–725. [CrossRef]
18. Yoo, O.J.; Menaker, M.; Takahashi, J.S. PERIOD2:LUCIFERASE real-time reporting of circadian dynamics reveals persistent circadian oscillations in mouse peripheral tissues. *Proc. Nat. Acad. Sci. USA* **2004**, *101*, 5339–5346. [CrossRef]
19. Welsh, D.K.; Yoo, S.H.; Liu, A.C.; Takahashi, J.S.; Kay, S.A. Bioluminescence imaging of individual fibroblasts reveals persistent independently phased circadian rhythms of clock gene expression. *Curr. Biol.* **2004**, *14*, 2289–2295. [CrossRef]
20. Metcalfe, D.D.; Peavey, R.D.; Gilfillan, A.M. Mechanisms of mast cell signaling in anaphylaxis. *J. Allergy Clin. Immunol.* **2009**, *124*, 639–646. [CrossRef]
21. Takatori, H.; Makita, S.; Ito, T.; Matsuki, A.; Nakajima, H. Regulatory Mechanisms of IL-33-ST2-Mediated Allergic Inflammation. *Front. Immunol.* **2018**, *9*, 2004. [CrossRef] [PubMed]
22. Gu, H.; Saito, K.; Klaman, L.D.; Shen, J.; Fleming, T.; Wang, Y.; Pratt, J.C.; Lin, G.; Lim, B.; Kinet, J.P.; et al. Essential role for Gab2 in the allergic response. *Nature* **2001**, *412*, 186–190. [CrossRef] [PubMed]
23. Sulli, G.; Manoogian, E.N.C.; Taub, P.R.; Panda, S. Training the Circadian Clock, Clocking the Drugs, and Drugging the Clock to Prevent, Manage, and Treat Chronic Diseases. *Trends Pharmacol. Sci.* **2018**, *39*, 812–827. [CrossRef] [PubMed]

24. Sato, S.; Sakurai, T.; Ogasawara, J.; Shirato, K.; Ishibashi, Y.; Oh-ishi, S.; Imaizumi, K.; Haga, S.; Hitomi, Y.; Izawa, T.; et al. Direct and indirect suppression of interleukin-6 gene expression in murine macrophages by nuclear orphan receptor REV-ERBα. *Sci. World J.* **2014**, *2014*, 685854. [CrossRef]
25. Wang, S.; Lin, Y.; Yuan, X.; Li, F.; Guo, L.; Wu, B. REV-ERBα integrates colon clock with experimental colitis through regulation of NF-κB/NLRP3 axis. *Nat. Commun.* **2018**, *9*, 4246. [CrossRef]
26. Song, C.; Tan, P.; Zhang, Z.; Wu, W.; Dong, Y.; Zhao, L.; Liu, H.; Guan, H.; Li, F. REV-ERB agonism suppresses osteoclastogenesis and prevents ovariectomy-induced bone loss partially via FABP4 upregulation. *FASEB J.* **2018**, *32*, 3215–3228. [CrossRef]
27. Dierickx, P.; Emmett, M.J.; Jiang, C.; Uehara, K.; Liu, M.; Adlanmerini, M.; Lazar, M.A. SR9009 has REV-ERB-independent effects on cell proliferation and metabolism. *Proc. Nat. Acad. Sci. USA* **2019**, *116*, 12147–12152. [CrossRef]
28. Matsushima, H.; Yamada, N.; Matsue, H.; Shimada, S. TLR3-, TLR7-, and TLR9-mediated production of proinflammatory cytokines and chemokines from murine connective tissue type skin-derived mast cells but not from bone marrow-derived mast cells. *J. Immunol.* **2004**, *173*, 531–541. [CrossRef]

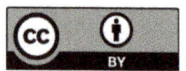 © 2019 by the authors. Licensee MDPI, Basel, Switzerland. This article is an open access article distributed under the terms and conditions of the Creative Commons Attribution (CC BY) license (http://creativecommons.org/licenses/by/4.0/).

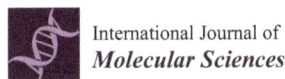

Article

Establishment and Characterization of a Murine Mucosal Mast Cell Culture Model

Aya Kakinoki [1], Tsuyoshi Kameo [1], Shoko Yamashita [2], Kazuyuki Furuta [2] and Satoshi Tanaka [3,*]

[1] Department of Immunobiology, Faculty of Pharmacy and Pharmaceutical Sciences, Okayama University, Tsushima naka 1-1-1, Kita-ku, Okayama 700-8530, Japan; ph20008@s.okayama-u.ac.jp (A.K.); plwv9rz8@s.okayama-u.ac.jp (T.K.)

[2] Department of Immunobiology, Okayama University Graduate School of Medicine, Dentistry, and Pharmaceutical Sciences, Tsushima naka 1-1-1, Kita-ku, Okayama 700-8530, Japan; ph421138@s.okayama-u.ac.jp (S.Y.); furutak@okayama-u.ac.jp (K.F.)

[3] Department of Pharmacology, Division of Pathological Sciences, Kyoto Pharmaceutical University, Misasagi Nakauchi-cho 5, Yamashina-ku, Kyoto 607-8414, Japan

* Correspondence: tanaka-s@mb.kyoto-phu.ac.jp; Tel.: +81-75-595-4667

Received: 6 December 2019; Accepted: 27 December 2019; Published: 29 December 2019

Abstract: Accumulating evidence suggests that mast cells play critical roles in disruption and maintenance of intestinal homeostasis, although it remains unknown how they affect the local microenvironment. Interleukin-9 (IL-9) was found to play critical roles in intestinal mast cell accumulation induced in various pathological conditions, such as parasite infection and oral allergen-induced anaphylaxis. Newly recruited intestinal mast cells trigger inflammatory responses and damage epithelial integrity through release of a wide variety of mediators including mast cell proteases. We established a novel culture model (IL-9-modified mast cells, MCs/IL-9), in which murine IL-3-dependent bone-marrow-derived cultured mast cells (BMMCs) were further cultured in the presence of stem cell factor and IL-9. In MCs/IL-9, drastic upregulation of *Mcpt1* and *Mcpt2* was found. Although histamine storage and tryptase activity were significantly downregulated in the presence of SCF and IL-9, this was entirely reversed when mast cells were cocultured with a murine fibroblastic cell line, Swiss 3T3. MCs/IL-9 underwent degranulation upon IgE-mediated antigen stimulation, which was found to less sensitive to lower concentrations of IgE in comparison with BMMCs. This model might be useful for investigation of the spatiotemporal changes of newly recruited intestinal mast cells.

Keywords: mast cell; IL-9; chymase; histamine; ATP

1. Introduction

Intestinal and respiratory tracts are constantly exposed to a wide variety of stimulatory factors and are in a continuous state of change. Immune cells located at these tracts have to adapt themselves to these changes in a timely manner. Mast cells are one of the most suitable immune cells that regulate immune responses at such interfaces because they express a diverse array of surface receptors and undergo flexible local transdifferentiation [1,2]. They were found not only to trigger inflammatory responses but also to be involved in immune suppression [3]. Accumulating evidence suggests that intestinal mast cells play critical roles in parasite expulsion through their multiple functions, including regulation of epithelial and endothelial functions and modulation of innate and adaptive immunity [4–6].

Interleukin-9 (IL-9), which was also found to be one of the critical mediators for worm expulsion, was first identified as a mast cell growth factor [7]. IL-9 transgenic mice exhibited rapid expulsion of the intestinal nematodes and local mastocytosis in epithelial layer of the gut, trachea and kidney [8–10].

The number of intestinal mast cells were unchanged in the gene-targeted mice lacking IL-9 or IL-9 receptor-α chain, whereas oral-antigen-induced accumulation of intestinal mast cells was impaired in these mice [11,12]. These findings indicate that IL-9 should trigger intestinal mastocytosis upon parasite infection and newly recruited mast cells should make a significant contribution towards worm expulsion. IL-9 was found to enhance stem cell factor (SCF)-mediated proliferation of murine bone-marrow-derived cultured mast cells, although IL-9 alone could not support mast cell growth and survival [13]. It remains largely unknown how transdifferentiation of intestinal mast cells should occur under the influence of IL-9 and SCF.

IL-3-dependent bone-marrow-derived cultured mast cells (BMMCs) have been investigated as a useful model of murine immature mast cells. BMMCs were initially regarded as a model of mucosal mast cells, because they stored chondroitin sulphate E, rather than heparin, in their granules and had lower amounts of histamine, both being characteristic of persistent mucosal mast cells [14]. However, accumulating evidence has suggested that there are many differences among BMMCs, resident mucosal mast cells and recruited mast cells upon parasite infection. IL-3 was found to play critical roles in parasite expulsion and intestinal mastocytosis [15]. Murine mucosal mast cells recruited upon parasite infection were found to highly express a series of chymase genes, such as *Mcpt1* [16], although little or no expression of these genes was confirmed in BMMCs. Furthermore, because the number of mucosal resident mast cells is quite small, they remain to be fully characterized. Because BMMCs are highly capable for further differentiation into mature mast cells, local reconstitution of BMMCs in recently developed mast-cell-deficient mice has been used as one of the best suitable approaches to clarify the functions of tissue mast cells [17]. We previously established a modified coculture method of BMMCs using murine fibroblastic cell line, Swiss 3T3, which shared many characteristics with murine cutaneous mast cells [18,19]. We tried to develop here a novel culture model, in which BMMCs were further cultured in the presence of IL-9 and SCF. This model at least partly reflected the characteristics of intestinally recruited mast cells and provided some insights into the process of transdifferentiation of newly recruited mast cells in intestinal tissues.

2. Results

2.1. Combination of IL-9 and SCF Induced Expression of Mcpt1 and Mcpt2 and Depleted Histamine in Murine BMMCs

Accumulating evidence suggests that SCF plays critical roles in growth and survival of murine tissue mast cells, which are enhanced by IL-9 in mucosal tissues. BMMCs, which are regarded as an immature mast cell population, were found to be obtained when murine bone marrow cells were cultured for about one month in the presence of IL-3. They have potential to undergo further differentiation in response to the environment changes. We first investigated the effects of IL-9 on BMMCs and found that IL-9 alone or in combination with IL-3 could not support the further survival of BMMCs. We, therefore, added SCF, which is responsible for growth and maturation of the connective-tissue-type mast cells and is also abundantly expressed in the intestinal tissues, to the culture to support survival of the cultured mast cells. Expression of *Mcpt1* and *Mcpt2*, both regarded as characteristic of mucosal mast cells [13], was drastically induced during the culture period in the presence of SCF and IL-9, whereas that of *Mcpt5* and *Cpa3* was upregulated and maintained (Figure 1a–d). It was noteworthy that a drastic downregulation of *Hdc*, which encodes the enzyme responsible for histamine synthesis, was unexpectedly observed (Figure 1e). We previously demonstrated that *Ptgr1*, which encodes the enzyme involved in inactivation of the eicosanoids, was expressed in the mucosal mast cells, not in the connective-tissue-type mast cells in murine stomach [20]. Expression of *Ptgr1* was found to be moderately upregulated in our system (Figure 1f). Surface expression levels of FcεRI and c-kit were significantly decreased in the presence of SCF and IL-9 (Figure 1g,h).

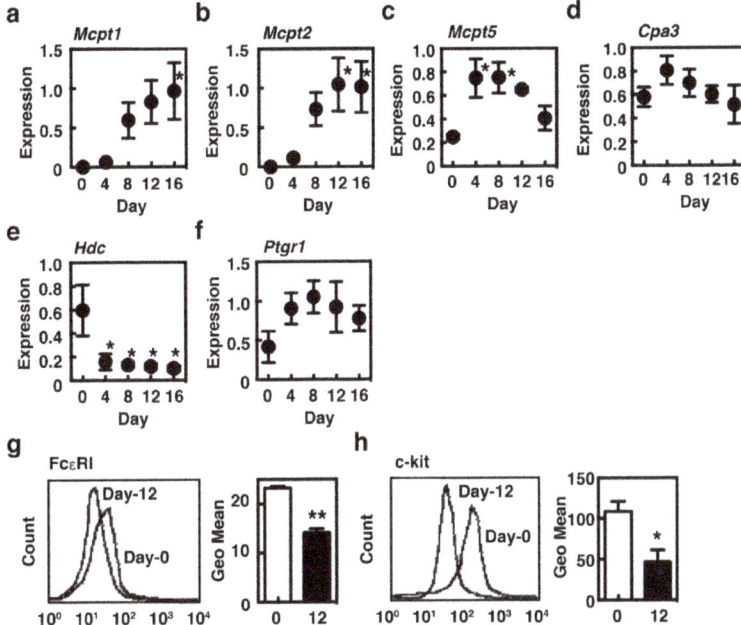

Figure 1. Induction of the characteristic genes of mucosal mast cells in the presence of interleukin-9 (IL-9) and stem cell factor (SCF). (**a–f**) Bone-marrow-derived cultured mast cells (BMMCs) were cultured in the presence of 10 ng/mL IL-9 and 30 ng/mL SCF for 16 days. Expression levels of mRNA of (**a**) *Mcpt1*, (**b**) *Mcpt2*, (**c**) *Mcpt5*, (**d**) *Cpa3*, (**e**) *Hdc* and (**f**) *Ptgr1* were measured by quantitative RT-PCR. The expression levels were normalized by measuring mRNA expression of *Gapdh*. The values are expressed as the means ± SEM ($n = 3$). Multiple comparisons were performed using one-way ANOVA with the Dunnett post-test. Values with * $p < 0.05$ are regarded as significant (vs. day 0). (**g,h**) Surface expression levels of (**g**) FcεRI and (**h**) c-kit of BMMCs (day 0, open columns) and MCs/IL-9 (day 12, closed columns) were measured by flow cytometry as described in Section 4. The mean fluorescence intensities are shown as the means ± SEM ($n = 3$, right panels). Statistical analysis was performed using Student's *t*-test. Values with * $p < 0.05$ and ** $p < 0.01$ are regarded as significant.

We then measured the enzymatic activities of the cultured mast cells. Chymotryptic activity was significantly increased in BMMCs cultured in the presence of SCF and IL-9 for 12 days (designed as IL-9-modified mast cells, MCs/IL-9), whereas tryptic activity was downmodulated (Figure 2a,b). Carboxypeptidase A activities varied greatly in MCs/IL-9 (Figure 2c). In agreement with the expression levels of *Hdc*, histamine synthesis was drastically suppressed in the presence of SCF and IL-9 (Figure 2d,e). Because tissue mast cells are often located next to cells expressing the membrane-bound form of SCF, we performed the coculture with a murine fibroblastic cell line, Swiss 3T3, in the presence of SCF and IL-9, and investigated the characteristics of the cocultured mast cells. The presence of fibroblasts enhanced the induction of chymotryptic activity (Figure 2f). Carboxypeptidase A activities were significantly induced in the cocultured MCs/IL-9 (Figure 2h). Regarding the tryptic activity and histamine synthesis, the presence of fibroblasts reversed the actions of SCF and IL-9 (Figure 2g,i,j).

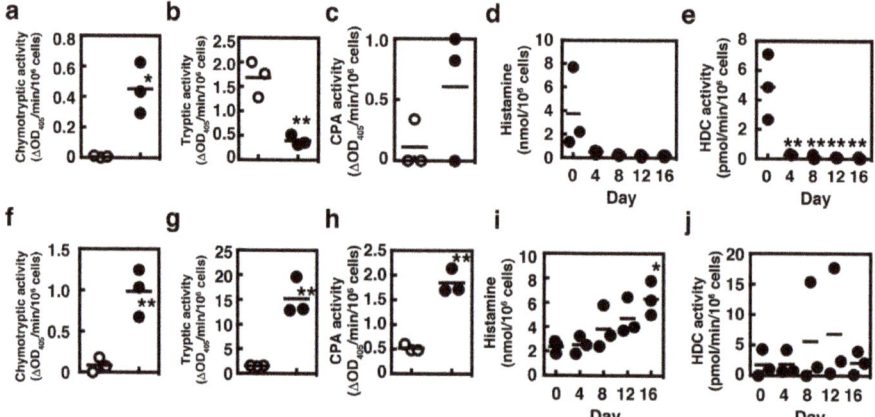

Figure 2. Effects of Swiss 3T3 fibroblastic cell line on the characteristic changes of the cultured mast cells in the presence of IL-9 and SCF. Enzymatic activities of (**a,f**) chymase, (**b,g**) tryptase and (**c,h**) carboxypeptidase A were measured in BMMCs (open circles, **a–c,f–h**) and in MCs cultured in the presence of IL-9 and SCF for 12 days (closed circles, **a–c**) and in MCs cocultured with Swiss 3T3 fibroblasts in the presence of IL-9 and SCF for 16 days (closed circles, **f–h**). Statistical analysis was performed using Student's *t*-test. Values with * $p < 0.05$ and ** $p < 0.01$ are regarded as significant. (**d,i**) Cellular contents of histamine and (**e,j**) enzymatic activities of HDC were measured (**d,e**) in MCs cultured in the presence of IL-9 and SCF and (**i,j**) in MCs cocultured with Swiss 3T3 fibroblasts in the presence of IL-9 and SCF, respectively. Statistical analysis was performed using one-way ANOVA with Dunnett's test. Values with * $p < 0.05$ and ** $p < 0.01$ are regarded as significant (compared with Day-0).

2.2. Antigen-Induced Degranulation Was Attenuated in MCs/IL-9 When They Were Sensitized with Lower Concentrations of IgE

Previous studies suggested that IL-9 alone should not be able to form a mast cell population from hematopoietic stem cells in the bone marrow but could support the expansion and maturation of a mucosal mast cell population [13]. We compared the characteristics of two model populations, BMMCs as a newly recruited immature population and MCs/IL-9 as a more differentiated mucosal population. MCs/IL-9 showed a similar profile to that of BMMCs in degranulation upon IgE-mediated antigen stimulation when they were sensitized with 1 µg/mL of IgE, whereas the levels of degranulation were significantly decreased in MCs/IL-9 when they were sensitized with 10 ng/mL IgE (Figure 3a,b). Decreases in the levels of degranulation were also found in MCs/IL-9 when they were stimulated with thapsigargin and A23187 (Figure 3c).

2.3. Degranulation of MCs/IL-9 in Response to ATP

Increased concentrations of ATP are often found in injured tissues and inflammatory sites. Several recent studies have indicated the significance of ATP-mediated activation of tissue mast cells [21]. Remarkable levels of degranulation (>50%) were found in BMMCs when they were stimulated with 0.3 mM ATP (Figure 4a). Such prominent responses were not observed in MCs/IL-9. We investigated the mRNA expression levels of several P_2X receptor subtypes that have been previously reported to be expressed in mast cells [22]. Moderate and high levels of expression of *P2rx1*, *P2rx4* and *P2rx7* along with very low levels of expression of *P2rx3* were detected both in BMMCs and in MCs/IL-9 (Figure 4b,e). The expression levels of *P2rx7* were slightly, but not significantly, elevated in MCs/IL-9.

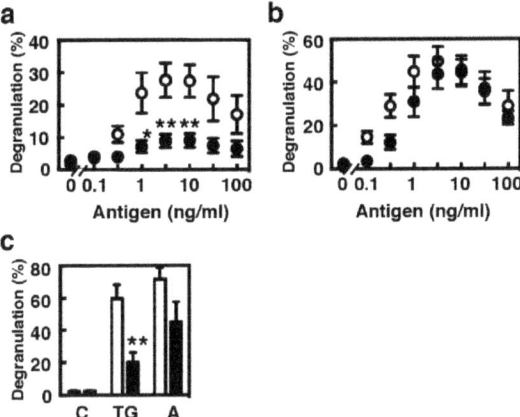

Figure 3. Comparison of the profiles of antigen-induced degranulation between BMMCs and MCs/IL-9. (**a**,**b**) BMMCs (open circles) or MCs/IL-9 (closed circles) were sensitized with (**a**) 10 ng/mL or (**b**) 1 μg/mL anti-TNP IgE (clone IgE-3) for 3 h at 37 °C. The cells were twice washed and stimulated with the indicated concentrations of the antigen (TNP-conjugated BSA). The levels of degranulation were determined by measuring the enzymatic activity of β-hexosaminidase. Values are presented as the means ± SEM ($n = 4$). Multiple comparisons were performed using two-way ANOVA with the Sidak test. Values with * $p < 0.05$ and ** $p < 0.01$ are regarded as significant. (**c**) BMMCs (open columns) or MCs/IL-9 (closed columns) were stimulated without (C, vehicle) or with 300 nM thapsigargin (TG) or 1 μM A23187 (A). The levels of degranulation were determined by measuring the enzymatic activity of β-hexosaminidase. Values are presented as the means ± SEM ($n = 4$). Statistical analysis was performed using Student's t-test. A value with ** $p < 0.01$ is regarded as significant.

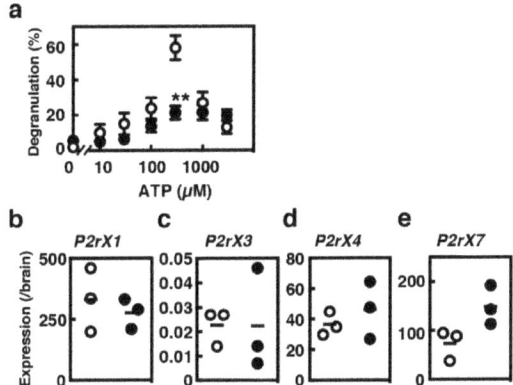

Figure 4. Comparison of the profiles of ATP-induced degranulation between BMMCs and MCs/IL-9. (**a**) BMMCs (open circles) and MCs/IL-9 (closed circles) were stimulated with the indicated concentrations of ATP. The levels of degranulation were determined by measuring the enzymatic activity of β-hexosaminidase. Values are presented as the means ± SEM ($n = 4$). Multiple comparisons were performed using two-way ANOVA with the Sidak test. A value with ** $p < 0.01$ is regarded as significant. (**b–e**) The levels of mRNA expression of (**b**) *P2rx1*, (**c**) *P2rx3*, (**d**) *P2rx4* and (**e**) *P2rx7* in BMMCs (open circles) and MCs/IL-9 (closed circles) were measured by quantitative RT-PCR.

2.4. Induction of the Inflammatory Cytokine Gene Expression in MCs/IL-9

Mast cells are known to be the sources of a wide variety of cytokines. We compared the cytokine gene expression profiles between BMMCs and MCs/IL-9, considering IL-4, -5, -6, -13 and TNF-α (Figure 5). Because TNF-α was found to be pre-formed in murine mast cells [23], the release of TNF-α protein may not reflect the changes of mRNA expression. Overall, MCs/IL-9 were found to be poor producers of these cytokines, which play critical roles in various intestinal inflammatory responses, in comparison with BMMCs. MCs/IL-9 were found to be incapable of IL-4 synthesis. Lipopolysaccharide (LPS) could induce the expression of proinflammatory cytokines such as IL-6 and TNF-α in BMMCs, whereas it could only induce marginal levels of IL-6 in MCs/IL-9. MCs/IL-9 had potential to produce IL-5, IL-6, IL-13 and TNF-α upon IgE-mediated antigen stimulation.

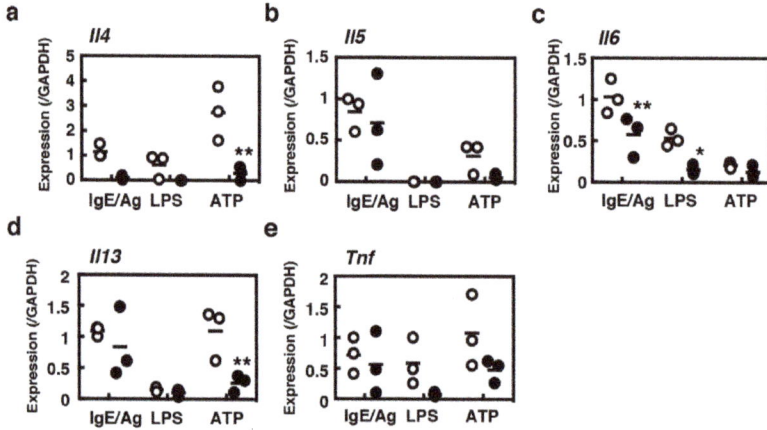

Figure 5. Comparison of transcriptional induction of various cytokines in between BMMCs and MCs/IL-9. BMMCs (open circles) or MCs/IL-9 (closed circles) were sensitized with 1 µg/mL anti-TNP IgE (clone IgE-3) for 3 h at 37 °C. The cells were twice washed and stimulated with the antigen (100 ng/mL, TNP-conjugated BSA) for 1 h (IgE/Ag). In parallel, BMMCs (open circles) or MCs/IL-9 (closed circles) were stimulated with LPS (1 µg/mL) or ATP (1 mM) for 1 h at 37 °C. Expression levels of mRNA of a series of cytokines ((**a**), IL-4; (**b**), IL-5; (**c**), IL-6; (**d**), IL-13; (**e**), TNF-α) were determined by quantitative RT-PCR. Statistical significance for comparison between BMMCs and MCs/IL-9 was determined by unpaired Student's *t*-test. Values with * $p < 0.05$ and ** $p < 0.01$ are regarded as significant.

3. Discussion

We characterized a novel bone-marrow-derived cultured mast cell model, which partly reflected the nature of newly recruited murine intestinal mast cells. Parasite infections or oral allergen-induced immediate responses cause drastic changes in the intestinal mucosa, whereas it remains largely unknown how local mast cells adapt themselves to these changes. We focused on the roles of SCF and IL-9, both of which were found to have major impacts on newly recruited intestinal mast cells. Accumulating evidence suggests that a large number of mast cells should be recruited into the intestinal tracts and that activated mast cells should play critical roles in pathology of inflammatory bowel diseases (IBD) and irritable bowel syndrome (IBS) [24–28], indicating that the characterization of intestinal mast cells should contribute to development of novel therapies for these chronic inflammatory diseases.

We previously found significant increases in histamine storage in BMMCs cocultured with Swiss 3T3 fibroblasts in the presence of SCF [18]. SCF alone was found to have a potential to induce histamine synthesis in BMMCs [29]. Here, histamine synthesis was abolished in the presence of SCF and IL-9, suggesting that IL-9 should be a potent suppressor of histamine synthesis. Histamine could profoundly affect the intestinal homeostasis through multiple pathways. It promotes increased vascular permeability and epithelial ion transport by acting on the H_1 receptors [30,31] and recruits neutrophils by acting on the H_4 receptors [32]. Forward et al. demonstrated in vitro that histamine could attenuate the suppressor functions of CD4$^+$CD25$^+$ T regulatory cells by acting on the H_1 receptors [33]. IL-9 may adequately control the intestinal environment through limiting the effects of mast-cell-derived histamine. Interestingly, contact with fibroblasts was found to cancel the effects of IL-9. Migration of newly recruited mast cells in the intestinal tissues may stimulate histamine synthesis and promote further inflammatory responses (Figure 6).

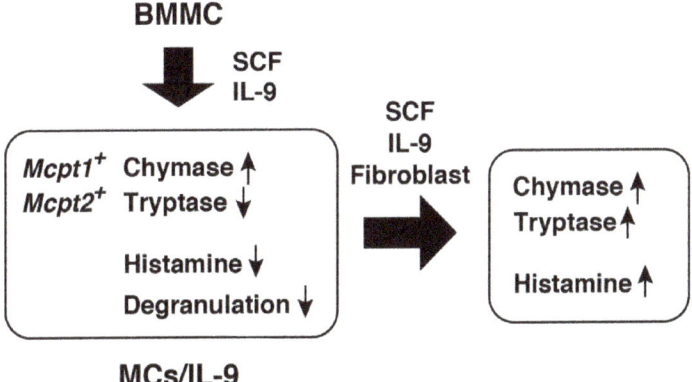

Figure 6. IL-9 has an impact on the characteristics of murine bone-marrow-derived cultured mast cells. The combination of SCF and IL-9 induced the expression of *Mcpt1* and *Mcpt2* in murine bone-marrow-derived cultured mast cells, as reported previously, and significantly suppressed the histamine synthesis and storage. IL-9-modified mast cells (MCs/IL-9) were less sensitive to ATP and the antigen in degranulation. The presence of fibroblasts recovered the histamine synthesis and tryptase expression.

IL-9 was found to induce the expression of *Mcpt1* and *Mcpt2* [13], which was often found during parasite infections and oral allergen-induced anaphylaxis [34,35]. Our findings are consistent with these findings. The gene-targeted mice lacking *Mcpt1* exhibited delayed expulsion of *Trichinella spiralis*, but not of *Nippostrongylus brasiliensis* [36]. Transcriptional induction of *Mcpt1* at the early phase should be required for efficient expulsion of *Trichinella spiralis*. Recently, mucosal mast cells were found to damage the epithelial barrier through release of Mcpt1 upon *Candida albicans* infection [37]. We noticed that tryptic activity was significantly decreased in the presence of SCF and IL-9, whereas this trend was entirely reversed by coculture with fibroblasts. This strict regulation of tryptase activity might reinforce the hypothesis that migration of recruited mast cells should regulate the intestinal epithelial integrity. In the jejunum of mice infected with *Trichinella spiralis*, Mcpt2$^+$ mast cells were accumulated in the mucosal layer at the early phase, with Mcpt2$^+$ and Mcpt6$^+$ mast cells being detected at the recovery phase [35]. Mast cells recruited in the intestinal tissues upon parasite infection were often resident after its complete expulsion and were involved in pathogenic changes of the epithelial integrity. The gene-targeted mice lacking *Mcpt6* exhibited less severe pathology than the wild-type mice in sodium dextran sulfate and trinitrobenzene sulfonic acid (TNBS) induced colitis model [38], indicating that Mcpt6 should be involved in disruption of the epithelial integrity.

A variety of cells were found to be involved in recruiting mast cells through the release of IL-9. CD4$^+$ IL-9 producing T cells (Th9) play critical roles in mast cell accumulation in allergic lung inflammation [39]. In the tolerant allografts, CD4$^+$CD25$^+$Foxp3$^+$ regulatory T cells were found to recruit mast cells through production of IL-9 [40]. Interestingly, the mast cell itself was found to be the source of IL-9, which was augmented by lipopolysaccharide [41–44]. These findings raised a possibility that the number of intestinal mast cells should be drastically increased via the positive feedback loop. CD1d-restricted NKT cells, which are also the source of IL-9, were found to be involved in the recruitment of mast cell progenitors to the lung upon the aerosolized antigen challenge [45]. In this model, IL-9 might be involved in the early step of pulmonary mastocytosis.

We characterized the stimulated mediator release of MCs/IL-9 in comparison with BMMCs. BMMCs were found to be more sensitive to lower concentrations of IgE and the other secretagogues than MCs/IL-9. Kurashima et al. demonstrated that extracellular ATP should play critical roles in the pathology of TNBS-induced colitis model by acting on P_2X_7 purinoreceptors in intestinal mast cells [46]. In our system, ATP induced expression of IL-4 and IL-13 in BMMCs, whereas little or no induction of cytokine genes were observed in MCs/IL-9, raising a possibility that mast-cell-derived inflammatory cytokines should function at a very early stage of inflammation. Intestinal mast cells under the influence of IL-9 may contribute to inflammatory responses mainly through the release of chymases, but not histamine and proinflammatory cytokines.

We here established a novel culture model, which might be useful for investigation of spatiotemporal changes of the newly recruited intestinal mast cells. It should be required to integrate the findings obtained in vitro and in vivo for in-depth understanding of mastocytosis in the intestinal tissues and phenotypic changes of the intestinal mast cells.

4. Materials and Methods

4.1. Materials

The following materials were commercially obtained from the sources indicated: ATP, an anti-dinitrophenyl IgE antibody (clone SPE-7), p-nitrophenyl-β-D-2-acetoamide-2-deoxyglucopyranoside, probenecid and N-succinyl-Ala-Ala-Pro-Phe-pNA from Sigma-Aldrich (St. Louis, MO, USA), fetal bovine serum (FBS) from Thermo Fisher Scientific (Waltham, MA, USA), an anti-trinitrophenyl IgE antibody (clone IgE-3), an FITC-conjugated rat anti-mouse IgE antibody, a phycoerythrin-conjugated rat anti-mouse CD117 antibody and Fc blocker (clone 2.4G2) from BD Biosciences (San Diego, CA, USA), trinitrophenyl bovine serum albumin (TNP-BSA) from LSL (Tokyo, Japan), H-D-Ile-Pro-Arg-pNA (S-2288) from Chromogenix (Milano, Italy), N-(4-methoxyphenylazoformyl)-Phe-OH potassium salt (M-2245) from Bachem AG (Bubendorf, Switzerland), thapsigargin from Merck Millipore (Billerica, MA, USA), Fura-2/AM from Dojindo Laboratories (Kumamoto, Japan), recombinant mouse IL-9 from PeproTech (Rocky Hill, NJ, USA) and recombinant mouse IL-3 from R & D Systems (Minneapolis, MN, USA). Murine SCF was prepared by baculovirus expression system with Sf9 cells according to the procedure described previously [16]. All other chemicals were commercial products of reagent grade.

4.2. Animals

Specific-pathogen-free, 8- to 10-week-old male BALB/c mice were obtained from Japan SLC (Hamamatsu, Japan) and were kept in a specific-pathogen-free animal facility at Okayama University. This study was approved by the Committee on Animal Experiments of Okayama University (approved #OKU2012218 and #OKU2015040).

4.3. Preparation of Bone-Marrow-Derived Cultured Mast Cells

Preparation of IL-3-dependent bone-marrow-derived cultured mast cells (BMMCs) was performed as previously described [47]. Bone marrow cells obtained from male BALB/c mice were cultured in the presence of 10 ng/mL murine recombinant IL-3 for ~30 days. More than 95% of the cells exhibited metachromasy by acidic toluidine blue (pH 3.3) staining and were FcεRI$^+$c-kit$^+$ on the flow cytometry. IL-9-modified mast cells (MCs/IL-9) were prepared by the culture of BMMCs in the presence of 10 ng/mL IL-9 and 30 ng/mL SCF. Subculture was performed every other day for 12 days. In some experiments, BMMCs were cocultured with Swiss 3T3 cells, which were pretreated with mitomycin c as described previously [18], in the presence of 10 ng/mL IL-9 and 30 ng/mL SCF.

4.4. Flowcytometry

The cultured cells were treated with 10 μg/mL Fc blocker (clone 2.4G2) for 10 min at 4 °C and then further incubated with 12.5 μg/mL IgE (clone SPE-7) for 50 min at 4 °C. The surface expression levels of FcεRI and c-kit were measured using FACSCalibur (BD Biosciences, San Diego, CA, USA) with an FITC-conjugated rat anti-mouse IgE antibody and a phycoerythrin-conjugated rat anti-CD117 antibody.

4.5. Measurement of Granule Protease Activities

The enzymatic activities of three kinds of granule proteases, i.e., chymase, tryptase and carboxypeptidase A, were measured using their specific substrates as described previously [18]. The cells were washed in phosphate-buffered saline (PBS), incubated in PBS containing 2 M NaCl and 0.5% Triton X-100 at 4 °C for 30 min and then centrifuged at 12,000× g for 30 min at 4 °C to obtain the supernatant fractions. Chymotryptic activity was measured in 33 mM Tris-HCl, pH 8.3, containing 3.3 mM $CaCl_2$ and 0.3 mM *N*-succinyl-Ala-Ala-Pro-Phe-*p*NA. Tryptic activity was measured in 33 mM Tris-HCl, pH 8.3, containing 2 mM S-2288. Carboxypeptidase A activity was measured in 33 mM Tris-HCl, pH 7.5, containing 0.6 mM M-2245. The enzymatic activity was calculated according to the changes of the values of OD_{405}.

4.6. Measurement of Enzymatic Activity of Histidine Decarboxylase

The cultured cells were homogenized in the lysis buffer (10 mM potassium phosphate, pH 6.8 containing 10 mM KCl, 1.5 mM $MgCl_2$, 1 mM EDTA, 1 mM EGTA, 0.2 mM dithiothreitol, 0.01 mM pyridoxal 5′-phosphate, 0.2 mM phenylmethylsulfonylfluoride, 0.1 mM benzamidine, 10 μg/mL aprotinin, 10 μg/mL leupeptin, 10 μg/mL E-64, 1 μg/mL pepstatin A and 0.1% Triton X-100) and centrifuged at 10,000× g for 30 min at 4 °C. The resultant supernatant was incubated in the assay buffer (0.1 M potassium phosphate, pH 6.8 containing 0.2 mM dithiothreitol, 0.01 mM pyridoxal 5′phosphate, 2% polyethylene glycol #300, 0.2 mM aminoguanidine and 0.8 mM L-histidine) at 37 °C for 4 h. The reaction was stopped by adding perchloric acid (3%). Histamine was fluorometrically measured by HPLC with a cation exchange column, WCX-1 (Shimadzu, Kyoto, Japan), after derivatization with *o*-phthalaldehyde [48].

4.7. Measurement of Degranulation

The cultured cells were suspended in PIPES-buffer (25 mM PIPES-NaOH, pH 7.4 containing 125 mM NaCl, 2.7 mM KCl, 1 mM $CaCl_2$, 5.6 mM glucose and 0.1% bovine serum albumin) and then stimulated with the antigen or ATP for 30 min at 37 °C. They were centrifuged at 800× g at 4 °C for 5 min to obtain the supernatants (extracellular fractions, E). The resultant pellets were resuspended in PIPES-buffer containing 0.5% Triton X-100 and were centrifuged at 10,000× g for 10 min to obtain the supernatants (cell-associated fractions, C). The enzymatic activities of β-hexosaminidase were measured using the specific substrate, *p*-nitrophenyl-β-D-2-acetoamide-2-deoxyglucopyranoside (3.4 mM) in 67 mM citrate, pH 4.5. The amounts of *p*-nitrophenol were determined by measuring the values of OD_{405}. The percentages of degranulation were calculated; E/(C + E) × 100 (%).

4.8. Quantitative RT-PCR

Total RNAs were extracted from the splenocytes using NucleoSpin RNA Kit (TaKaRa Bio Inc., Kusatsu, Japan) and reverse transcribed using PrimeScript™ RT Reagent Kit (TaKaRa Bio Inc.). First strand DNAs were subjected to quantitative PCR using KOD SYBR qPCR Mix (TOYOBO, Osaka, Japan) or SYBR Green PCR Master Mix (Thermo Fisher Scientific) with the specific primer pairs as follows. *Mcpt1*: 5′-GCA CTT CTC TTG CCT TCT GG-3′, 5′-TAA GGA CGG GAG TGT GGT CT-3′;

Mcpt2: 5′-GCA CTT CTT TTG CCT TCT GG-3′, 5′-TAA GGA CGG GAG TGT GGT TT-3′; *Mcpt5*: 5′-AGA ACT ACC TGT CGG C-3′, 5′-GTC GTG GAC AAC CAA AT-3′; *Cpa3*: 5′-GAT GTC TCG TGG GAC T-3′, 5′-GCC GTA GAT GTA ACG GG-3′; *Hdc*: 5′-TGC ACG CCT ACT ATC CTG CTC TTA C-3′, 5′-TCT GTG CAA GCT GGG CTA GAT G-3′; *Ptgr1*: 5′-CAT CGT GAA TCG GTG G-3′; *Il4*: 5′-TCG GCA TTT TGA ACG AGG TC-3′, 5′-GAA AAG CCC GAA AGA GTC TC-3′; *Il5*: 5′- ATG GAG ATT CCC ATG AGC AC-3′, 5′-GTC TCT CCT CGC CAC ACT TC-3′; *IL6*: 5′-TGG AGT CAC AGA AGG AGT GGC TAA G-3′, 5′-TCT GAC CAC AGT GAG GAA TGT CCA C-3′; *Il13*: 5′- CAG CTC CCT GGT TCT CTC AC-3′, 5′-CCA CAC TCC ATA CCA TGC TG-3′; *Tnf*: 5′-AAG CCT GTA GCC CAC GTC GTA-3′, 5′-GGC ACC ACT AGT TGG TTG TCT TTG-3′; *P2rx1*: 5′-CCA GGA CTT CCG AAG CCT TGC-3′, 5′-AGA ACT GTG GCC ACT CCA AAG ATG-3′; *P2rx3*: 5′-TCT TGC ACG AGA AGG CCT ACC AA-3′, 5′-GAT CTC ACA GGT CCG ACG GAC A-3′; *P2rx4*: 5′-GTG ACG TCA TAG TCC TCT ACT GT-3′, 5′-TGC TCG TAG TCT TCC ACA TAC TT-3′; *P2rx7*: 5′-AGC CTG TTA TCA GCT CCG TGC A-3′, 5′-TCA GGA CAC AGC GTC TGC ACT T-3′; *Gapdh*: 5′-TGT GTC CGT CGT GGA TCT GA-3′, 5′-TTG CTG TTG AAG TCG CAG GAG-3′.

4.9. Statistics

Statistical significance between two independent groups was determined by unpaired Student's *t*-test. Statistical significance among multiple groups was determined using one-way ANOVA. Post-tests were performed with the Dunnett multiple comparison test for comparison with the control groups or the Tukey–Kramer multiple comparison test for all pairs of column comparison.

Author Contributions: Conceptualization, K.F. and S.T.; investigation, A.K., T.K. and S.Y.; writing—original draft preparation, A.K., T.K., S.T.; writing—review and editing, K.F. and S.T.; project administration, S.T.; funding acquisition, S.T. All authors have read and agreed to the published version of the manuscript.

Funding: This research was funded by grants from the JSPS KAKENHI Grant Number 23590077 and 16K08231.

Conflicts of Interest: The authors declare no conflict of interest.

Abbreviations

ANOVA	Analysis of variance
BMMC	IL-3-dependent bone-marrow-derived cultured mast cell
FBS	Fetal bovine serum
MC/IL-9	IL-9-modified mast cell
PCR	Polymerase chain reaction
SCF	Stem cell factor (c-kit ligand)

References

1. Kitamura, Y. Heterogeneity of mast cells and phenotypic changes between subpopulations. *Annu. Rev. Immunol.* **1989**, *7*, 59–76. [CrossRef] [PubMed]
2. Galli, S.J.; Borregaard, N.; Wynn, T.A. Phenotypic and functional plasticity of cells of innate immunity: Macrophages, mast cells and neutrophils. *Nat. Immunol.* **2011**, *12*, 1035–1044. [CrossRef] [PubMed]
3. Galli, S.J.; Grimbaldeston, M.; Tsai, M. Immunomodulatory mast cells: negative, as well as positive, regulators of immunity. *Nat. Rev. Immunol.* **2008**, *8*, 478–486. [CrossRef] [PubMed]
4. Woodbury, R.G.; Miller, H.R.; Huntley, J.F.; Newlands, G.F.; Palliser, A.C.; Wakelin, D. Mucosal mast cells are functionally active during spontaneous expulsion of intestinal nematode infections in rat. *Nature* **1984**, *312*, 450–452. [CrossRef] [PubMed]
5. Bischoff, S.C. Role of mast cells in allergic and non-allergic immune responses: comparison of human and murine data. *Nat. Rev. Immunol.* **2007**, *7*, 93–104. [CrossRef]
6. Albert-Bayo, M.; Paracuellos, I.; González-Castro, A.M.; Rodriguez-Urrutia, A.; Rodríguez-Lagunas, M.J.; Alonso-Cotoner, C.; Santos, J.; Vicario, M. Intestinal mucosal mast cells: key modulators of barrier function and homeostasis. *Cells* **2019**, *8*, E135. [CrossRef]

7. Hültner, L.; Druez, C.; Moeller, J.; Uyttenhove, C.; Schmitt, E.; Rüde, E.; Dörmer, P.; van Snick, J. Mast cell growth-enhancing activity (MEA) is structurally related and functionally identical to the novel mouse T cell growth factor P40/TCGFIII (interleukin 9). *Eur. J. Immunol.* **1990**, *20*, 1413–1416. [CrossRef]
8. Faulkner, H.; Humphreys, N.; Renauld, J.C.; Van Snick, J.; Grencis, R. Interleukin-9 is involved in host protective immunity to intestinal nematode infection. *Eur. J. Immunol.* **1997**, *27*, 2536–2540. [CrossRef]
9. Godfrained, C.; Louahed, J.; Faulkner, H.; Vink, A.; Warnier, G.; Grencis, R.; Renauld, J.C. Intraepithelial infiltration by mast cells with both connective tissue-type and mucosal-type characteristics in gut, trachea, and kidneys of IL-9 transgenic mice. *J. Immunol.* **1998**, *160*, 3989–3996.
10. Faulkner, H.; Renauld, J.C.; Van Snick, J.; Grencis, R.K. Interleukin-9 enhances resistance to the intestinal nematode Trichuris muris. *Infect. Immun.* **1998**, *66*, 3832–3840.
11. Townsend, J.M.; Fallon, G.P.; Matthews, J.D.; Smith, P.; Jolin, E.H.; McKenzie, N.A. IL-9-deficient mice establish fundamental roles for IL-9 in pulmonary mastocytosis and goblet cell hyperplasia but not T cell development. *Immunity* **2000**, *13*, 573–583. [CrossRef]
12. Osterfeld, H.; Ahrens, R.; Strait, R.; Finkelman, F.D.; Renauld, J.C.; Hogan, S.P. Differential roles for the IL-9/IL-9 receptor a-chain pathway in systemic and oral antigen–induced anaphylaxis. *J. Allergy Clin. Immunol.* **2010**, *125*, 469–476. [CrossRef] [PubMed]
13. Eklund, K.K.; Ghildyal, F.; Austen, K.F.; Stevens, R.L. Induction by IL-9 and suppression by IL-3 and IL-4 of the levels of chromosome 14-derived transcripts that encode late-expressed mouse mast cell proteases. *J. Immunol.* **1993**, *151*, 4266–4273. [PubMed]
14. Nakahata, T.; Kobayashi, T.; Ishuguro, A.; Tsuji, K.; Naganuma, K.; Ando, O.; Yagi, Y.; Tadokoro, K.; Akabane, T. Extensive proliferation of mature connective-tissue type mast cells in vitro. *Nature* **1986**, *324*, 65–67. [CrossRef] [PubMed]
15. Lantz, C.S.; Boesiger, J.; Song, C.H.; Mach, N.; Kobayashi, T.; Mulligan, R.C.; Nawa, Y.; Dranoff, G.; Galli, S.J. Role for interleukin-3 in mast cell and basophil development and in immunity to parasites. *Nature* **1998**, *392*, 90–93. [CrossRef]
16. Scudamore, C.L.; McMillan, L.; Thornton, E.M.; Wright, S.H.; Newlands, G.F.J.; Miller, H.R.P. Mast cell heterogeneity in the gastrointestinal tract: variable expression of mouse mast cell protease-1 (mMCP-1) in intraepithelial mucosal mast cells in nematode-infected and normal BALB/c mice. *Am. J. Pathol.* **1997**, *150*, 1661–1672.
17. Reber, L.L.; Marichal, T.; Galli, S.J. New models for analyzing mast cell functions in vivo. *Trends Immunol.* **2012**, *33*, 613–625. [CrossRef]
18. Takano, H.; Nakazawa, S.; Okuno, Y.; Shirata, N.; Tsuchiya, S.; Kainoh, T.; Takamatsu, S.; Furuta, K.; Taketomi, Y.; Naito, Y.; et al. Establishment of the culture model system that reflects the process of terminal differentiation of connective tissue-type mast cells. *FEBS Lett.* **2008**, *582*, 1444–1450. [CrossRef]
19. Yamada, K.; Sato, H.; Sakamaki, K.; Kamada, M.; Okuno, Y.; Fukuishi, N.; Furuta, K.; Tanaka, S. Suppression of IgE-independent degranulation of murine connective tissue-type mast cells by dexamethasone. *Cells* **2019**, *8*, 112. [CrossRef]
20. Tsuchiya, S.; Tachida, Y.; Segi-Nishida, E.; Okuno, Y.; Tamba, S.; Tsujimoto, G.; Tanaka, S.; Sugimoto, Y. Characterization of gene expression profiles for different types of mast cells pooled from mouse stomach subregions by an RNA amplification method. *BMC Genom.* **2009**, *10*, 35. [CrossRef]
21. Gao, Z.G.; Jacobson, K.A. Purinergic signaling in mast cell degranulation and asthma. *Front. Pharmacol.* **2017**, *8*, 947. [CrossRef] [PubMed]
22. Yoshida, K.; Ito, M.; Hoshino, Y.; Matsuoka, I. Effects of dexamethasone on purinergic signaling in murine mast cells: Selective suppression of P2X7 receptor expression. *Biochem. Biophys. Res. Commun.* **2017**, *493*, 1587–1593. [CrossRef] [PubMed]
23. Gordon, J.R.; Galli, S.J. Release of both preformed and newly synthesized tumor necrosis factor alpha (TNF-alpha)/cachectin by mouse mast cells stimulated via the Fc epsilon RI. A mechanism for the sustained action of mast cell-derived TNF-alpha during IgE-dependent biological responses. *J. Exp. Med.* **1991**, *174*, 103–107. [CrossRef] [PubMed]
24. Andoh, A.; Deguchi, Y.; Inatomi, O.; Yagi, Y.; Bamba, S.; Tsujikawa, T.; Fujiyama, Y. Immunohistochemical study of chymase-positive mast cells in inflammatory bowel disease. *Oncol. Rep.* **2006**, *16*, 103–107. [CrossRef]

25. Han, W.; Lu, X.; Jia, X.; Zhou, T.; Guo, C. Soluble mediators released from PI-IBS patients' colon induced alteration of mast cells: involvement of reactive oxygen species. *Dig. Dis. Sci.* **2012**, *57*, 311–319. [CrossRef]
26. De Winter, B.Y.; van den Wijngaard, R.M.; de Jonge, W.J. Intestinal mast cells in gut inflammation and motility disturbances. *Biochim. Biophys. Acta* **2012**, *1822*, 66–73. [CrossRef]
27. Wouters, M.M.; Vicario, M.; Santos, J. The role of mast cells in functional GI disorders. *Gut* **2016**, *65*, 155–168. [CrossRef]
28. Bischoff, S.C. Mast cells in gastrointestinal disorders. *Eur. J. Pharmacol.* **2016**, *778*, 139–145. [CrossRef]
29. Tsai, M.; Takeishi, T.; Thompson, H.; Langley, K.E.; Zsebo, K.M.; Metcalfe, D.D.; Geissler, E.N.; Galli, S.J. Induction of mast cell proliferation, maturation, and heparin synthesis by the rat c-kit ligand, stem cell factor. *Proc. Natl. Acad. Sci. USA* **1991**, *88*, 6382–6386. [CrossRef]
30. Mortillaro, N.A.; Granger, D.N.; Kvietys, P.R.; Rutill, G.; Taylor, A.E. Effects of histamine and histamine antagonists on intestinal capillary permeability. *Am. J. Physiol.* **1981**, *240*, G381–G386. [CrossRef]
31. Keely, S.J.; Stack, W.A.; O'Donoghue, D.P.; Baird, A.W. Regulation of ion transport by histamine in human colon. *Eur. J. Pharmacol.* **1995**, *279*, 203–209. [CrossRef]
32. Wechsler, J.B.; Szabo, A.; Hsu, C.L.; Krier-Burris, R.A.; Schroeder, H.A.; Wang, M.Y.; Carter, R.G.; Velez, T.E.; Aguiniga, L.M.; Brown, J.B.; et al. Histamine drives severity of innate inflammation via histamine 4 receptor in murine experimental colitis. *Mucosal Immunol.* **2018**, *11*, 861–870. [CrossRef] [PubMed]
33. Forward, N.A.; Furlong, S.J.; Yang, Y.; Lin, T.J.; Hoskin, D.W. Mast cells down-regulate CD4$^+$CD25$^+$ T regulatory cell suppressor function via histamine H_1 receptor interaction. *J. Immunol.* **2009**, *183*, 3014–3022. [CrossRef] [PubMed]
34. Forbes, E.E.; Groschwitz, K.; Abonia, J.P.; Brandt, E.B.; Cohen, E.; Blanchard, C.; Ahrens, R.; Seidu, L.; McKenzie, A.; Strait, R.; et al. IL-9- and mast cell-mediated intestinal permeability predisposes to oral antigen hypersensitivity. *J. Exp. Med.* **2008**, *205*, 897–913. [CrossRef] [PubMed]
35. Friend, D.S.; Ghildyal, N.; Gurish, M.F.; Hunt, J.; Hu, X.; Austen, K.F.; Stevens, R.L. Reversible expression of tryptases and chymases in the jejunum mast cells of mice infected with Trichinella spiralis. *J. Immunol.* **1998**, *160*, 5537–5545.
36. Knight, P.A.; Wright, S.H.; Lawrence, C.E.; Paterson, Y.Y.W.; Miller, H.R.P. Delayed expulsion of the Nematode *Trichinella spiralis* in mice lacking the mucosal mast cell-specific granule chymase, mouse mast cell protease-1. *J. Exp. Med.* **2000**, *192*, 1849–1856. [CrossRef]
37. Renga, G.; Moretti, S.; Oikonomou, V.; Borghi, M.; Zelente, T.; Paolicelli, G.; Costantini, C.; De Zuani, M.; Villella, V.R.; Raia, V.; et al. IL-9 and mast cells are key players of Candida albicans commensalism and pathogenesis in the gut. *Cell Rep.* **2018**, *23*, 1767–1778. [CrossRef]
38. Hamilton, M.J.; Sinnamon, M.J.; Lyng, G.D.; Glickman, J.N.; Wang, X.; Xing, W.; Krilis, S.A.; Blumberg, R.S.; Adachi, R.; Lee, D.M.; et al. Essential role for mast cell tryptase in acute experimental colitis. *Proc. Natl. Acad. Sci. USA* **2011**, *108*, 290–295. [CrossRef]
39. Sehra, S.; Yao, W.; Nguyen, E.T.; Glosson-Byers, N.L.; Akhtar, N.; Zhou, B.; Kaplan, M.H. TH9 cells are required for tissue mast cell accumulation during allergic inflammation. *J. Allergy Clin. Immunol.* **2015**, *136*, 433–440. [CrossRef]
40. Lu, L.F.; Lind, E.F.; Gondek, D.C.; Bennett, K.A.; Gleeson, M.W.; Pino-Lagos, K.; Scott, Z.A.; Coyle, A.J.; Reed, J.L.; Van Snick, J.; et al. Mast cells are essentials intermediaries in regulatory T-cell tolerance. *Nature* **2006**, *442*, 997–1002. [CrossRef]
41. Hültner, L.; Kölsch, S.; Stassen, M.; Kaspers, U.; Kremer, J.P.; Mailhammer, R.; Moeller, J.; Broszeit, H.; Schmitt, E. In activated mast cells, IL-1 up-regulates the production of several Th2-related cytokines including IL-9. *J. Immunol.* **2000**, *164*, 5556–5563. [CrossRef] [PubMed]
42. Stassen, M.; Arnold, M.; Hültner, L.; Müller, C.; Neudörfl, C.; Reineke, T.; Schmitt, E. Murine bone marrow-derived mast cells as potent producers of IL-9: Costimulatory function of IL-10 and kit ligand in the presence of IL-1. *J. Immunol.* **2000**, *164*, 5549–5555. [CrossRef] [PubMed]
43. Stassen, M.; Müller, C.; Arnold, M.; Hültner, L.; Klein-Hessling, S.; Neudörfl, C.; Reineke, T.; Serfling, E.; Schmitt, E. IL-9 and IL-13 production by activated mast cells is strongly enhanced in the presence of lipopolysaccharide: NF-kappa B is decisively involved in the expression of IL-9. *J. Immunol.* **2001**, *166*, 4391–4398. [CrossRef] [PubMed]

44. Chen, C.Y.; Lee, J.B.; Liu, B.; Ohta, S.; Wang, P.Y.; Kartashov, A.V.; Mugge, L.; Abonia, J.P.; Barski, A.; Izuhara, K.; et al. Induction of interleukin-9-producing mucosal mast cells promotes susceptibility to IgE-mediated experimental food allergy. *Immunity* **2015**, *43*, 788–802. [CrossRef]
45. Jones, T.G.; Hallgren, J.; Humbles, A.; Burwell, T.; Finkelman, F.D.; Alcaide, P.; Austen, K.F.; Gurish, M.F. Antigen-induced increases in pulmonary mast cell progenitor numbers depend on IL-9 and CD1d-restircted NKT cells. *J. Immunol.* **2009**, *183*, 5251–5260. [CrossRef]
46. Kurashima, Y.; Amiya, T.; Nohi, T.; Fujisawa, K.; Haraguchi, T.; Iba, H.; Tsutsui, H.; Sato, S.; Nakajima, S.; Iijima, H.; et al. Extracelluar ATP mediates mast cell-dependent intestinal inflammation through P_2X_7 purinoreceptors. *Nat. Cummun.* **2012**, *3*, 1034. [CrossRef]
47. Tanaka, S.; Takasu, Y.; Mikura, S.; Satoh, N.; Ichikawa, A. Antigen-independent induction of histamine synthesis by immunoglobulin E in mouse bone marrow-derived mast cells. *J. Exp. Med.* **2002**, *196*, 229–235. [CrossRef]
48. Yamatodani, A.; Fukuda, H.; Wada, H.; Iwaeda, T.; Watanabe, T. High-performance liquid chromatographic determination of plasma and brain histamine without previous purification of biological samples: Cation-exchange chromatography coupled with post-column derivatization fluorometry. *J. Chrmatogr.* **1985**, *344*, 115–123. [CrossRef]

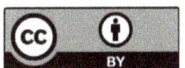

© 2019 by the authors. Licensee MDPI, Basel, Switzerland. This article is an open access article distributed under the terms and conditions of the Creative Commons Attribution (CC BY) license (http://creativecommons.org/licenses/by/4.0/).

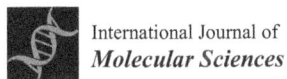

Communication

Clinical Significance of Cytoplasmic IgE-Positive Mast Cells in Eosinophilic Chronic Rhinosinusitis

Yuka Gion [1,2], Mitsuhiro Okano [3,4,*], Takahisa Koyama [3], Tokie Oura [1], Asami Nishikori [1], Yorihisa Orita [5], Tomoyasu Tachibana [6], Hidenori Marunaka [3], Takuma Makino [3], Kazunori Nishizaki [3] and Yasuharu Sato [1,2,*]

[1] Division of Pathophysiology, Okayama University Graduate School of Health Sciences, Okayama 700-8558, Japan; gion@okayama-u.ac.jp (Y.G.); pe0r79kv@s.okayama-u.ac.jp (T.O.); asami.kei@s.okayama-u.ac.jp (A.N.)
[2] Department of Pathology, Okayama University Graduate School of Medicine, Dentistry and Pharmaceutical Sciences, Okayama 700-8558, Japan
[3] Department of Otolaryngology of Head and Neck Surgery, Okayama University Graduate School of Medicine, Dentistry and Pharmaceutical Sciences, Okayama 700-8558, Japan.; koyatakaco@gmail.com (T.K.); marunaka@okayama-u.ac.jp (H.M.); takmak0617@yahoo.co.jp (T.M.); nishizak@cc.okayama-u.ac.jp (K.N.)
[4] Department of Otorhinolaryngology, International University of Health and Welfare Graduate School of Medicine, Narita 286-8686, Japan
[5] Department of Otolaryngology, Head and Neck Surgery, Kumamoto University Graduate School, Kumamoto 860-8556, Japan; y.orita@live.jp
[6] Department of Otolaryngology, Japanese Red Cross Society Himeji Hospital, Himeji 670-8540, Japan; tomoyasutachibana@hotmail.co.jp
* Correspondence: mokano@iuhw.ac.jp (M.O.); sato-y@okayama-u.ac.jp (Y.S.); Tel.: +81-86-235-7150 (Y.S.); Fax: +81-86-235-7156 (Y.S.)

Received: 16 January 2020; Accepted: 5 March 2020; Published: 7 March 2020

Abstract: Cross-linking of antigen-specific IgE bound to the high-affinity IgE receptor (FcεRI) on the surface of mast cells with multivalent antigens results in the release of mediators and development of type 2 inflammation. FcεRI expression and IgE synthesis are, therefore, critical for type 2 inflammatory disease development. In an attempt to clarify the relationship between eosinophilic chronic rhinosinusitis (ECRS) and mast cell infiltration, we analyzed mast cell infiltration at lesion sites and determined its clinical significance. Mast cells are positive for c-kit, and IgE in uncinated tissues (UT) and nasal polyps (NP) were examined by immunohistochemistry. The number of positive cells and clinicopathological factors were analyzed. Patients with ECRS exhibited high levels of total IgE serum levels and elevated peripheral blood eosinophil ratios. As a result, the number of mast cells with membranes positive for c-kit and IgE increased significantly in lesions forming NP. Therefore, we classified IgE-positive mast cells into two groups: membrane IgE-positive cells and cytoplasmic IgE-positive cells. The amount of membrane IgE-positive mast cells was significantly increased in moderate ECRS. A positive correlation was found between the membrane IgE-positive cells and the radiological severity score, the ratio of eosinophils, and the total serum IgE level. The number of cytoplasmic IgE-positive mast cells was significantly increased in moderate and severe ECRS. A positive correlation was observed between the cytoplasmic IgE-positive cells and the radiological severity score, the ratio of eosinophils in the blood, and the total IgE level. These results suggest that the process of mast cell internalization of antigens via the IgE receptor is involved in ECRS pathogenesis.

Keywords: mast cell; eosinophilic chronic rhinosinusitis; c-kit; IgE

1. Introduction

Chronic rhinosinusitis (CRS) is a condition characterized by chronic mucosal inflammation in paranasal sinuses for more than 12 weeks, which ultimately causes nasal obstruction, rhinorrhea, and posterior nasal discharge. CRS is a disease with various etiologies and pathologies and is often accompanied by headaches and olfactory disorders. One type of CRS is refractory eosinophilic chronic rhinosinusitis (ECRS). Many patients with non-ECRS are cured by antibiotic administration or surgery. However, ECRS forms multiple nasal polyps (NP) in a bilateral nature and tends to relapse even after surgery [1,2]. This disease is relieved by steroid administration, and steroid therapy is considered to be the most effective treatment [3,4]. ECRS lesions are characterized by an infiltration of numerous eosinophils. Furthermore, in these patients, increases in peripheral blood allergic factors are observed, including an increase in eosinophils and IgE. Additionally, this disease frequently occurs in patients with aspirin intolerance, in which aspirin causes asthma [5].

Mast cells have a wide variety of functional molecules expressed on their surface, which facilitate cell activation via chemical mediators that synthesize and secrete various cytokines during allergic or innate immune responses, both of which are heavily influenced by the involvement of the acquired immune system [6–8]. Mast cells have also been shown to interact with immune cells, such as T-cells, B-cells, and dendritic cells, and to participate in transplant rejection and tumor immunity [9,10] while also assisting in protection against viral and bacterial infection via Toll-like receptors (TLRs) [11,12]. Regarding allergies, it has been confirmed that mast cells interact with B-cells in the nasal mucosa and bronchial mucosa at the time of allergic inflammation leading to the promotion of local IgE production, suggesting the existence of an allergic exacerbation cycle [13]. Further, mast cells activated by local inflammation express CD40L (CD154) and produce Th2 cytokines such as interleukin (IL)-4 and IL-13. It has also been shown that IgE production is induced by co-culturing nasal mucosal mast cells from allergic rhinitis patients with B-cells in vitro [13]. This IgE produced in inflamed regions serves to enhance high-affinity IgE receptor (FcεRI) expression on the surface of mast cells and markedly increases sensitivity to this antigen [14]. Thus, it seems that the allergic exacerbation cycle, responsible for further promoting the inflammatory response, will be initiated in the local area of allergic inflammation. Herein, we focused on the fact that many patients with ECRS had a predisposition to allergies, and thus, the current study sought to investigate mast cell expression and its clinical significance in ECRS lesions.

2. Results

2.1. Patients' Characteristics

Clinical features are shown in Table 1. Prior to surgery, each CRS patient was examined for serum levels of IgE, eosinophil ratio, and 1-s forced expiratory volume/forced vital capacity (FEV_1/FVC) ratio. Serum IgE levels were found to be high in severe cases of ECRS (median; 476.2 IU/mL, $n = 10$), while moderate and severe ECRS cases showed an increased eosinophil count in the peripheral blood. Specifically, the mean blood eosinophil ratio was 5.6% for moderate ECRS and 10.8% for severe ECRS. Further, the mean cognitive threshold in the baseline olfactory examination was particularly high in patients with ECRS. Among 71 CRS patients, 57 patients exhibited nasal polyps (CRSwNP), with the remainder exhibiting no visible NP in the middle meatus (CRSsNP; $n = 14$). Samples were divided into six groups according to the CRS phenotype: uncinated process tissues (UT) from non-CRS ($n = 13$), UT from CRSsNP ($n = 14$), NP from non-ECRS ($n = 27$), NP from mild ECRS ($n = 8$), NP from moderate ECRS ($n = 12$), and NP from severe ECRS ($n = 10$) (Figure 1).

Table 1. Subjects' characteristics.

Groups	Non-CRS (UT)	CRSsNP (UT)	Non-ECRS (NP)	Mild ECRS (NP)	Moderate ECRS (NP)	Severe ECRS (NP)
Number	13	14	27	8	12	10
Age (years old)	61.4 (41–92)	60.5 (35–75)	57.6 (36–84)	56.8 (34–70)	52.5 (32–78)	49.5 (33–74)
Sex (female/male)	9/4	6/8	8/19	2/6	5/7	3/7
Blood eosinophil rate (%)	2.1 (0–5.9)	2.5 (0.8–8.6)	3.2 (0.1–7.3)	3.8 (2.6–4.7)	5.6 (1.7–7.9)	10.8 (4.6–22.8)
Serum total IgE (IU/mL)	34.5 (2–99)	141.7 (4–923)	164.6 (4–1322)	150.4 (10–452)	256.4 (34–1768)	476.2 (34–1899)
FEV1/FVC ratio (%)	83.8 (68.7–92.7)	77.3 (66.5–84.7)	78.3 (47.2–91.9)	76.3 (73.2–86.4)	76.0 (49.2–92.3)	72.8 (52.6–89.5)
CT grading score (Lund–Mackay)	1.9 (1–3)	6.5 (1–14)	13.4 (3–24)	14.3 (8–22)	13.4 (7–21)	16.6 (10–24)
Comorbidity of asthma (n)	0	0	5	0	5	10
Comorbidity of NSAIDs intolerance (n)	0	0	2	0	1	3

CRS, chronic rhinosinusitis; ECRS, eosinophilic chronic rhinosinusitis; CRSsNP, chronic rhinosinusitis without nasal polyps; UT, uncinated tissues; NP, nasal polyps; FEV1/FVC ratio, 1-s forced expiratory volume/forced vital capacity ratio; NSAIDs, nonsteroidal anti-inflammatory drugs.

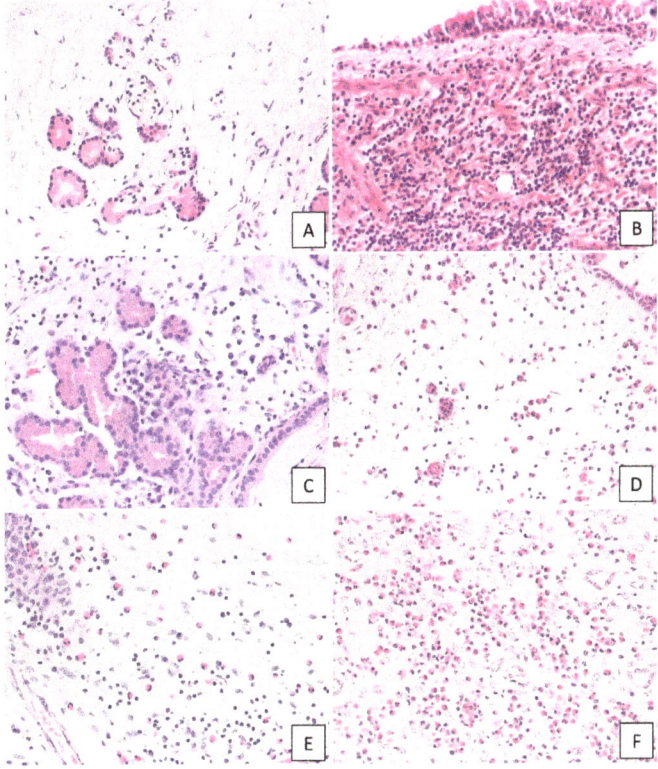

Figure 1. Histological findings of non-chronic rhinosinusitis (CRS), CRS, and eosinophilic chronic rhinosinusitis (ECRS). Hematoxylin and eosin staining at 400× magnification (high-powered field, HPF). (**A**) non-CRS, (**B**) CRS with no visible NP in the middle meatus (CRSsNP), (**C**) non-ECRS, (**D**) mild ECRS, (**E**) moderate ECRS, and (F) severe ECRS. In ECRS, infiltration of eosinophils under the mucosa was observed.

2.2. Histological Evaluation and Pathophysiological Significance of c-Kit-Positive Cells

The c-kit-positive mast cells were observed in each group (Figure 2), with the number of c-kit-positive cells in UT and NP ranging from 0–18 (median: 5.3 cells/HPF) and from 2–36 (median: 9.6 cells/HPF), respectively, per high-power field (HPF). The number of c-kit-positive cells was significantly higher in NP than in UT ($p < 0.001$; Figure 3A), which was then compared between the six study groups. No significant differences were observed between the UT from the non-CRS group and the CRSsNP group; however, the c-kit-positive cells were significantly increased in the groups forming NP as compared to CRSsNP. The Kruskal–Wallis test revealed a significant difference in the number of infiltrating c-kit-positive cells among these groups ($p < 0.0001$). However, no significant difference was observed between non-ECRS and each ECRS group. In addition, the severity of ECRS and the number of c-kit-positive cells were not directly related.

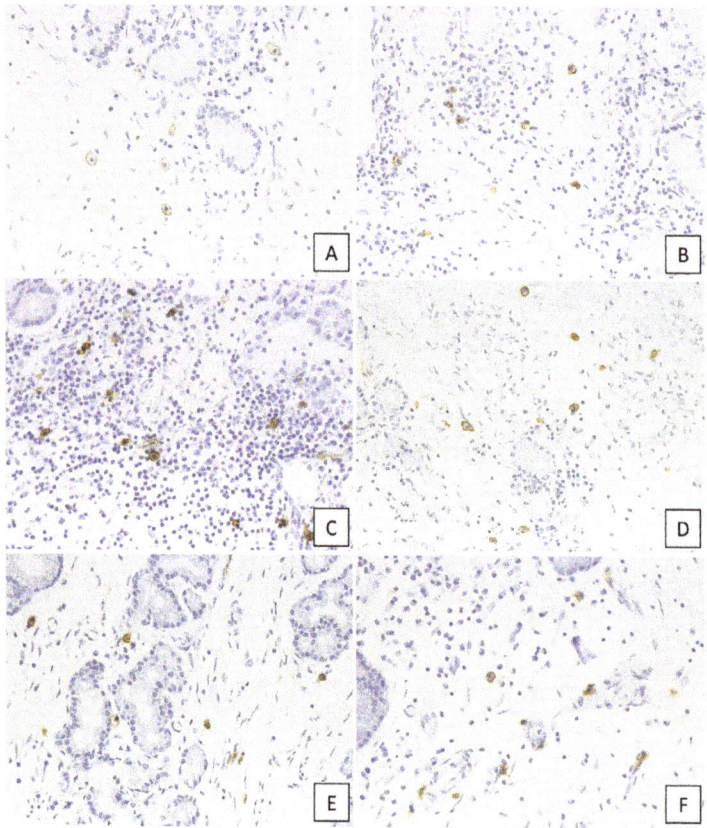

Figure 2. Immunohistochemical staining of c-kit in the diseased tissue. (**A**) non-CRS, (**B**) CRSsNP, (**C**) non-ECRS, (**D**) mild ECRS, (**E**) moderate ECRS, and (**F**) severe ECRS. The surface membrane of mast cells was positive for c-kit (400× magnification).

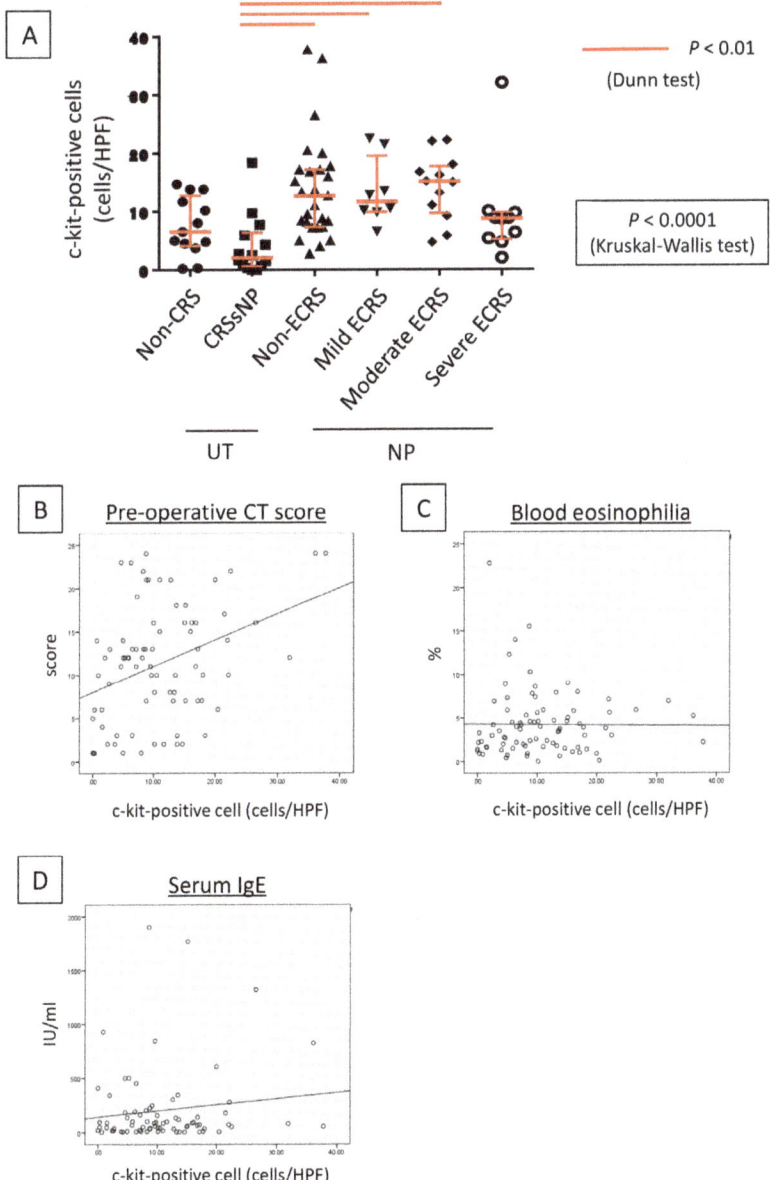

Figure 3. Lesion infiltration by c-kit-positive cells and the number of c-kit-positive cells. (**A**) Examination of the number of c-kit positive cells in the hotspot of each case. The number of c-kit-positive cells increased in the nasal polyp groups ($p < 0.0001$, Kruskal–Wallis test). Relationship between the number of c-kit positive cells and the preoperative CT score (**B**), eosinophil ratio in peripheral blood (**C**), and total serum IgE level (**D**).

Next, we pathophysiologically characterized the degree of c-kit-positive cell infiltration in sinonasal tissues. A significant positive correlation was found between the number of infiltrating c-kit-positive cells and the radiological severity of CRS ($r = 0.309$, $p = 0.006$; Figure 3B). Conversely, no correlation was observed between the number of infiltrating c-kit-positive cells and peripheral blood eosinophilia (r = 0.123, p = 0.265; Figure 3C) or total serum IgE level (r = 0.043, p = 0.710; Figure 3D).

2.3. Histological Evaluation and Pathophysiological Significance of IgE-Positive Cells

IgE-positive mast cells were observed in each group (Figure 4) and classified into two types: mast cells that showed IgE-positive only in the membrane were termed "membrane IgE-positive mast cells", while mast cells with IgE positivity in the cytoplasm were designated "cytoplasmic IgE-positive mast cells". The number of each cell type was enumerated.

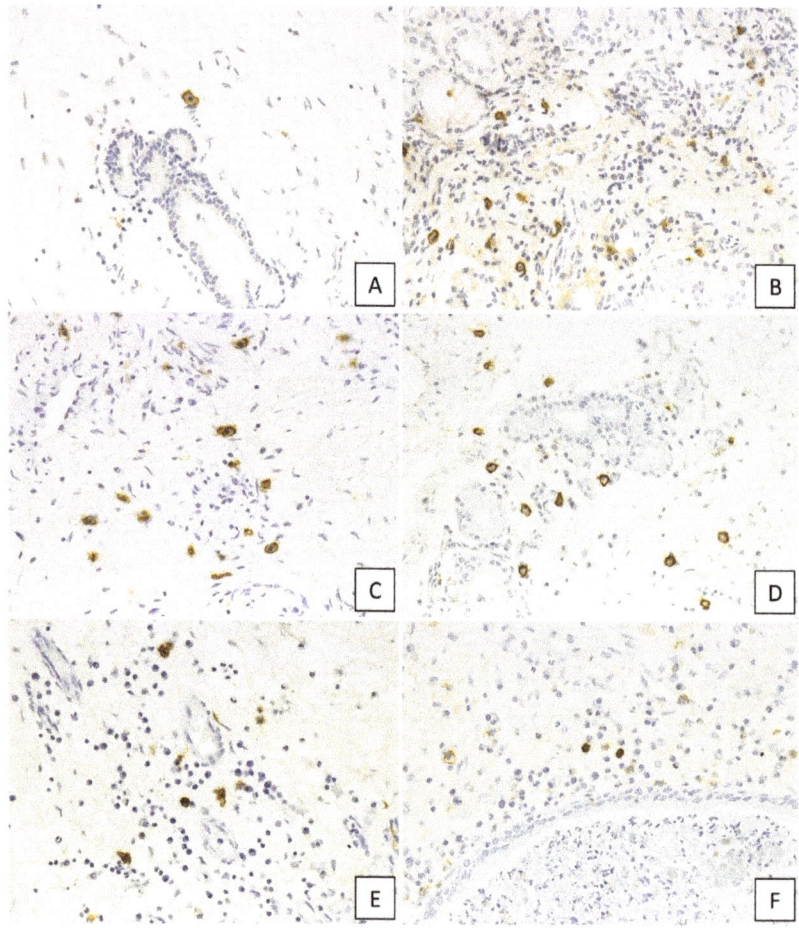

Figure 4. Immunohistochemical findings of IgE in the diseased tissue. (**A**) non-CRS, (**B**) CRSsNP, (**C**) non-ECRS, (**D**) mild ECRS, (**E**) moderate ECRS, and (**F**) severe ECRS. IgE-positive cells increased in the diseased tissue (400× magnification).

A higher number of membrane IgE-positive mast cells was observed in cases with NP compared to those without, with the numbers of membrane IgE-positive mast cells in the UT and NP ranging from 0–16 (median: 5.2 cells/HPF) and from 0–27 (median: 9.5 cells/HPF), respectively, per HPF. The Kruskal–Wallis test further demonstrated that, although the number was not different between UT from non-CRS and UT from CRSsNP, membrane IgE-positive mast cells increased in NP-forming groups. In addition, moderate ECRS showed a statistically significant increase compared to non-CRS and CRSsNP (UT from non-CRS: $p < 0.05$; UT from non-ECRS: $p < 0.05$) (Figure 5A). However, no significant difference was observed between non-ECRS and ECRS. Furthermore, comparing the clinical data with membrane IgE-positive cells revealed that the number of membrane IgE-positive mast cells was also positively correlated with radiological severity of CRS ($r = 0.470$, $p < 0.001$; Figure 5B), peripheral blood eosinophilia ($r = 0.327$, $p = 0.002$; Figure 5C), and the total serum IgE level ($r = 0.458$, $p < 0.001$; Figure 5D).

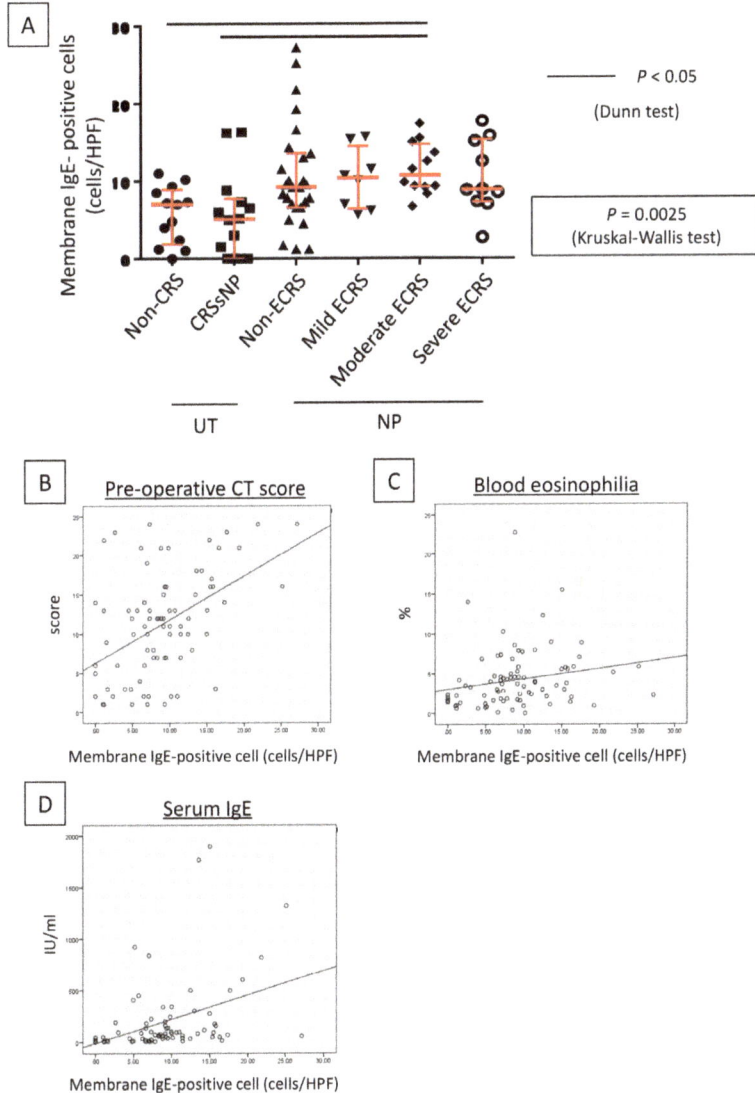

Figure 5. Lesion infiltration by membrane IgE-positive cells and the number of IgE-positive cells. (**A**) Determination of membrane IgE-positive cell number in the hotspot of each case. The number of membrane IgE-positive cells increased in the nasal polyp groups ($p < 0.0025$, Kruskal–Wallis test). Relationships between the number of membrane IgE-positive cells and the preoperative CT score (**B**), eosinophil ratio in peripheral blood (**C**), and total serum IgE level (**D**).

Furthermore, cytoplasmic IgE-positive mast cells were found in lesions of moderate and severe ECRS (Figure 6A–F). The number of these cells was statistically higher in moderate and severe ECRS than in the other groups ($p < 0.05$ and $p < 0.01$, respectively; Figure 6G). The number of cytoplasmic IgE-positive mast cells was also significantly correlated to radiological severity of CRS ($r = 0.280$, $p = 0.012$; Figure 6H), peripheral blood eosinophilia ($r = 0.404$, $p < 0.001$; Figure 6I), and total serum IgE ($r = 0.500$, $p < 0.001$; Figure 6J).

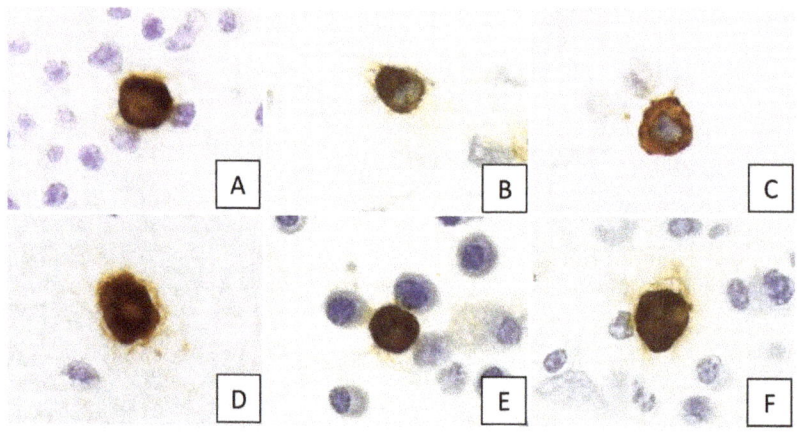

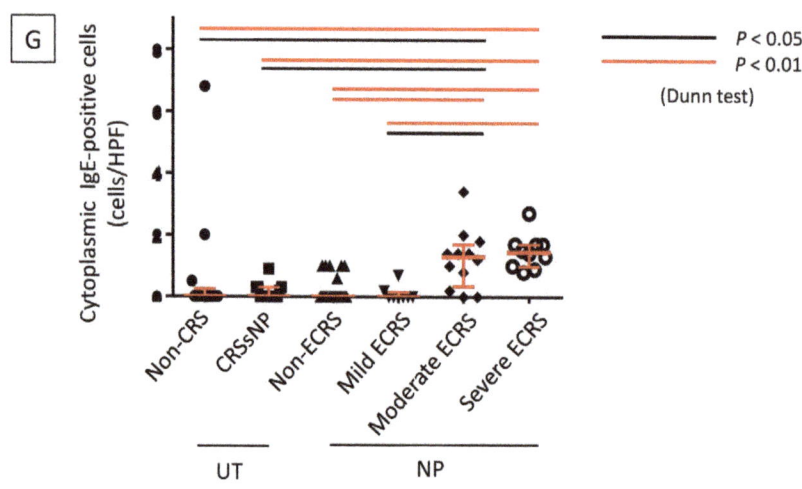

Figure 6. *Cont.*

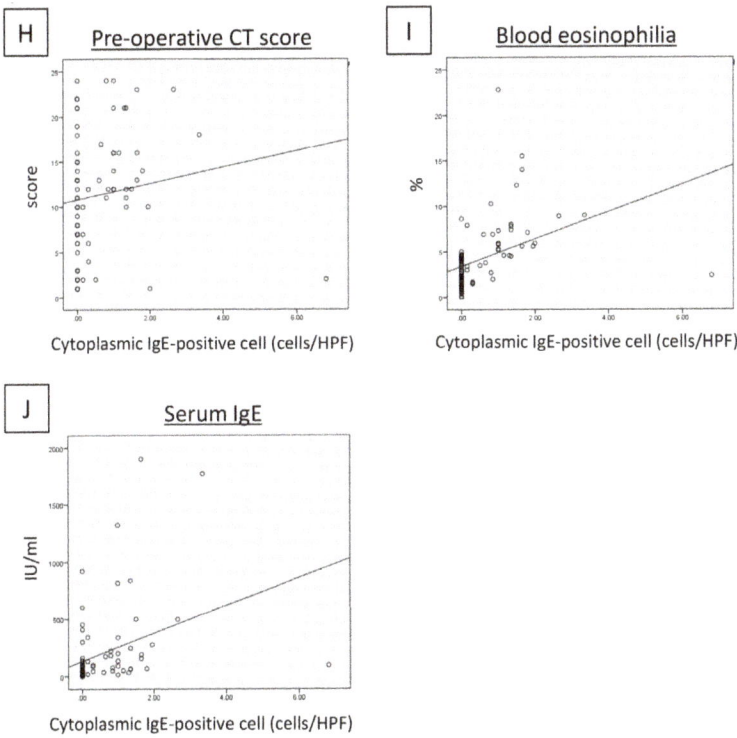

Figure 6. Lesion infiltration by cytoplasmic IgE-positive cells in each lesion. (**A**) non-CRS, (**B**) CRSsNP, (**C**) non-ECRS, (**D**) mild ECRS, (**E**) moderate ECRS, and (**F**) severe ECRS. (**G**) Cytoplasmic IgE-positive mast cells were significantly increased in moderate and severe ECRS lesions ($p < 0.05$ and $p < 0.01$, respectively). Relationships between the number of cytoplasmic IgE-positive cells and the preoperative CT score (**H**), eosinophil ratio in peripheral blood (**I**), and total serum IgE level (**J**).

3. Discussion

In this study, an increase in mast cells was observed in non-ECRS and ECRS lesions. Two types of human mast cells have been described: mast cells that express both tryptase and chymase, found in the subcutaneous connective tissue (TC-type mast cells; MC_{TC}), and mast cells that express only tryptase, found in the airway mucosa and intestinal mucosa (T-type mast cells; MC_T) [15]. Baba et al. reported increased numbers of MC_{TC} in the epithelium, glands, and submucosa of ECRS polyps, as well as increased numbers of MC_T in the glands and submucosa of non-ECRS polyps [16]. Furthermore, it was suggested that the distribution of IgE-positive mast cell subtypes differs between ECRS and non-ECRS [16]. As the present study did not analyze production of tryptase and chymase, it is unclear which type of mast cells increased. However, it is presumed that MC_T increased with non-ECRS and MC_{TC} increased with ECRS. In our study, the number of c-kit-positive cells and the number of membrane IgE-positive mast cells increased in cases where NP were formed. In addition, moderate and severe ECRS exhibited an increase in the number of cytoplasmic IgE-positive mast cells. Mast cell endocytosis is caused by strong antigen stimulation and is a phenomenon in which FcεRI and IgE antibodies on the membrane surface are taken into the cytoplasm. Mast cell endocytosis is considered to be the cause of positive cytoplasmic IgE. Increased levels of IgE are believed to increase the amount of FcεRI, which in turn induces increased levels of endocytosis [17]. In patients with ECRS, IgE-positive cells are increased due to an allergic predisposition. In severe cases of ECRS, the majority of patients have asthma, and excessive endocytosis may further activate the allergic reaction.

In addition, sustained mucosal inflammation causes the cells to be susceptible to infection from bacteria and viruses, resulting in strong antigen stimulation and further activation of the immune response. The accumulation of these factors results in the activation of mast cells, which further increases IgE levels. As such, we speculate that moderate or severe ECRS lesions may result in an increase in mast cells positive for cytoplasmic IgE. In the present study, cytoplasmic IgE-positive mast cells were significantly increased in moderate and severe ECRS, suggesting that the status of ECRS is primarily allergic, involving activation of mast cells.

As an internal immune mechanism, mast cells are activated upon antigen stimulation to release cytokines, such as IL-4, IL-13, and IL-5, which are classified as type 2 cytokines and are involved in the production of IgE as well as the differentiation/proliferation of eosinophils, thus promoting eosinophil expansion and production of IgE antibody by plasma cells. With increased severity of ECRS, mucosal rupture may continuously occur, resulting in enhanced and sustained antigenic stimulation and further mast cell activation, which subsequently cause an enhanced expression of FcεRI. Propagation of this cycle is considered to lead to endocytosis of mast cells. In this study, since the patients' blood samples were not preserved due to the nature of the study being retrospective, it was not possible to quantify Th2 cytokines in the blood. In addition, the quantification of these cytokines in tissues was not possible due to the small amount of FFPE samples.

In addition, it has been reported that staphylococcal enterotoxin is likely to be involved in eosinophilic inflammation of the nasal mucosa as a superantigen or as an adjuvant [18]. The staphylococcal enterotoxin of *Staphylococcus aureus* has been detected in NP and mucins, and specific IgE against *S. aureus* enterotoxins has also been detected. Furthermore, the polyclonal increase of nonspecific IgE in the nasal cavity is considered to be important for nasal polyp formation [19], while also inducing differentiation of precursor cells to eosinophils and contributing to proliferation. Furthermore, it has been reported that anti-IgE antibody therapy is an effective treatment for ECRS accompanied by NP [20–22]. It has also been reported that anti-IL-5 antibodies were effective against eosinophil-dominated NP [23]. IL-5 is an important cytokine for eosinophil migration and activation. Taken together, it has been suggested that mast cells are involved in the mechanism of ECRS accompanied by the formation of NP.

In a recent study, it has been reported that IgG4-positive cells increase significantly in severe ECRS [24]. Particularly in allergic diseases, IgG4 is considered to act as a blocking agent for IgE antibodies induced by the antigen. Furthermore, mast cells positive for cytoplasmic IgE have been reported in IgG4-related disease (IgG4-RD) [17]. In addition, it has been shown that the number of endocytic mast cells also increases in the lesions of IgG4-RD [17]. Severe cases of IgG4-RD often have multiorgan lesions. Similarly, multiple organ lesions, such as eosinophilic esophagitis, have been reported in severe cases of ECRS [25,26]. While the precise pathogenesis of these diseases is unclear, there may be a link to family predisposition and allergic diseases [27,28].

In conclusion, it is suggested that mast cells that receive antigen stimulation are involved in the pathogenesis of ECRS.

4. Materials and Methods

4.1. Patients

Seventy-one Japanese patients with CRS (47 males and 24 females; mean age, 55.8 years) were enrolled. Among these, 57 patients exhibited NP, and the remainder demonstrated no visible NP in the middle meatus ($n = 14$) [24]. Patients with CRSwNP were divided into non-ECRS ($n = 27$) and ECRS ($n = 30$) groups based on the Japanese Epidemiological Survey of Refractory Eosinophilic Chronic Rhinosinusitis (JESREC) criteria [5]. In brief, the JESREC scoring system assesses whether it is a unilateral or bilateral disease, the presence of NP, degree of blood eosinophilia, and the dominant shadow of ethmoid sinus in computed tomography (CT) scans. Herein, a case was diagnosed as ECRS if it showed a JESREC score of ≥ 1, and tissue eosinophilia ≥ 70 per HPF; ×400). The severity of ECRS was further determined by the JESREC algorithm using factor A (presence of both blood eosinophilia equal to or greater than 5% and an ethmoid-dominant shadow on a CT scan) and factor B (comorbid bronchial asthma or nonsteroidal anti-inflammatory drug intolerance) as follows: cases negative for both factor A and B, cases positive for either factor A or B, or cases positive for both factor A and B were grouped into mild, moderate, or severe ECRS groups, respectively [5]. Using this algorithm, 30 ECRS patients were categorized as mild ($n = 8$), moderate ($n = 12$), or severe ($n = 10$) ECRS subgroups. All CRSsNP patients were diagnosed as being non-ECRS using these criteria. During surgery, NP and UT were taken from patients with CRSwNP and CRSsNP, respectively. Serum samples were collected from 17 patients (non-ECRS: $n = 6$; mild ECRS: $n = 4$; moderate ECRS: $n = 2$; severe ECRS: $n = 5$). As the control, 13 non-CRS patients (e.g., patients with blowout fractures, posterior ethmoidal cysts, or sphenoidal cysts) with normal UT at inspection were enrolled (four males and nine females; mean age, 61.4 years). After surgery, CRS patients received medications, including macrolides and mucolytic agents for 2 months, together with saline douching, which was continued as long as they could. In addition, NP patients received systemic corticosteroids (prednisolone: started with 20 mg/day, then gradually decreased over 1 month) followed by intranasal corticosteroids. Furthermore, ECRS patients standardly received oral antileukotrienes.

Informed consent for participation in the study was obtained from each patient, and the study was approved by the Human Research Committee of the Okayama University Graduate School of Medicine and Dentistry (reference number 1505-030).

4.2. Histological Examination and Immunohistochemistry

All samples used in this study were surgically resected specimens. The surgically removed tissues were fixed in 10% formaldehyde and embedded in paraffin. Serial 3-μm-thick sections were cut from the blocks and stained with hematoxylin and eosin (H&E); the sections were immunohistochemically stained using an automated BOND III stainer (Leica Biosystems, Wetzlar, Germany). Primary antibodies against the following antigens were used: c-kit (diluted antibody; Nichirei Biosciences Inc., Tokyo, Japan) and IgE (1:200; DAKO, Glostrup, Denmark).

4.3. Histological Evaluation of c-Kit and IgE-Positive Cell

Mast cells are defined as cells that express both high-affinity IgE receptors and the stem cell factor receptor, c-kit; therefore, we analyzed the number of mast cells by immunostaining for these markers. As dendritic cells also express FcεRI, they also stain positive for IgE immunohistochemistry; however, their shape is significantly different from that of mast cells, allowing us to only quantify cells that could be distinguished as mast cells.

Cell counts were performed by two independent researchers, and the average number was calculated. The cells were counted in three hotspot fields with an HPF (×400), and the average per field was determined. In the hotspot area of c-kit-positive cells, the number of c-kit-positive cells was counted for each specimen. In the hotspot area of IgE-positive cells, the numbers of cells showing IgE-positive in the membrane and cytoplasm were counted separately.

4.4. Statistical Analysis

Values are given as the median. The nonparametric Mann-Whitney U test was used to compare data between groups, and Wilcoxon's signed-rank test was used to analyze data within each group. A Kruskal–Wallis test, followed by a Dunn test, was used for multiple comparisons. Correlation analyses were performed using Spearman's rank correlation. Statistical analyses were performed with GraphPad Prism 6 software (GraphPad Software, Inc., La Jolla, CA, USA). The p-values for sensitivity and specificity were calculated using JMP Pro 13.2 (SAS Institute Inc., Cary, NC, USA), and logistic regression analyses were conducted using STATA 12.1 (StataCorp, College Station, TX, USA). A p value less than 0.05 (two-tailed) was considered to be statistically significant.

To compare the c-kit-positive cells and IgE-positive cells among eosinophilic sinusitis, nonsinusitis, chronic sinusitis, and noneosinophilic sinusitis, the Kruskal–Wallis test method, using IBM-SPSS statistics software (version 24; IBM, Armonk, NY, USA), was applied. A p value < 0.05 was considered statistically significant.

Author Contributions: Conceptualization, M.O. and Y.S.; Methodology, Y.G. and Y.S.; Validation, Y.G. and T.K.; Formal Analysis, Y.G., T.O. and A.N.; Investigation, Y.O., T.T., H.M. and T.M.; Resources, K.N.; Data Curation, T.K.; Writing-Original Draft Preparation, Y.G.; Writing-Review & Editing, Y.S. and M.O.; Supervision, Y.S. and M.O.; Project Administration, M.O. All authors have read and agreed to the published version of the manuscript.

Funding: This work was partially supported by the Grant-in-Aid for Young Scientists (JSPS KAKENHI grant number 19K16586), from the Japan Society for the Promotion of Science.

Conflicts of Interest: The authors declare no conflict of interest.

References

1. Matsuwaki, Y.; Ookushi, T.; Asaka, D.; Mori, E.; Nakajima, T.; Yoshida, T.; Kojima, J.; Chiba, S.; Ootori, N.; Moriyama, H. Chronic rhinosinusitis: Risk factors for the recurrence of chronic rhinosinusitis based on 5-year follow-up after endoscopic sinus surgery. *Int. Arch. Allergy Immunol.* **2008**, *146*, 77–81. [CrossRef]
2. Fujieda, S.; Imoto, Y.; Kato, Y.; Ninomiya, T.; Tokunaga, T.; Tsutsumiuchi, T.; Yoshida, K.; Kidoguchi, M.; Takabayashi, T. Eosinophilic chronic rhinosinusitis. *Allergol. Int.* **2019**, *68*, 403–412. [CrossRef]
3. Ishitoya, J.; Sakuma, Y.; Tsukuda, M. Eosinophilic chronic rhinosinusitis in Japan. *Allergol. Int.* **2010**, *59*, 239–245. [CrossRef]
4. Takeno, S.; Hirakawa, K.; Ishino, T. Pathological mechanisms and clinical features of eosinophilic chronic rhinosinusitis in the Japanese population. *Allergol. Int.* **2010**, *59*, 247–256. [CrossRef]
5. Tokunaga, T.; Sakashita, M.; Haruna, T.; Asaka, D.; Takeno, S.; Ikeda, H.; Nakayama, T.; Seki, N.; Ito, S.; Murata, J.; et al. Novel scoring system and algorithm for classifying chronic rhinosinusitis: The JESREC study. *Allergy* **2015**, *70*, 995–1003. [CrossRef]
6. Bradding, P.; Holgate, S.T. Immunopathology and human mast cell cytokines. *Crit. Rev. Oncol. Hematol.* **1999**, *31*, 119–133.
7. Henz, B.M.; Maurer, M.; Lippert, U.; Worm, M.; Babina, M. Mast cells as initiators of immunity and host defense. *Exp. Dermatol.* **2001**, *10*, 1–10.
8. Metcalfe, D.D.; Baram, D.; Mekori, Y.A. Mast cells. *Physiol. Rev.* **1997**, *77*, 1033–1079. [CrossRef]
9. Galli, S.J.; Nakae, S.; Tsai, M. Mast cells in the development of adaptive immune responses. *Nat. Immunol.* **2005**, *6*, 135–142. [CrossRef]
10. Lu, L.F.; Lind, E.F.; Gondek, D.C.; Bennett, K.A.; Gleeson, M.W.; Pino-Lagos, K.; Scott, Z.A.; Coyle, A.J.; Reed, J.L.; Van Snick, J.; et al. Mast cells are essential intermediaries in regulatory T-cell tolerance. *Nature* **2006**, *442*, 997–1002. [CrossRef]
11. Supajatura, V.; Ushio, H.; Nakao, A.; Okumura, K.; Ra, C.; Ogawa, H. Protective roles of mast cells against enterobacterial infection are mediated by Toll-like receptor 4. *J. Immunol.* **2001**, *167*, 2250–2256.
12. Supajatura, V.; Ushio, H.; Nakao, A.; Akira, S.; Okumura, K.; Ra, C.; Ogawa, H. Differential responses of mast cell Toll-like receptors 2 and 4 in allergy and innate immunity. *J. Clin. Investig.* **2002**, *109*, 1351–1359. [CrossRef]
13. Pawankar, R.; Okuda, M.; Yssel, H.; Okumura, K.; Ra, C. Nasal mast cells in perennial allergic rhinitics exhibit increased expression of the Fc epsilonRI, CD40L, IL-4, and IL-13, and can induce IgE synthesis in B cells. *J. Clin. Investig.* **1997**, *99*, 1492–1499. [CrossRef]
14. Fattakhova, G.V.; Masilamani, M.; Narayanan, S.; Borrego, F.; Gilfillan, A.M.; Metcalfe, D.D.; Coligan, J.E. Endosomal trafficking of the ligated FcvarepsilonRI receptor. *Mol. Immunol.* **2009**, *46*, 793–802. [CrossRef]
15. Irani, A.A.; Schechter, N.M.; Craig, S.S.; DeBlois, G.; Schwartz, L.B. Two types of human mast cells that have distinct neutral protease compositions. *Proc. Natl. Acad. Sci. USA* **1986**, *83*, 4464–4468.
16. Baba, S.; Kondo, K.; Suzukawa, M.; Ohta, K.; Yamasoba, T. Distribution, subtype population, and IgE positivity of mast cells in chronic rhinosinusitis with nasal polyps. *Ann. Allergy Asthma Immunol.* **2017**, *119*, 120–128. [CrossRef]

17. Nishida, K.; Gion, Y.; Takeuchi, M.; Tanaka, T.; Kataoka, T.R.; Yoshino, T.; Sato, Y. Mast cells exhibiting strong cytoplasmic staining for IgE and high affinity IgE receptor are increased in IgG4-related disease. *Sci. Rep.* **2018**, *8*, 4656. [CrossRef]
18. Bachert, C.; Zhang, N.; Holtappels, G.; De Lobel, L.; van Cauwenberge, P.; Liu, S.; Lin, P.; Bousquet, J.; Van Steen, K. Presence of IL-5 protein and IgE antibodies to staphylococcal enterotoxins in nasal polyps is associated with comorbid asthma. *J. Allergy Clin. Immunol.* **2010**, *126*, 962–968.e6. [CrossRef]
19. Patou, J.; Gevaert, P.; Van Zele, T.; Holtappels, G.; van Cauwenberge, P.; Bachert, C. Staphylococcus aureus enterotoxin B, protein A, and lipoteichoic acid stimulations in nasal polyps. *J. Allergy Clin. Immunol.* **2008**, *121*, 110–115. [CrossRef]
20. Grundmann, S.A.; Hemfort, P.B.; Luger, T.A.; Brehler, R. Anti-IgE (omalizumab): A new therapeutic approach for chronic rhinosinusitis. *J. Allergy Clin. Immunol.* **2008**, *121*, 257–258.
21. Bobolea, I.; Barranco, P.; Fiandor, A.; Cabanas, R.; Quirce, S. Omalizumab: A potential new therapeutic approach for aspirin-exacerbated respiratory disease. *J. Investig. Allergol. Clin. Immunol.* **2010**, *20*, 448–449.
22. Okano, M.; Kariya, S.; Ohta, N.; Imoto, Y.; Fujieda, S.; Nishizaki, K. Association and management of eosinophilic inflammation in upper and lower airways. *Allergol. Int.* **2015**, *64*, 131–138. [CrossRef]
23. Gevaert, P.; Van Bruaene, N.; Cattaert, T.; Van Steen, K.; Van Zele, T.; Acke, F.; De Ruyck, N.; Blomme, K.; Sousa, A.R.; Marshall, R.P.; et al. Mepolizumab, a humanized anti-IL-5 mAb, as a treatment option for severe nasal polyposis. *J. Allergy Clin. Immunol.* **2011**, *128*, 989–995.e8. [CrossRef]
24. Koyama, T.; Kariya, S.; Sato, Y.; Gion, Y.; Higaki, T.; Haruna, T.; Fujiwara, T.; Minoura, A.; Takao, S.; Orita, Y.; et al. Significance of IgG4-positive cells in severe eosinophilic chronic rhinosinusitis. *Allergol. Int.* **2018**. [CrossRef]
25. Padia, R.; Curtin, K.; Peterson, K.; Orlandi, R.R.; Alt, J. Eosinophilic esophagitis strongly linked to chronic rhinosinusitis. *Laryngoscope* **2016**, *126*, 1279–1283. [CrossRef]
26. Wise, S.K.; Lin, S.Y.; Toskala, E.; Orlandi, R.R.; Akdis, C.A.; Alt, J.A.; Azar, A.; Baroody, F.M.; Bachert, C.; Canonica, G.W.; et al. International consensus statement on allergy and rhinology: Allergic rhinitis. *Int. Forum. Allergy Rhinol.* **2018**, *8*, 108–352. [CrossRef]
27. Alexander, E.S.; Martin, L.J.; Collins, M.H.; Kottyan, L.C.; Sucharew, H.; He, H.; Mukkada, V.A.; Succop, P.A.; Abonia, J.P.; Foote, H.; et al. Twin and family studies reveal strong environmental and weaker genetic cues explaining heritability of eosinophilic esophagitis. *J. Allergy Clin. Immunol.* **2014**, *134*, 1084–1092.e1. [CrossRef]
28. Karkos, P.D.; Srivastava, R.; Kaptanis, S.; Vaughan, C. Eosinophilic esophagitis for the otolaryngologist. *Int. J. Otolaryngol.* **2012**, *2012*, 181402. [CrossRef]

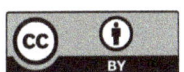

© 2020 by the authors. Licensee MDPI, Basel, Switzerland. This article is an open access article distributed under the terms and conditions of the Creative Commons Attribution (CC BY) license (http://creativecommons.org/licenses/by/4.0/).

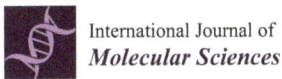

Article

Highly Selective Cleavage of TH2-Promoting Cytokines by the Human and the Mouse Mast Cell Tryptases, Indicating a Potent Negative Feedback Loop on TH2 Immunity

Zhirong Fu, Srinivas Akula, Michael Thorpe and Lars Hellman *

Department of Cell and Molecular Biology, Uppsala University, SE-75124 Uppsala, Sweden; fuzhirong.zju@gmail.com (Z.F.); srinivas.akula@icm.uu.se (S.A.); getmeinahalfpipe@gmail.com (M.T.)
* Correspondence: Lars.Hellman@icm.uu.se; Tel.: +46-0-18-471-4532

Received: 25 September 2019; Accepted: 15 October 2019; Published: 17 October 2019

Abstract: Mast cells (MC) are resident tissue cells found primarily at the interphase between tissues and the environment. These evolutionary old cells store large amounts of proteases within cytoplasmic granules, and one of the most abundant of these proteases is tryptase. To look deeper into the question of their in vivo targets, we have analyzed the activity of the human MC tryptase on 69 different human cytokines and chemokines, and the activity of the mouse tryptase (mMCP-6) on 56 mouse cytokines and chemokines. These enzymes were found to be remarkably restrictive in their cleavage of these potential targets. Only five were efficiently cleaved by the human tryptase: TSLP, IL-21, MCP3, MIP-3b, and eotaxin. This strict specificity indicates a regulatory function of these proteases and not primarily as unspecific degrading enzymes. We recently showed that the human MC chymase also had a relatively strict specificity, indicating that both of these proteases have regulatory functions. One of the most interesting regulatory functions may involve controlling excessive TH2-mediated inflammation by cleaving several of the most important TH2-promoting inflammatory cytokines, including IL-18, IL-33, TSLP, IL-15, and IL-21, indicating a potent negative feedback loop on TH2 immunity.

Keywords: mast cell; tryptase; chymase; serine protease; human chymase; cleavage specificity; cytokine; chemokine; TH2

1. Introduction

Mast cells are resident tissue cells of hematopoietic origin that primarily are found at the interphase between tissues and environment such as skin, intestinal mucosa, lungs, and close to blood vessels and nerves. These cells store massive amounts of immune mediators in cytoplasmic granules. A large fraction of the proteins stored in these granules are serine proteases, and all of these belong to the large family of trypsin/chymotrypsin-related serine proteases [1–5]. This protease family also includes several coagulation factors, complement factors, and the pancreatic digestive enzymes. The members of this family that are expressed by hematopoietic cells have been named hematopoietic serine proteases. They are primarily found in mast cells (MCs), neutrophils, natural killer (NK) cells, and cytotoxic T cells (Tc), where they are stored in their active forms in the granules for rapid release. Very high amounts of these proteases are found in these cells; the levels in mast cells can reach 35% of the total cellular protein [6]. hMCs express one chymotryptic enzyme, the MC chymase (HC), one enzyme with tryptic specificity, the tryptase and sometimes an enzyme, cathepsin G (hCG), which is otherwise primarily found in neutrophils.

The various granule proteins of the hematopoietic cells have been shown to have a number of important immune functions including antibacterial, antiparasitic, general inflammatory, anti-inflammatory or apoptosis-inducing activity. For example, the mouse counterpart of the HC, mouse mast cell protease-4 (mMCP-4) has been shown to be very potent in inactivating several snake, bee, and scorpion toxins, indicating an important role in defense against potentially life threatening toxins, a function that is probably evolutionary very old [7]. Recently, some of the hematopoietic serine proteases have been shown to cleave, and thereby inactivate, various cytokines and chemokines. For example, mMCP-4 cleaves and inactivates tumor necrosis factor-alpha (TNF-α), thereby limiting the inflammatory response [8]. The HC also cleaves and activates IL-1β and IL-18, as well as cleaving the region just outside of the membrane of membrane bound stem cell factor (SCF), which releases it from the cell [9–11]. The release of SCF from the cell surface makes it able to move more freely in the tissue, which may then be of importance for attracting progenitor cells, primarily MC progenitors, from the blood. In addition, HC has been found to cleave two chemotactic substances: active chemerin and eotaxin-3 (CCL26) [12,13]. The degradation of IL-33, an IL-1-related cytokine, by mMCP-4 and HC indicates that they potentially have a role in limiting inflammation [14,15]. Another of the hMC enzymes, the tryptase, has also been shown to efficiently degrade the chemokine eotaxin [16]. Numerous examples on the role of these enzymes in the degradation of inflammatory mediators have been described, indicating that this may be one of the important functions of these enzymes. In order to study the potential roles of these in limiting inflammation by cleaving cytokines and chemokines in more general terms, we recently performed an extensive analysis of the cleavage of 51 different human cytokines and chemokines by the HC and hCG. The results showed a remarkable selectivity for both enzymes but primarily for the HC. Only significant cleavage in 3–4 of the 51 studied cytokines and chemokines for this enzyme was detected [17]. The cleavage by both enzymes of two IL-1-related cytokines, IL-18 and IL-33, which act as alarmins, indicated a role of these enzymes in limiting excessive inflammation. As a continuation of these studies, here we present a similar study of the human and the mouse mast cell tryptases. The tryptase found in human MCs is a homo or heterotetramer of four closely related proteases the α, β1, β2, and β3 tryptases [1]. Interestingly the formation of a heteroteramer between the proteolytically inactive α-tryptase and one of the active β-tryptases changes both the stability and specificity of the β-tryptase [18]. The mouse counterpart is named mouse mast cell proteases 6 (mMCP-6) [19]. Interestingly, the active sites of these four subunits are positioned in the center of the tetramer, making them less accessible for larger substrates [20].

The human tryptase was found to be even more specific than the HC and we could only observe cleavage of five out of 69 different cytokines and chemokines. The cytokines that were efficiently degraded were TSLP and IL-21 and the chemokines MCP3, MIP-1b, and eotaxin. Interestingly, when combining the cleavage of the two of the major proteolytic enzymes of hMCs, the tryptase and the chymase, we can now see that together they cleave three of the most potent TH2 promoting cytokines, IL-18, TSLP, and IL-33. Interestingly, also IL-15 and IL-21, which both are efficiently cleaved by HC and the tryptase, respectively, have been indicated in either promoting TH2 immunity or inhibiting TH1 immunity [21–23]. This indicates that one major function of the MC proteases is to limit excessive TH2 driven inflammation. They may act together as a negative feedback loop by cleaving and thereby inactivating early TH2 promoting inflammatory cytokines.

2. Results

2.1. Analysis of the Purity and Activity of the Recombinant Human and Mouse Mast Cell Tryptases

To determine the activity and purity of the recombinant human tryptase, the enzyme was dissolved in assay buffer and a sample of approximately 2 μg was separated on a 4–12% SDS-PAGE gel (Figure 1a). The figure showed several bands that most likely originate from heterogenous glycosylation (Figure 1a). Expression in fungal expression systems like the *Pichia pastoris* often generates heterogenous glycosylation. However, deglycosylation of proteins produced in this system, using the same purification strategy as this commercial enzyme have shown high purity and that all the diverse bands observed on gels originate from differently glycosylated tryptase [24].

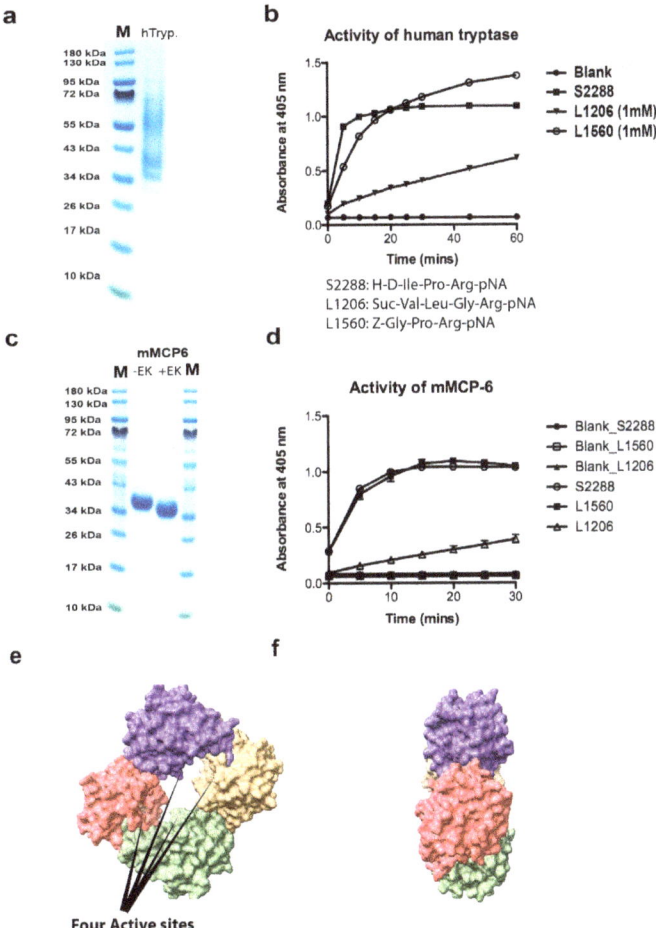

Figure 1. Analysis of the recombinant human and mouse mast cell tryptases used for the substrate analysis by SDS-PAGE and chromogenic substrate assay. (**a**) Approximately two micrograms of the recombinant human tryptase was separated on a 4–12% gradient SDS-PAGE gel and stained with colloidal Coomassie blue solution. Several bands starting at approximately 36 kDa up to almost 70 kDa were seen, indicating heterogenous glycosylation. (**b**) The activity of the human recombinant tryptase was assayed against three different chromogenic substrates. All three are substrates for tryptic enzymes due to the Arg in the P1 position. The human tryptase showed good activity against all three, but the best activity against the two substrates occurred when the Arg was preceded by a Pro residue. (**c**) The purified recombinant mouse mast cell tryptase (mMCP-6) before and after enterokinase cleavage. (**d**) The activity of the mouse recombinant tryptase was assayed against three different chromogenic substrates. The substrate preference for the mouse enzyme was almost identical to its human counterpart shown in (**b**). (**e**,**f**) Three-dimensional structural models of the human tryptase tetramer (PDB No: 2fs9). The space filling model of the human MC tryptase is shown from two angles, from the front looking into the tetramer and from the side [20]. The four active sites in the middle of the tetramer are marked by four arrows. The pictures were visualized in the UCSF Chimera program.

The activity of this recombinant tryptase was then tested on three different chromogenic substrates and the enzyme was found to be highly active against all three of these low molecular weight substrates, which shows the enzyme has a high proteolytic activity (Figure 1b). The mouse mast cell tryptase, mMCP-6 was produced in the human cell line HEK293-EBNA, and after purification on Ni^{+2} chelating IMAC columns activated by cleavage by enterokinase, lowering the pH to 6.0, and adding heparin, as previously described (Figure 1c) [19].

The activities of both enzymes were analyzed against three chromogenic tryptase substrates (Figure 1b,d).

2.2. Analysis of Cleavage Sensitivity against a Panel of 69 Cytokines and Chemokines by the Recombinant Human Tryptase

The cleavage activity on 69 different recombinant human cytokines and chemokines by the recombinant human tryptase was analyzed in 11 µL cleavage reactions with approximately 1.2 µg of cytokine and chemokine and 13 ng of the tryptase (Figure 2). To confirm the initial results, the experiment was repeated under the same conditions as previously described. The results were the same as the first experiment (data not shown). In both experiments the enzyme to target ratio was the same, approximately 1:92.

Most of the 69 cytokines and chemokines analyzed were not cleaved by this enzyme. Of the cytokines analyzed, only two were efficiently cleaved, TSLP and IL-21, and we could only observe efficient cleavage of three chemokines, MCP3, MIP-3b, and eotaxin (Figure 2). A minor N or C terminal trimming of IFN-γ, IL-8, and IP-10, and a minor degrading effect on IL-7, SDF-1β, and CTGF could also be detected (Figure 2). By using a three-fold increase in the amount of enzyme, we observed a more pronounced degrading effect on CTGF, and also cleavage of IGF-1, IGF-2, and FGF-1, indicating that some more targets appear with increasing enzyme to target ratio. However, generally, the tryptase was remarkably restrictive in its cleavage of this large panel of cytokines and chemokines (Figure 2a,b). Interestingly, where cleavage occurred, it appeared as if it degraded the target almost completely as only very faint bands for fragments could be detected for three of the most sensitive targets, TSLP, IL-21, eotaxin, and MIP-3b and there were no traces of MCP3 after cleavage (Figure 2).

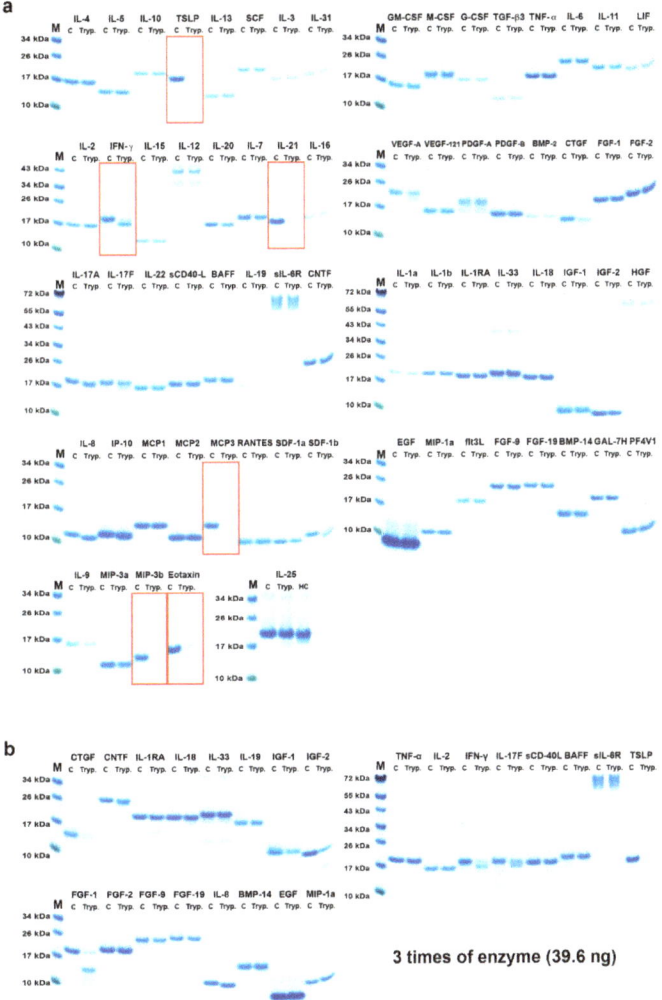

Figure 2. Cleavage analysis of a panel of 69 recombinant human cytokines and chemokines. The various recombinant cytokines and chemokines were divided into two separate tubes. One was kept as negative control (C) where PBS (no enzyme) was added and one was cleaved with the human tryptase. The cleavage was performed at 37 °C in PBS buffered solution (pH 7.3) for 2.5 h. The samples were separated on 4–12% SDS-PAGE gels under reducing conditions. Size markers are found at the left side of each gel. The gels were stained in colloidal Coomassie blue solution. (**a**) Cleavage with 13 ng of tryptase. (**b**) Cleavage using three times higher enzyme concentration. The cytokines and chemokines that were efficiently cleaved or trimmed are marked by red rectangles.

2.3. Analysis of Cleavage Sensitivity against a Panel of 56 Cytokines and Chemokines by the Recombinant Mouse Tryptase, mMCP-6

The cleavage activity on 56 different recombinant mouse cytokines and chemokines by the recombinant mouse tryptase, mMCP-6, was performed (two times with identical result) under the same conditions as described for the human tryptase (Figure 3).

Most of the 56 cytokines and chemokines analyzed were not cleaved by this enzyme. Of the cytokines and growth factors analyzed, only eight were efficiently cleaved, IL-13, IL-9, IL-21, IL-33, VEGF-A, PDGF-B, IL-17C, and IGF-1 (Figure 3), and we could only observe efficient cleavage of five chemokines, IP-10, MCP-1, MIP-3a, MIP-3b, and eotaxin (Figure 3). A minor N or C terminal trimming of IFN-γ, IL-6, IL-11, and IL-17F, and a minor degrading effect on IL-7 and SDF-1α could also be detected (Figure 3).

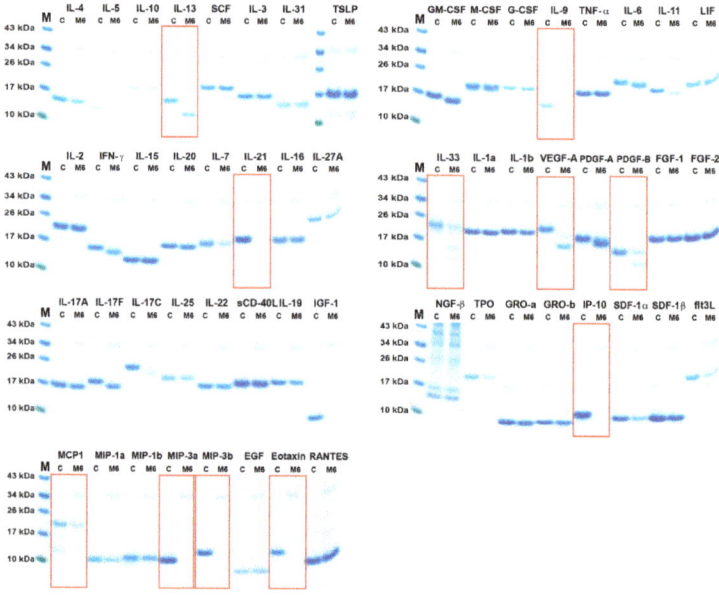

Figure 3. Cleavage analysis of a panel of 56 recombinant mouse cytokines and chemokines. The various recombinant cytokines and chemokines in buffer solution were divided into two separate tubes. One was kept as negative control (C) where PBS (no enzyme) was added and one was cleaved with the mouse tryptase (mMCP-6). The cleavage was performed at 37 °C in PBS at pH 7.3 for 2.5 h. The samples were separated on 4–12% SDS-PAGE gels under reducing conditions. Size markers are found at the left side of each gel. The gels were stained in colloidal Coomassie blue solution. The cytokines and chemokines that were efficiently cleaved or trimmed are marked by red rectangles.

2.4. Analysis of Structural Similarities between the Three Efficiently Cleaved Cytokines and Chemokines

To try to understand why a few of the cytokines and chemokines were efficiently cleaved and why the remaining majority were almost totally unaffected by this enzyme, we wanted to see if there were any structural characteristics in common between the three cleaved cytokines and chemokines. After analyzing the sequence, all three contained positively charged patches (Figure 4). Human TSLP was probably the most extreme in this case, with seven basic amino acids in a row (KKRRKRK) (Figure 4). Interestingly this sequence is lacking in both rat and mouse TSLP but present in human and dog TSLP (Figure 4). In order to study if this difference affected the efficiency in cleavage by the human tryptase, we tested cleavage of both human and mouse TSLP. Human TSLP was very efficiently cleaved and was totally degraded by 13 ng of tryptase, whereas mouse TSLP was not cleaved at all, even when using 10 times higher enzyme concentration, 136 ng, which clearly indicates that this positively charged patch is of importance for the cleavage (Figure 5a). This sequence (KKRRKRK) is not found in any other cytokine of chemokine in the entire human proteome. All other human cytokines and chemokines analyzed in this study also lacked a positive patch except VEGF-A, PDGF-A and B. A C-terminal patch of positively charged amino acids were also seen in IFN-γ. Interestingly IFN-γ is trimmed most likely in the C-terminal (Figure 2). However, no cleavage by the human tryptase of VEGF-A, PDGF-A and B was observed, indicating that also higher order structure of the protein is of importance. Interestingly mMCP-6 did cleave mouse VEGF-A, PDGF-A and B, indicating that even minor differences in the structure of the protease or of the target may affect this selectivity. It should be noted that these three cytokines are highly homologous and almost identical in the regions of interest, possibly except VEGF-A where the mouse protein has a big C-terminal deletion, which did not affect the positively charged region. The deletion may possibly enhance the accessibility of this charged region, making it a better target for mMCP-6. Higher order structures most likely play an important role in the selectivity, if the positively charged region is exposed or not on the surface of the protein. Cleavage may also occur only if the protein has an unstructured region accessibly for cleavage by the tryptase. Two structural requirements may therefore have to be fulfilled, a positive patch for targeting and a loose structure to allow targeting by the enzymes.

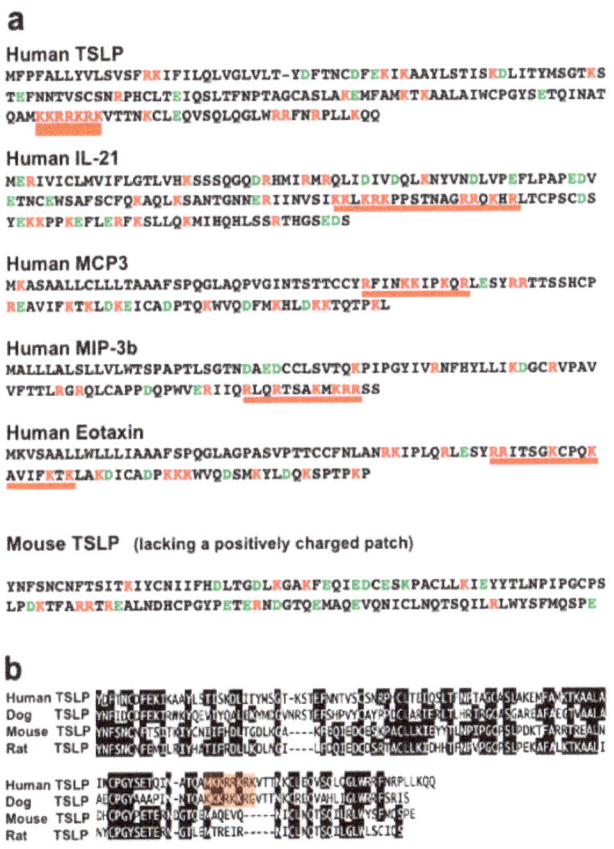

Figure 4. (**a**) Analysis of the primary amino acid sequences of human TSLP, IL-21, MCP3, MIP-1b, eotaxin, and mouse TSLP. The amino acid sequences of the five cytokines and chemokines that were efficiently cleaved by the human skin tryptase are shown in one letter code. Negatively charged residues are marked in green and positively charged in red. The regions that are highly positively charged and that may act as targets for the tryptase are marked by a red thick line. In (**b**) an alignment of human, dog, mouse, and rat TSLP is presented. The conserved residues between the majority of the four sequences are marked in black. The positively charged patch found in human and dog TSLP is marked in red for more easy identification.

2.5. Analysis of the Effect of Spermine on Tryptase Activity

As indicated from previous sections, a high positive charge, as exemplified by the KKRRKRK sequence in human TSLP, seems to be an important factor for the selectivity of the tryptase. To look deeper into this selectivity, we decided to analyze the effect on cleavage by a potential low molecular weight competitor. Spermine appeared as a good candidate. It has a molecular weight of only 202.34 g/mol and at physiological pH all of its four amino groups are charged. The spermine solutions were made fresh from powder just before use and pH adjusted to pH 7.2. Spermine and tryptase were first mixed in the reaction buffer and left to equalize for a few minutes before starting the experiment by addition of the chromogenic substrate. No effect on the cleavage of the chromogenic substrate was seen at concentrations of spermine from 0.1 to 3 mM, indicating that spermine has no effect on the cleavage on low molecular weight substrates (Figure 5b). However, when we analyzed the cleavage of human TSLP the effect of spermine was quite dramatic (Figure 5c). Already at a concentration of 0.5 mM, the cleavage was reduced by approximately 20%, at 1 mM the cleavage was inhibited by approximately 50%, and at 3 mM almost totally inhibited, which shows a strong inhibitory effect of spermine on the cleavage of the positively charged target human TSLP by the human tryptase (Figure 5c).

2.6. Cleavage of other Substrates by Human Tryptase

Several proteins have previously been shown to be trimmed or degraded by human tryptase including fibrinogen and fibronectin [26,27]. To confirm these results and look at potential mechanisms, we performed a cleavage reaction with purified human fibrinogen and human fibronectin (Figure 5d). We could not detect any cleavage of fibronectin and only minor trimming of fibrinogen (Figure 5d). It is known that the N terminal tails of fibrinogen α and β chains are relatively unstructured and open for cleavage by thrombin (Figure 5e) [25]. The cleavage of the ends of the α and β chains of fibrinogen by thrombin results in the polymerization of fibrinogen into fibrin clots. It is highly possible that these loose unstructured ends make them accessible for cleavage also by the human tryptase, whereas the more tightly structured remaining parts of fibrinogen are more difficult for the tryptase to access.

In marked contrast to the tryptase, both human and opossum chymases did cleave both fibronectin and fibrinogen quite efficiently (Figure 5d). Furthermore, the cleavage patterns generated were quite similar indicating a conservation in target specificity over more than 150 million years of mammalian evolution.

2.7. Cleavage Selectivity of Wild Type (WT) and Mutant Human Tryptase

By a detailed analysis of the amino acid sequence of the human tryptase we observed a region just C-terminally of the Asp of the active site of the enzyme in a panel of tryptases. All had negatively charged amino acids, whereas a panel of chymases in the same region was positively charged (Figure 6a). To test if this region was involved in guiding positively charged substrates into the tetramer for efficient cleavage, we produced wt and mutant human tryptase involving these two residues (Figure 6a,b). We exchanged two glutamic acid residues of the tryptase into lysines, the amino acids found in these positions in the chymases (Figure 6a). The wt and mutant tryptases were produced in the human cell line HEK-293 EBNA and tested for their activity against three chromogenic substrates and against recombinant human TSLP (Figure 6c,d). To our surprise, both enzymes were equally active against all of these substrates, showing that this region of the protease has no effect on the selectivity of the tryptase (Figure 6c,d).

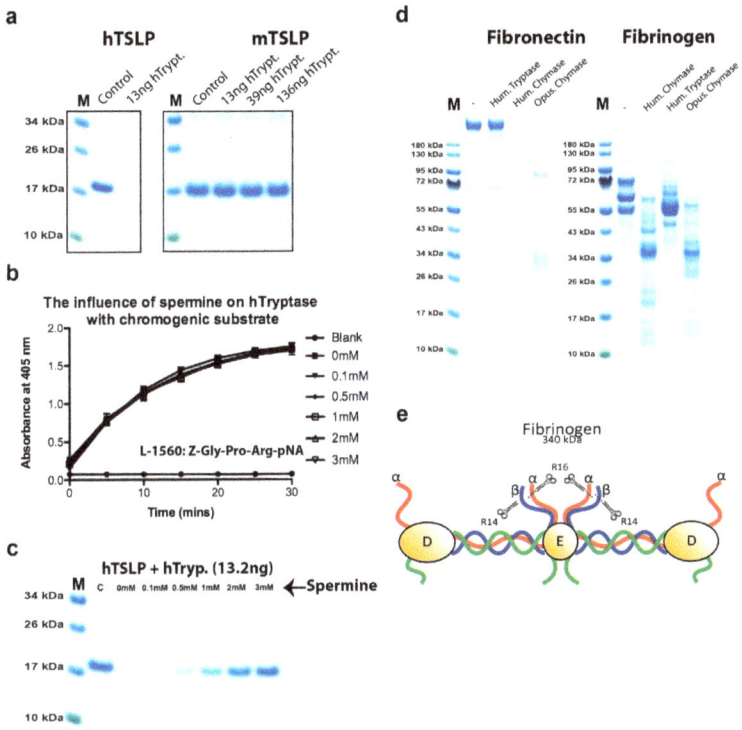

Figure 5. Cleavage analysis of human and mouse TSLP, the analysis of the effect by spermine on tryptase activity, and the cleavage of human fibrinogen and fibronectin by human tryptase, HC, and opossum chymase. In (**a**), 2.4 micrograms of active human TSLP was divided into two tubes and in one of the tubes human tryptase was added. The two tubes were incubated at 37 °C for 2.5 h. Following addition of sample buffer and beta mercaptoethanol, the samples were separated on a 4–12% SDS PAGE gel. A similar analysis was performed on mouse TSLP, which lacks the positively charged patch that is present in human and dog TSLP (Figure 4). In (**b**,**c**), the effect of spermine on cleavage by the human tryptase was analyzed by adding spermine to the cleavage reaction at different concentrations ranging from 0.1 to 3 mM and tested against both a chromogenic substrate (**b**) and a macromolecule as represented by human TSLP (**c**). As can be seen from the figure, spermine had no effect on the cleavage of the chromogenic substrate, but a potent effect on the cleavage of human TSLP. In (**d**), the cleavage of human fibrinogen and fibronectin by human tryptase, HC, and opossum chymase have been analyzed. Purified human fibrinogen and fibronectin were cleaved with three different enzymes, human tryptase, human chymase, and opossum chymase. In (**d**), we can see that no cleavage could be detected with the tryptase on fibronectin, but a very potent effect on this target by both human and opossum chymase. We can also see that human tryptase trims the ends of fibrinogen, whereas both human and opossum chymase has a much more pronounced effect on this target by also cleaving into the more tightly folded parts of fibrinogen. In (**e**), a schematic presentation of the overall structure of fibrinogen is presented [25]. The small scissors and R14 and R16 represent the cleavage sites in these regions of the α and β chains of fibrinogen by the coagulation enzyme thrombin.

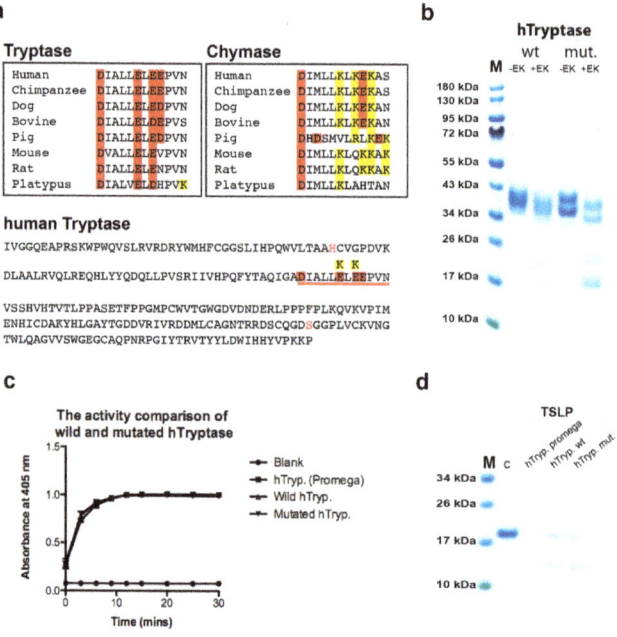

Figure 6. The effect on cleavage by mutating two negatively charged residues close to the active site of human tryptase. By analysis of the primary structure of the human tryptase we have observed a marked difference concerning charge close to the active site between tryptases and chymases. C-terminally of the asparagine residue of the catalytic triad all tryptases have a negative patch of three negatively charged residues (**a**). This region including the Asp of the catalytic triad and the three negatively charged residues is underlined in red in the sequence of the entire human tryptase shown in the bottom panel of (**a**). In this region, all chymases instead have two positively charged residues and one negatively charged amino acid (**a**). Could this region be involved in target selection? Two residues that differ between tryptases and chymases in the human tryptase was therefore mutated to study their involvement on cleavage (**a**). The wt and mutant enzymes were produced in HK-293-EBNA cells and activated by enterokinase cleavage, lowering the pH to 6.0, and adding heparin. (**b**) SDS-PAGE gel analysis of wt and mutant enzyme before and after enterokinase cleavage. (**c**) Cleavage of chromogenic substrates and (**d**) the cleavage of human TSLP by the pichia produced enzyme and the wt and mutated tryptase produced in mammalian cells.

3. Discussion

In a recent study, we have shown that both HC and hCG show a relatively selective cleavage of a panel of human cytokines and chemokines [17]. This finding contradicted the previously dominating view of the hematopoietic serine proteases as being relatively unspecific and cleaving almost any substrate if allowed to do so for extended periods of time. In order to broaden this analysis, here we have studied another dominating serine protease of human MCs, namely the tryptase. Here, we can see that this enzyme is even more restrictive. For the human tryptase, we could observe efficient cleavage of only five cytokines and chemokines out of the 69 tested (Figure 2). All of the five that were efficiently cleaved had one interesting characteristic in common, the presence of one or several patches of highly positively charged residues (Figure 4). If that patch was not present, as tested by cleavage of mouse TSLP, this protein was totally resistant to cleavage even with 10 times more enzyme (Figure 5a). Mouse TSLP is similar in its overall structure to its human counterpart but lacks this positive patch. Human TSLP was also very efficiently cleaved and almost no traces of the target could be seen on the SDS-PAGE gel, indicating that if the substrate enters the tetramer it becomes fully degraded (Figures 1e and 2). This shows clear similarities with the general cytoplasmic proteasome, which primarily cleaves polyubiquinated substrates [28,29]. The tryptase also show similarities to the coagulation protease thrombin, where positively charged patches on the enzyme, so called exosites, attract negatively charged regions on the substrate and thereby bring the target close to the active site [30].

The question is what region on the tryptase acts as an exosite? One very interesting candidate is heparin, which is not part of the enzyme itself but is attached to the tryptase, acting as a stabilizer and activator of the enzyme. When producing the tryptase as a recombinant protein, the enzyme is inactive before adding heparin [19]. Heparin then assists the tetramerization of the enzyme. At neutral pH, tetramerization is most likely essential for activity and here heparin is part of this activation step [19]. Heparin is the most negatively charged molecule in the human body and is thereby a likely candidate for the selectivity of tryptase for positively charged substrates [31,32]. Interestingly, a similar effect has previously been observed for the other dominating proteolytic enzyme of human connective tissue MCs, the chymase. Chymase needs heparin for efficient targeting of several targets including fibronectin, thrombin, and plasmin [33,34]. The mechanism is probably very similar to the proposed effect on tryptase, where heparin acts as a binding surface to attract the target and increase the target concentration close to the active site. These findings add additional support for the very important role of heparin and other highly negatively charged proteoglycans such as different chondroitin sulfates in MC biology [31,32].

In order to test the importance of the positive patch for the target selectivity of the human tryptase, we analyzed the effect of a spermine on the cleavage of chromogenic substrates and of human TSLP. We observed no effect by spermine on the cleavage of a low molecular weight chromogenic substrate, which contains no positive patch; however, a potent effect by spermine on the cleavage of human TSLP was observed (Figure 5b,c). This latter potent inhibitory effect by spermine on the cleavage of a positively charged substrate indicates that the interaction between a positively charged substrate and the enzyme, with its attached negatively charged heparin, is inhibited by the presence of a positively charged molecule like spermine, which supports the role of a positive patch on the substrate for the targeting by the tryptase.

Upon detailed analysis of a panel of tryptases and a panel of MC chymases, we also observed a striking difference. In a region just C-terminally of the asparagine of the catalytic triad, there were several positively charged residues in all the chymases, whereas in all tryptases this region was negatively charged (Figure 6a). To test the possibility that this region was responsible for guiding positively charged substrates into the mouth of the tryptase, we produced wt and mutant human tryptase, where the mutant had two of the negatively charged amino acids of the tryptases exchanged for the corresponding positively charged residues of the chymases (Figure 6a). Interestingly, both wt and mutant enzymes were equally active against both chromogenic substrates and on human TSLP, indicating that these residues had nothing to do with the selectivity for positively charged substrates (Figure 6c,d). This adds additional support for the idea that it is not the enzyme itself but heparin that is the prime reason for this selectivity, as there are no other regions with strong negative charge on the enzyme.

In addition to targets with a positive patch, proteins that have unstructured regions and are therefore more accessible to enter the tetramer may still be cleaved, as seen for fibrinogen, where only the relatively unstructured ends were cleaved (Figure 5d,e).

Many of the potential targets identified for the human tryptase are actually also small peptide hormones, like vasoactive intestinal peptide (VIP) and several airway neuropeptides [1,35,36]. These may more easily enter the tetramer (Figure 1e).

When we look at the panel of cytokines cleaved by the two MC enzymes, one striking feature appears; these two enzymes together cleave several of the most potent TH2 promoting cytokines, including IL-18, IL-33, and TSLP (Table 1). This finding indicates that these MC enzymes have a prominent role in dampening a TH2 driven inflammation, and inflammation at least partly is initiated by the same cells, namely MCs and basophils. This points towards a negative feedback loop by these enzymes on a TH2 dependent inflammatory response.

Table 1. Summary of the results from the cleavage analysis of cytokines and chemokines by the human and mouse tryptases and the hMC chymase (HC).

Cytokine	hTryp.	M6	HC	Cytokine	hTryp.	M6	HC
IL-4	−	−	−	IL-1α	−	−	
IL-5	−	−	−	IL-1β	−	−	−
IL-10	−	−	−	IL-1RA	+		
TSLP	++++	−	+	IL-33	−	+	++++
IL-13	−	+++	+	IL-18	−		+++
SCF	−	−	−	IGF-1	−	++++	
IL-3	−	−	+	IGF-2	−		
IL-31	−	−	−	HGF	−		
GM-CSF	−	+	−	IL-8	++		
M-CSF	−	−		IP-10	−	++++	−
G-CSF	−	−	−	MCP-1	−	+	−
TGF-β3	−			MCP-2	−		−
TNF-α	−	−	−	MCP-3	++++		−
IL-6	−	+	++	RANTES	−	−	−
IL-11	−	+	+	SDF-1α	−	++	−
LIF	−	−	+	SDF-1β	+	−	−
IL-2	−	−	−	EGF	−	−	−
IFN-γ	+++	+	+	MIP-1α	−	−	-
IL-15	−	−	++++	flt3L	−	+	++
IL-12	−		−	FGF-9	−		
IL-20	+	−	−	FGF-19	−		
IL-7	+	+	−	BMP-14	−		
IL-21	++++	++++	−	GAL-7H	−		
IL-16	−	−		pF4V1	−		
VEGF-A	+	++++	−	IL-25	−	−	−
VEGF-121	−			IL-9	−	++++	
PDGF-A	−	+	−	MIP-3a	−	++++	
PDGF-B	−	+++	−	MIP-3b	++++	++++	
BMP-2	−			Eotaxin	+++	++++	
CTGF	++		+	IL-27A	−		-
FGF-1	+	−	+	IL17C	−	++++	
FGF-2	−	+	+	NGF-β	−	−	
IL-17A	+	−	−	TPO	−	+	
IL-17F	+	+	−	GRO-a	−	−	
IL-22	−	−	−	GRO-b	−	−	
CD40L	−	+	−	MIP-1b	−	−	
BAFF	−		+				
IL-19	−	−	−				
sIL-6R	−						
CNTF	−						

All the results concerning the MC chymase originate from an earlier study [17]. The analysis is based on the SDS-PAGE analysis in Figures 2 and 3. (−) no cleavage activity was observed. (+) showed minor activity, (++) and (+++) partial cleavage. (++++) complete or almost complete cleavage by the enzyme.

In a parallel project, we have been working on the development of therapeutic vaccines against allergy, and there focused on a few early TH2-inducing cytokines as potential targets for an allergy vaccine [37–39]. Interestingly, both of these projects have resulted in the identification of the same three cytokines, TSLP, IL-18, and IL-33 (Figures 2, 3 and 7). The interest for these early TH2-inducing cytokines from completely different origins does, in our mind, strongly favor a role of the MC proteases to limit excessive TH2-driven inflammation by cleavage, and thereby inactivation, of several of these early TH2-promoting inflammatory cytokines (Figure 7). The MC proteases may thereby act as a negative feedback loop to regulate the inflammation partly initiated by the same cell.

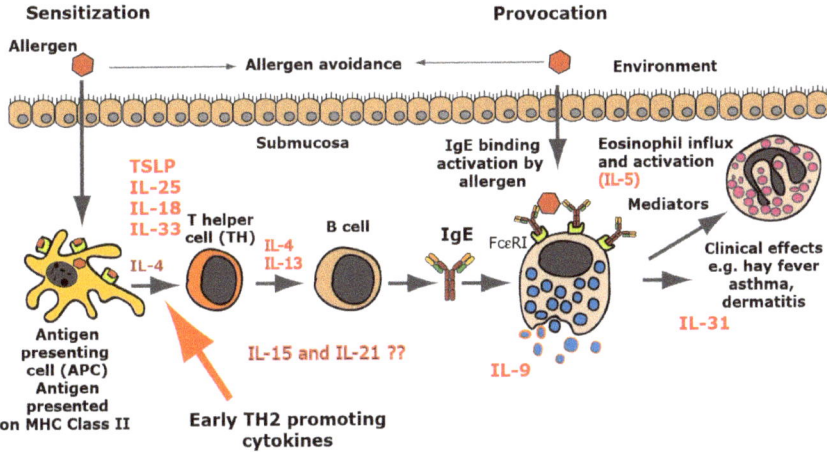

Figure 7. TH2-inducing cytokines in allergy development. A number of cytokines have been shown to be potent inducers of TH2-mediated immunity. The most well characterized are thymic stromal lymphopoietin (TSLP), IL-33, IL-18, IL-25, and IL-4. IL-18 has been shown to be a potent inducer of TH2-mediated immunity when present alone and not in combination with IL-12. Interestingly when present together with IL-12, IL-18 acts instead as an enhancer of TH1-mediated immunity [40]. IL-4 and IL-13 are the only two cytokines known to induce isotype switching in B cells to IgE [41]. IL-5 is important for eosinophil infiltration activation and proliferation, and IL-31 acts as an inducer of itch in skin with atopic dermatitis. IL-9 is, in mice, an inducer of mucosal mast cell differentiation [42]. Both IL-15 and IL-21 have been found to have TH2-promoting activity as described in the text. Cleavage of the TH2-initiating early cytokines would most likely result in a dampening effect on TH2-mediated immunity.

We also observed efficient cleavage of IL-15 by the HC and of IL-21, MCP3, and eotaxin by the tryptase, indicating an even broader anti-inflammatory effect of these two MC enzymes, when they act together. IL-15 is an important cytokine for NK cell activation, and cleavage of this cytokine by the chymase can thereby also have a dampening effect on NK cell activity [43]. However, and interestingly, Il-15 has been shown to enhance TH2 immunity and blocking IL-15 has been shown to prevent the induction of allergen-specific T cells and allergic inflammation in vivo, indicating that IL-15 can also act as a potent TH2-promoting cytokine [21,22]. IL-21, which was also efficiently cleaved by the tryptase, has been shown to downregulate TH1-mediated immunity, indicating that it may act as a TH2 cytokine [23]. HC and the human tryptase thereby seem to act together in a potential negative feedback loop on TH2-mediated immunity by cleavage of TSLP, IL18, IL-33, IL-15, and IL-21. The potent cleavage of two of the most important chemokines for eosinophil and basophil influx into an area of inflammation, eotaxin and MCP3, further supports the role of these two enzymes in controlling excessive TH2 immunity.

Several studies on the potential role of these enzymes or cytokines in vivo have been performed, which gives strong support the role of these mast cell proteases in controlling excessive TH2 immunity. One very important study is a study of the mouse counterpart of the human mast cell chymase, mMCP-4. Knock out of mMCP-4 shows a strong effect on both sensitization and IgE levels [14]. This study gives a strong indication that the cleavage of IL-33 and potentially also IL-18 and IL-15 by mMCP-4 is important for the control of excessive TH2-mediated immunity in mice and most likely also in humans. Two important studies on the effect of blocking IL-15 in vivo have also been published [21,22]. Blocking IL-15 in vivo has been shown to prevent the induction of allergen-specific T cells and allergic inflammation, which further substantiates the effect of reducing the levels of these cytokines on allergic sensitization. Also, IL-21 has been shown in vivo to act as a TH2 cytokine by suppressing the induction of a TH1 response [23]. There are a number of important in vivo studies that support the role of these enzymes in regulating TH2 immunity by cleavage and thereby reduction in the in vivo levels of these selected cytokines and thereby on allergic sensitization. What also is remarkable is the high selectivity of the HC and human tryptase on these TH2 cytokines and almost no effect on the majority of all the other cytokines or chemokines tested.

Interestingly, concerning the roles of MC proteases in cytokine regulation, is the fact that human TSLP was degraded but not mouse TSLP, indicating different functions between different species. A similar phenomenon was seen in our previous analysis of the HC. Here, the human enzyme was seen not to cleave the inflammatory cytokine TNF-α, which is in marked contrast to its mouse counterpart mMCP-4, which efficiently cleaves mouse TNF-α [8,17]. This clearly indicates that the targets may vary quite extensively between relatively closely related species, but that the effects may still be quite similar, in this case an anti-inflammatory effect. The same was seen for the mouse and human tryptases. Both efficiently cleaved IL-21, MIP-3B, and eotaxin; however, they differ in the cleavage of two other TH2 cytokines. The human tryptase cleaves TSLP, whereas mMCP-6, the mouse tryptase, instead cleaves IL-13 (Figures 2 and 3). Both of these cytokines are important TH2 cytokines whose effect may be similar even if some of the targets may differ.

In summary, our analysis of this broad panel of 69 different active human cytokines and chemokines for their sensitivity to cleavage by the human MC tryptase showed a remarkably restrictive cleavage. Only five out of 69 were efficiently cleaved. This is together with the knowledge that the HC has previously been shown to be highly selective in its cleavage of cytokines and chemokines, and together they act on a few inflammatory cytokines including several of the most prominent TH2-inducing cytokines, IL-18, IL-33, TSLP, IL-21, and IL-15. These findings concerning the potent activity on TH2-inducing cytokines by these two prominent MC enzymes needs to be taken into careful consideration when studying the effects of protease inhibitors targeting chymase or tryptase in allergy treatment. Interestingly, the mouse counterpart of the human tryptase, mMCP-6, was almost as restrictive in its cleavage. It also cleaved almost all the cytokines and chemokines cleaved by the human enzyme, except TSLP. However, to compensate for this loss in activity on TSLP, mMCP-6 instead cleaves two other important TH2 cytokines, IL-13 and IL-9.

4. Materials and Methods

4.1. Enzymes and other Reagents

The recombinant human tryptase was purchased from Promega Biotech (Madison, WI, USA). This enzyme was expressed in a fungal (*Pichia pastoris*) expression system. Purified human fibrinogen (natural human) and fibronectin (from human plasma) were purchased from Abcam (Cambridge, UK) and Gibco-Life Technologies (Frederick MD, USA), respectively. Spermine was purchased from Sigma Aldrich (S3236) (Saint Louis, MO, USA). mMCP-6, the human and opossum chymases, and the wt and mutant human tryptase were produced in the mammalian cell line HEK293-EBNA with the vector pCEP-Pu2 according to previously published procedures [44–46]. The coding regions for full-length enzymes containing an N-terminal 6-histidine purification tag were order as designer genes from Genscript (Piscataway, NJ, USA), and the proteins were purified from conditioned media from transfected HEK293-EBNA cells on Ni-chelating IMAC agarose (Qiagen, Hilden, Germany).

Recombinant Human and Mouse Cytokines and Chemokines

Sixty-six recombinant human (rh) cytokines and chemokines, and 56 mouse cytokines and chemokines were purchased from Immuno Tools (Friesoythe, Germany). rhIL-25 from R&D systems

(Abingdon, UK) rhIL-18 from MBL (MBL International, Woburn, MA, USA), rhIL-33 from GIBCO (Invitrogen Corporation, Camarillo, CA, USA).

4.2. Analysis of the Sensitivity to Cleavage by the Recombinant Human and Mouse Tryptase

The cytokines and chemokines were dissolved in PBS or sterile water, according to the recommendations of the supplier (Immuno Tools, Friesoythe, Germany), to get an approximate concentration of 0.13 µg/µL. Subsequently, 9 µL (~1.2 µg) of the cytokine was mixed with 2 µL of the recombinant human tryptase (~13 ng) or in-house produced mMCP-6 and incubated for 2.5 h at 37 °C. Two µL of PBS was used as control. The cleavage was performed in 1× PBS at pH 7.3. After incubation, the reactions were stopped with the addition of 3 µL of 4x sample buffer. Half a microliter of β-mercaptoethanol was then added to each sample followed by heating for 7 min at 85 °C. The reaction mixtures were then analyzed on 4–12% precast SDS-PAGE gels (Novex, Invitrogen, Camarillo, CA, USA). To visualize the proteins, the gels were stained overnight in colloidal Coomassie staining solution and destained with 25% (*v/v*) methanol in ddH$_2$O for 4 h [47]. The analysis was completely repeated and the result was identical between the two independent experiments.

4.3. Analysis of the Cleavage of Human Fibrinogen and Fibronectin

Human fibronectin: 6 µg per lane was cleaved with three different enzymes for 30 min at 37 °C, with the following amounts of enzyme: human tryptase 136 ng, HC 272 ng and the opossum chymase 500 ng. Human fibrinogen: 4 µg per lane was cleaved with three different enzymes for 30 min at 37 °C, with the following amounts of enzyme, human tryptase 136 ng, HC 136 ng, and opossum chymase 500 ng. After incubation, the reactions were stopped with the addition of 3 µL of 4× sample buffer. Half a microliter of β-mercaptoethanol was then added to each sample followed by heating for 7 min at 85 °C. The reaction mixtures were then analyzed on 4–12% precast SDS-PAGE gels (Novex, Invitrogen, Camarillo, CA, USA). To visualize the proteins, the gels were stained overnight in colloidal Coomassie staining solution and destained with 25% (*v/v*) methanol in ddH$_2$O for 4 h [47].

Author Contributions: Conceptualization, Z.F., S.A. and L.H.; Investigation, Z.F., S.A. Data curation, Z.F., S.A. and L.H.; Funding acquisition, Supervision and Writing original draft, L.H.; Language editing M.T.

Funding: This study was supported by the Knut and Alice Wallenberg Foundation (KAW 2017-0022).

Conflicts of Interest: The authors declare no conflict of interest.

References

1. Hallgren, J.; Pejler, G. Biology of mast cell tryptase. An inflammatory mediator. *Febs. J.* **2006**, *273*, 1871–1895. [CrossRef]
2. Korkmaz, B.; Moreau, T.; Gauthier, F. Neutrophil elastase proteinase 3, cathepsin G: Physicochemical properties activity physiopathological functions. *Biochimie* **2008**, *90*, 227–242. [CrossRef]
3. Pejler, G.; Rönnberg, E.; Waern, I.; Wernersson, S. Mast cell proteases: Multifaceted regulators of inflammatory disease. *Blood* **2010**, *115*, 4981–4990. [CrossRef]
4. Caughey, G.H. Mast cell proteases as protective and inflammatory mediators. *Single Mol. Single Cell Seq.* **2011**, *716*, 212–234.
5. Hellman, L.; Thorpe, M. Granule proteases of hematopoietic cells, a family of versatile inflammatory mediators – an update on their cleavage specificity, in vivo substrates, and evolution. *Boil. Chem.* **2014**, *395*, 15–49. [CrossRef]
6. Schwartz, L.B.; Irani, A.M.; Roller, K.; Castells, M.C.; Schechter, N.M. Quantitation of histamine, tryptase, and chymase in dispersed human T and TC mast cells. *J. Immunol.* **1987**, *138*, 2611–2615.
7. Galli, S.J.; Starkl, P.; Marichal, T.; Tsai, M. Mast cells and IgE in defense against venoms: Possible "good side" of allergy? *Allergol. Int.* **2016**, *65*, 3–15. [CrossRef]
8. Piliponsky, A.M.; Chen, C.C.; Rios, E.J.; Treuting, P.M.; Lahiri, A.; Abrink, M.; Pejler, G.; Tsai, M.; Galli, S.J. The chymase mouse mast cell protease 4 degrades TNF, limits inflammation, and promotes survival in a model of sepsis. *Am. J. Pathol.* **2012**, *181*, 875–886. [CrossRef]

9. Mizutani, H.; Schechter, N.; Lazarus, G.; Black, R.A.; Kupper, T.S. Rapid and specific conversion of precursor interleukin 1 beta (IL-1 beta) to an active IL-1 species by human mast cell chymase. *J. Exp. Med.* **1991**, *174*, 821–825. [CrossRef]
10. Omoto, Y.; Tokime, K.; Yamanaka, K.; Habe, K.; Morioka, T.; Kurokawa, I.; Tsutsui, H.; Yamanishi, K.; Nakanishi, K.; Mizutani, H. Human mast cell chymase cleaves pro-IL-18 and generates a novel and biologically active IL-18 fragment. *J. Immunol.* **2006**, *177*, 8315–8319. [CrossRef]
11. Longley, B.J.; Tyrrell, L.; Ma, Y.; Williams, D.A.; Halaban, R.; Langley, K.; Lu, H.S.; Schechter, N.M. Chymase cleavage of stem cell factor yields a bioactive, soluble product. *Proc. Natl. Acad. Sci. USA* **1997**, *94*, 9017–9021. [CrossRef]
12. Guillabert, A.; Wittamer, V.; Bondue, B.; Godot, V.; Imbault, V.; Parmentier, M.; Communi, D. Role of neutrophil proteinase 3 and mast cell chymase in chemerin proteolytic regulation. *J. Leukoc. Boil.* **2008**, *84*, 1530–1538. [CrossRef]
13. Gela, A.; Kasetty, G.; Jovic, S.; Ekoff, M.; Nilsson, G.; Mörgelin, M.; Kjellstrom, S.; Pease, J.E.; Schmidtchen, A.; Egesten, A. Eotaxin-3 (CCL26) exerts innate host defense activities that are modulated by mast cell proteases. *Allergy* **2015**, *70*, 161–170. [CrossRef]
14. Waern, I.; Lundequist, A.; Pejler, G.; Wernersson, S. Mast cell chymase modulates IL-33 levels and controls allergic sensitization in dust-mite induced airway inflammation. *Mucosal Immunol.* **2013**, *6*, 911–920. [CrossRef]
15. Roy, A.; Ganesh, G.; Sippola, H.; Bolin, S.; Sawesi, O.; Dagälv, A.; Schlenner, M.S.; Feyerabend, T.; Rodewald, R.H.; Kjellén, L.; et al. Mast cell chymase degrades the alarmins heat shock protein 70, biglycan, HMGB1, and interleukin-33 (IL-33) and limits danger-induced inflammation. *J. Biol. Chem.* **2014**, *289*, 237–250. [CrossRef]
16. Pang, L.; Nie, M.; Corbett, L.; Sutcliffe, A.; Knox, A.J. Mast cell beta-tryptase selectively cleaves eotaxin and RANTES and abrogates their eosinophil chemotactic activities. *F1000 Post Publ. Peer Rev. Biomed. Lit.* **2006**, *176*, 3788–3795.
17. Fu, Z.; Thorpe, M.; Alemayehu, R.; Roy, A.; Kervinen, J.; De Garavilla, L.; Abrink, M.; Hellman, L. Highly selective cleavage of cytokines and chemokines by the human mast cell chymase and neutrophil cathepsin G. *J. Immunol.* **2017**, *198*, 1474–1483. [CrossRef]
18. Le, Q.T.; Lyons, J.J.; Naranjo, A.N.; Olivera, A.; Lazarus, A.R.; Metcalfe, D.D.; Milner, J.D.; Schwartz, L.B. Impact of naturally forming human alpha/beta-tryptase heterotetramers in the pathogenesis of hereditary alpha-tryptasemia. *J. Exp. Med.* **2019**, *216*, 2348–2361. [CrossRef]
19. Hallgren, J.; Karlson, U.; Poorafshar, M.; Hellman, L.; Pejler, G.; Martinsson, J.H. Mechanism for activation of mouse mast cell tryptase: Dependence on heparin and acidic pH for formation of active tetramers of mouse mast cell protease 6†. *Biochemistry* **2000**, *39*, 13068–13077. [CrossRef]
20. Pereira, P.J.; Bergner, A.; Macedo-Ribeiro, S.; Huber, R.; Matschiner, G.; Fritz, H.; Sommerhoff, C.P.; Bode, W. Human beta-tryptase is a ring-like tetramer with active sites facing a central pore. *Nature* **1998**, *392*, 306–311. [CrossRef]
21. Rückert, R.; Herz, U.; Paus, R.; Ungureanu, D.; Pohl, T.; Renz, H.; Bulfone-Paus, S. IL-15-IgG2b fusion protein accelerates and enhances a Th2 but not a Th1 immune response in vivo, while IL-2-IgG2b fusion protein inhibits both. *Eur. J. Immunol.* **1998**, *28*, 3312–3320. [CrossRef]
22. Rückert, R.; Brandt, K.; Braun, A.; Hoymann, H.-G.; Herz, U.; Budagian, V.; Dürkop, H.; Renz, H.; Bulfone-Paus, S. Blocking IL-15 prevents the induction of allergen-specific T cells and allergic inflammation in vivo. *J. Immunol.* **2005**, *174*, 5507–5515. [CrossRef] [PubMed]
23. Wurster, A.L.; Rodgers, V.L.; Satoskar, A.R.; Whitters, M.J.; Young, D.A.; Collins, M.; Grusby, M.J. Interleukin 21 is a T helper (Th) cell 2 cytokine that specifically inhibits the differentiation of naive Th cells into interferon gamma-producing Th1 cells. *J. Exp. Med.* **2002**, *196*, 969–977. [CrossRef] [PubMed]
24. Niles, A.L.; Maffitt, M.; Haak-Frendscho, M.; Wheeless, C.J.; Johnson, D.A. Recombinant human mast cell tryptase beta: Stable expression in Pichia pastoris and purification of fully active enzyme. *Biotechnol. Appl. Biochem.* **1998**, *28*, 125–131. [PubMed]
25. Doolittle, R.F. Structural basis of the fibrinogen-fibrin transformation: Contributions from X-ray crystallography. *Blood Rev.* **2003**, *17*, 33–41. [CrossRef]

26. Schwartz, L.B.; Bradford, T.R.; Littman, B.H.; Wintroub, B.U. The fibrinogenolytic activity of purified tryptase from human lung mast cells. *J. Immunol.* **1985**, *135*, 2762–2767.
27. Kaminska, R.; Helisalmi, P.; Harvima, R.J.; Horsmanheimo, M.; Harvima, I.T.; Naukkarinen, A. Focal Dermal–epidermal separation and fibronectin cleavage in basement membrane by human mast cell tryptase. *J. Investig. Dermatol.* **1999**, *113*, 567–573. [CrossRef]
28. Im, E.; Chung, K.C. Precise assembly and regulation of 26S proteasome and correlation between proteasome dysfunction and neurodegenerative diseases. *BMB Rep.* **2016**, *49*, 459–473. [CrossRef]
29. Vanderlinden, R.T.; Hemmis, C.W.; Yao, T.; Robinson, H.; Hill, C.P. Structure and energetics of pairwise interactions between proteasome subunits RPN2, RPN13, and ubiquitin clarify a substrate recruitment mechanism. *J. Boil. Chem.* **2017**, *292*, 9493–9504. [CrossRef]
30. Chahal, G.; Thorpe, M.; Hellman, L. The importance of exosite interactions for substrate cleavage by human thrombin. *PLoS ONE* **2015**, *10*, e0129511. [CrossRef]
31. Forsberg, E.; Pejler, G.; Ringvall, M.; Lunderius, C.; Tomasini-Johansson, B.; Kusche-Gullberg, M.; Eriksson, I.; Ledin, J.; Hellman, L.; Kjellén, L. Abnormal mast cells in mice deficient in a heparin-synthesizing enzyme. *Nature* **1999**, *400*, 773–776. [CrossRef]
32. Pejler, G.; Sadler, J.E. Mechanism by which heparin proteoglycan modulates mast cell chymase activity†. *Biochemistry* **1999**, *38*, 12187–12195. [CrossRef]
33. Tchougounova, E.; Forsberg, E.; Angelborg, G.; Kjellén, L.; Pejler, G. Altered processing of fibronectin in mice lacking heparin. a role for heparin-dependent mast cell chymase in fibronectin degradation. *J. Biol. Chem.* **2001**, *276*, 3772–3777. [CrossRef]
34. Tchougounova, E. Regulation of extravascular coagulation and fibrinolysis by heparin-dependent mast cell chymase. *FASEB J.* **2001**, *15*, 2763–2765. [CrossRef]
35. Caughey, G.H.; Leidig, F.; Viro, N.F.; A Nadel, J. Substance P and vasoactive intestinal peptide degradation by mast cell tryptase and chymase. *J. Pharmacol. Exp. Ther.* **1988**, *244*, 133–137.
36. Tam, E.K.; Caughey, G.H. Degradation of airway neuropeptides by human lung tryptase. *Am. J. Respir. Cell Mol. Boil.* **1990**, *3*, 27–32. [CrossRef]
37. Hellman, L. Regulation of IgE homeostasis, and the identification of potential targets for therapeutic intervention. *Biomed. Pharmacother.* **2007**, *61*, 34–49. [CrossRef]
38. Hellman, L. Therapeutic vaccines against IgE-mediated allergies. *Expert Rev. Vaccines* **2008**, *7*, 193–208. [CrossRef]
39. Lei, Y.; Boinapally, V.; Zoltowska, A.; Adner, M.; Hellman, L.; Nilsson, G. Vaccination against IL-33 inhibits airway hyperresponsiveness and inflammation in a house dust mite model of asthma. *PLoS ONE* **2015**, *10*, e0133774. [CrossRef]
40. Nakanishi, K. Unique action of interleukin-18 on T cells and other immune cells. *Front. Immunol.* **2018**, *9*, 763. [CrossRef]
41. Punnonen, J.; Aversa, G.; Cocks, B.G.; McKenzie, A.N.; Menon, S.; Zurawski, G.; Malefyt, R.D.W.; De Vries, J.E. Interleukin 13 induces interleukin 4-independent IgG4 and IgE synthesis and CD23 expression by human B cells. *Proc. Natl. Acad. Sci. USA* **1993**, *90*, 3730–3734. [CrossRef]
42. Miller, H.R.; Wright, S.H.; Knight, P.A.; Thornton, E.M. A novel function for transforming growth factor-beta1: Upregulation of the expression and the IgE-independent extracellular release of a mucosal mast cell granule-specific beta-chymase, mouse mast cell protease-1. *Blood* **1999**, *93*, 3473–3486. [CrossRef]
43. Waldmann, T.A.; Tagaya, Y. The multifaceted regulation of interleukin-15 expression and the role of this cytokine in NK cell differentiation and host response to intracellular pathogens 1. *Annu. Rev. Immunol.* **1999**, *17*, 19–49. [CrossRef]
44. Vernersson, M. Generation of therapeutic antibody responses against IgE through vaccination. *FASEB J.* **2002**, *16*, 875–877. [CrossRef]
45. Reimer, J.M.; Enoksson, M.; Samollow, P.B.; Hellman, L. Extended substrate specificity of opossum chymase—Implications for the origin of mast cell chymases. *Mol. Immunol.* **2008**, *45*, 2116–2125. [CrossRef]

46. Andersson, M.K.; Enoksson, M.; Gallwitz, M.; Hellman, L. The extended substrate specificity of the human mast cell chymase reveals a serine protease with well-defined substrate recognition profile. *Int. Immunol.* **2009**, *21*, 95–104. [CrossRef]
47. Neuhoff, V.; Arold, N.; Taube, D.; Ehrhardt, W. Improved staining of proteins in polyacrylamide gels including isoelectric focusing gels with clear background at nanogram sensitivity using Coomassie Brilliant Blue G-250 and R-250. *Electrophoresis* **1988**, *9*, 255–262. [CrossRef]

 © 2019 by the authors. Licensee MDPI, Basel, Switzerland. This article is an open access article distributed under the terms and conditions of the Creative Commons Attribution (CC BY) license (http://creativecommons.org/licenses/by/4.0/).

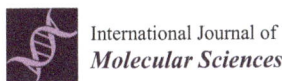

Article

Mouse Tryptase Gene Expression is Coordinately Regulated by GATA1 and GATA2 in Bone Marrow-Derived Mast Cells

Kinuko Ohneda [1,*], Shin'ya Ohmori [1] and Masayuki Yamamoto [2]

1. Department of Pharmacy, Faculty of Pharmacy, Takasaki University of Health and Welfare, Takasaki 370-0033, Japan; omori@takasaki-u.ac.jp
2. Department of Medical Biochemistry, Tohoku University Graduate School of Medicine, Sendai 980-8573, Japan; masiyamamoto@med.tohoku.ac.jp
* Correspondence: kohneda@megabank.tohoku.ac.jp; Tel.: +81-22-274-5990

Received: 16 July 2019; Accepted: 11 September 2019; Published: 17 September 2019

Abstract: Mast cell tryptases have crucial roles in allergic and inflammatory diseases. The mouse tryptase genes represent a cluster of loci on chromosome 16p3.3. While their functional studies have been extensively performed, transcriptional regulation of tryptase genes is poorly understood. In this study, we examined the molecular basis of the tryptase gene expression in bone marrow-derived mast cells (BMMCs) of C57BL/6 mice and in MEDMC-BRC6 mast cells. The expression of the *Tpsb2* and *Tpsg1* genes, which reside at the 3'-end of the tryptase locus, is significantly decreased by the reduction of the GATA transcription factors GATA1 or GATA2. Chromatin immunoprecipitation assays have shown that the GATA factors bind at multiple regions within the locus, including 1.0 and 72.8 kb upstream of the *Tpsb2* gene, and that GATA1 and GATA2 facilitate each other's DNA binding activity to these regions. Deletion of the −72.8 kb region by genome editing significantly reduced the *Tpsb2* and *Tpsg1* mRNA levels in MEDMC-BRC6 cells. Furthermore, binding of CTCF and the cohesin subunit Rad21 was found upstream of the −72.8 kb region and was significantly reduced in the absence of GATA1. These results suggest that mouse tryptase gene expression is coordinately regulated by GATA1 and GATA2 in BMMCs.

Keywords: mast cell; tryptase; gene transcription

---

1. Introduction

Mast cell tryptases are expressed abundantly and are the major component in secretory granules. In humans, elevated levels of tryptase in serum are associated with anaphylaxis [1] and systemic mastocytosis [2]. Mice lacking mast cell tryptase mMCP6 show impaired immunoprotective activity against bacteria [3] and parasite [4] infection, suggesting its important role in host defense.

The genes encoding mast cell tryptase form a cluster of loci on chromosome 16p3.3 and 17A3.3 in humans and mice, respectively. Human tryptase loci contain four genes expressed in mast cells: *TPSG1*, *TPSB2*, *TPSAB1* and *TPSD1*. *TPSG1* encodes γ-tryptase, the only membrane-anchored member of the family. In humans, there are three soluble tryptases—α-, β- (βI, βII and βIII) and δ-tryptase—that are transcribed from three genes, *TPSB2*, *TPSAB1* and *TPSD1*. The βII and βIII isoforms are transcribed from the *TPSB2* gene, whereas the α and βI isoforms are transcribed from the *TPSAB1* gene. In mice, the transcripts from the *Tpsg1*, *Tpsb2* and *Tpsab1* genes are mTMT, mMCP6 and mMCP7, respectively. The mTMT is membrane-anchored, whereas mMCP6 and mMCP7 are soluble tryptases.

A strong linkage disequilibrium has been demonstrated between the *TPSAB1* and *TPSB2* genes, and the expression of these genes is polymorphic [5,6]. In mice, no murine counterpart of the human *TPSD1* gene has been found. Although the overall structure and number of tryptase genes have been well conserved in mammals [7], genomic deletions, mutations and copy number abnormalities are frequently found in both mice and humans [5,8–10]. For instance, the expression of mMCP7 is dependent on strain background and is disrupted in C57BL/6 mice [8]. Recently, germline duplications and triplications in the *TPSAB1* gene have been identified, and an increased copy number of the *TPSAB1* gene leads to an elevated basal serum tryptase concentration, which is associated with multisystem disorders in humans [10].

However, while genetic and functional studies have been extensively performed, transcriptional regulation of tryptase genes is less well defined [11]. A basic helix–loop–helix transcription factor, microphthalmia-associate transcription factor (MITF), was shown to activate the transcription of the *Tpsb2* [12,13], *Tpsab1* [14] and *Tpsg1* [15] genes. Whereas direct binding of MITF to the proximal promoter region was shown for *Tpsb2* and *Tpsg1* [12,15], the *Tpsab1* activation by MITF was mediated by the activation of c-Jun [14]. Regarding the *Tpsb2* activation, polyomavirus enhancer binding protein 2 (PEBP2) physically interacts with MITF and synergistically activates the *Tpsb2* gene transcription [13]. The MITF mRNA and protein levels were recently shown to be reduced upon copper-mediated phosphorylation of MEK1/2 [16].

In addition to MITF, we previously reported that the GATA transcription factors GATA1 and GATA2 are also involved in the tryptase gene regulation [17,18]. We showed that conditional ablation of GATA2 in bone marrow-derived mast cells (BMMCs) resulted in the reduced expression of a number of mast cell-specific genes, including the mast cell tryptase genes *Tpsb2* and *Tpsg1* [18]. In contrast, GATA1-deficient BMMCs unexpectedly exhibited minor phenotypic changes, although a reduction in the expression of *Tpsb2* and *Tpsg1* was also observed [17]. Furthermore, we found a 500-kb region containing seven GATA sites in the 5′ of the tryptase loci at chromosome 17A3.3. This region, referred to as "region A", was bound by both GATA1 and GATA2 in ChIP assays [17]. However, the molecular mechanisms underlying the GATA factor-mediated tryptase gene activation are largely unknown.

In the present study, we investigated how GATA1 and GATA2 regulate tryptase gene expression in BMMCs. Because region A resides at the 5′-end of the locus, we hypothesized that the genes on this locus might be coordinately regulated by the GATA factors.

2. Results

2.1. The Introduction of siRNA Targeting Either GATA1 or GATA2 into BMMCs Leads to a Significant Reduction in Mast Cell Tryptase Gene Expression

To precisely evaluate the contribution of GATA1 and GATA2 to mast cell protease gene expression, siRNA targeting either GATA1 or GATA2 was introduced into BMMCs, and the mRNA levels of mast cell protease genes were assessed by reverse transcription quantitative polymerase chain reaction (qRT-PCR). The introduction of GATA1 and GATA2 siRNAs led to a significant reduction in the corresponding GATA factor expression at both the mRNA and protein levels at 24 h after transfection (Figure 1A,B). In our previous study, the persistent loss of GATA2 led to the dedifferentiation of BMMCs to immature myeloid-like cells with the induction of the myeloid transcription factor C/EBPα [18]. However, at 24 h after siRNA transduction, the C/EBPα mRNA level was not increased by GATA2 ablation (Figure 1C). The MITF mRNA level was moderately but significantly reduced in both GATA1 and GATA2 knockdown cells (Figure 1C). Because the mRNA levels of mast cell proteases at the steady state vary widely, we utilized our previously published RNA sequencing (RNA-seq) data of control BMMCs [18] and checked the reads per kilobase million (RPKM) values of several mast cell proteases (Figure 1D). This revealed that mRNA transcripts from the *Cpa3* gene were the most abundant, followed by those from the *Cma1* and *Tpsb2* genes.

We then examined the mRNA levels of mast cell protease genes at 24 h after GATA1 or GATA2 siRNA transduction (Figure 1E). Consistent with our previous observation in the conditional GATA2 knockout BMMCs [18], the downregulation of GATA2 resulted in a significant reduction in all mast cell protease genes compared to those transfected with the control siRNA (Figure 1E). In contrast, the downregulation of GATA1 did not affect the expression of *Cpa3* or protease genes located on chromosome 14 (*Mcpt4*, *Mcpt8*, *Cma1* and *Ctsg*). In contrast, consistent with our previous findings for GATA1 knockout BMMCs [17], the expression of mast cell tryptases (*Tpsb2* and *Tpsg1*) was significantly reduced in the GATA1 knockdown cells (Figure 1E). These results support our previous conclusion that GATA2 plays a more important role than GATA1 in the regulation of the mast cell gene expression. GATA1 may have a unique role that cannot be compensated for by GATA2 in the regulation of mast cell tryptase genes.

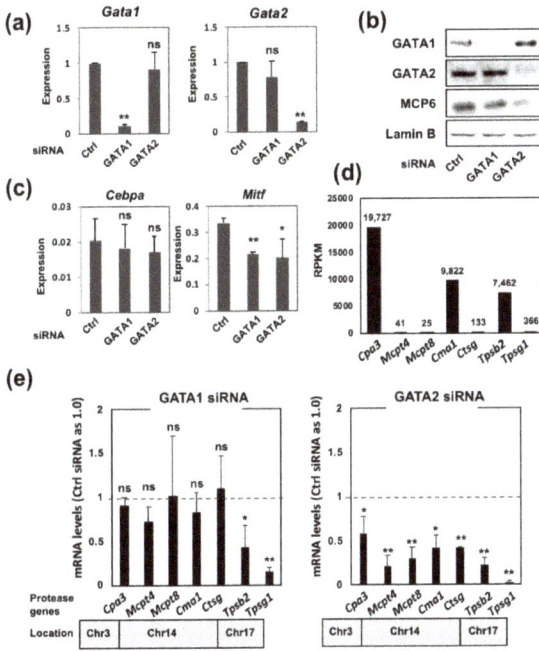

Figure 1. The expression of the mast cell protease gene in the bone marrow-derived mast cells (BMMCs) transfected with either GATA1 or GATA2 siRNA. (**a**) The results of qRT-PCR of GATA1 and GATA2 in the BMMCs transfected with either control, GATA1 or GATA2 siRNA. (**b**) Western blot analyses of GATA1, GATA2, MCP6 and Lamin B (loading control) in the BMMCs transfected with either control, GATA1 or GATA2 siRNA. (**c**) The results of qRT-PCR of C/EBPα and microphthalmia-associate transcription factor (MITF) in the BMMCs transfected with either control, GATA1 or GATA2 siRNA. (**d**) The reads per kilobase million (RPKM) values of mast cell proteases obtained from RNA-seq data of control BMMCs [18]. (**e**) The results of qRT-PCR of mast cell proteases in the BMMCs transfected with the GATA1 or GATA2 siRNAs. The values from the control siRNA-transduced BMMCs were set at 1.0. The bottom bar indicates the localization of protease genes on mouse chromosome. *, $p < 0.05$; **, $p < 0.01$; n.s., not significant. $n = 3$.

2.2. Overexpression of MITF Failed to Restore the Reduced Tpsb2 Transcript Level in the GATA1/GATA2 Double-Knockdown BMMCs

Since the MITF mRNA level was reduced in the GATA factor knockdown cells (Figure 1C), we considered that GATA factors might indirectly regulate the *Tpsb2* gene expression through MITF. The mouse *Mitf* gene is transcribed into multiple RNA species by alternative splicing (Figure 2A). These variants differ in their amino termini and are expressed in cell type-specific manners [19]. RT-PCR using a forward primer specific to each alternative first exon and a common reverse primer set at exon 2 revealed that MITF-A and MITF-MC, transcribed from exons 1a and 1mc, respectively, are expressed in BMMCs (Figure 2B). The mRNA levels of both MITF-A and MITF-MC were reduced in GATA1 or GATA2 knockdown BMMCs, although the reduction of MITF-MC mRNA in the GATA1 knockdown cells was not statistically significant (Figure 2C). Simultaneous knockdown of GATA1 and GATA2 in BMMCs (GATA1/GATA2 KD BMMCs) further decreased the MITF-A and MITF-MC mRNA levels, indicating that GATA1 and GATA2 coordinately regulate the *Mitf* gene expression (Figure 2C). To examine whether or not GATA factors regulate the *Tpsb2* gene expression through MITF, MITF-A or MITF-MC cDNA was overexpressed into the GATA1/GATA2 KD BMMCs, and the transcript level of *Tpsb2* gene was examined by qRT-PCR. To this end, the expression plasmids were constructed by using the bicystronic pIRES2 DsRed-Express2 vector, and MITF-A and MITF-MC protein expression was confirmed by Western blot analysis in 293T cells (Figure 2D). These plasmids were co-transfected with the GATA1 and GATA2 siRNAs, and the cells expressing DsRed were sorted for the analysis. This revealed that the overexpression of neither MITF-A nor MITF-MC cDNA affected the *Tpsb2* transcript level in the GATA1/GATA2 KD BMMCs (Figure 2E). These results suggest that GATA1 and GATA2 activate the *Tpsb2* gene expression independent of MITF.

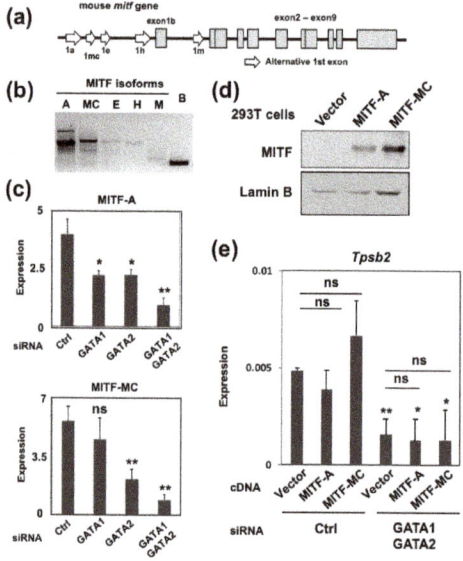

Figure 2. The GATA factor-mediated *Tpsb2* gene repression is independent of MITF. (**a**) A schematic diagram of the mouse MITF gene. Shaded boxes indicate exon 1b and exons 2–8, and open arrows indicate alternative first exons. (**b**) The results of RT-PCR of the MITF isoforms in BMMCs. (**c**) The results of qRT-PCR of MITF-A and MITF-MC isoforms in the BMMCs transfected with the indicated siRNAs. (**d**) Western blot analyses of MITF and Lamin B (loading control) in the 293T cells transfected with either MITF-A or MITF-MC cDNA. (**e**) The results of qRT-PCR of MCP6 in the BMMCs co-transfected with the indicated siRNAs and pIRES2 DsRed-Express2 plasmids. *, $p < 0.05$; **, $p < 0.01$; n.s., not significant. $n = 3$.

2.3. GATA1 and GATA2 Bind to Three Genomic Regions Upstream of the Tpsb2 Gene

To identify cis-acting elements required for the GATA factor-mediated mast cell tryptase gene regulation, we used publicly available ChIP-seq data for GATA2 binding and two histone modifications (H3K27Ac and H3K4me1) that are known to be associated with active enhancers [20,21]. As shown in Figure 3A, several GATA2 binding peaks were observed at the tryptase gene locus on mouse Chr.17A3.3. Some of these peaks were found to overlap with the H3K27Ac and H3K4me1 marks, suggesting that these regions might contribute to the GATA factor-mediated tryptase gene expression. This locus contains six genes (*Prss34*, *Prss28*, *Prss29*, *Tpsab1*, *Tpsb2* and *Tpsg1*) within a region of less than 80 kb. We evaluated the mRNA levels of these genes by qRT-PCR in BMMCs and quantified the relative expression level to that of KIT (Figure 3B). The *Tpsb2* gene was found to be expressed the most abundantly, whereas the *Tpsg1* transcript was detected at a much lower level. Transcripts from the *Prss34*, *Prss28*, *Prss29* and *Tpsab1* genes were undetectable in BMMCs. We named the GATA2 binding peaks of the ChIP-seq data after the distance from the *Tpsb2* gene transcription start site (Figure 3A). Region A, which was bound by GATA1 in our previous report [17], was renamed as the −72.8 kb region in the present study (Figure 3A).

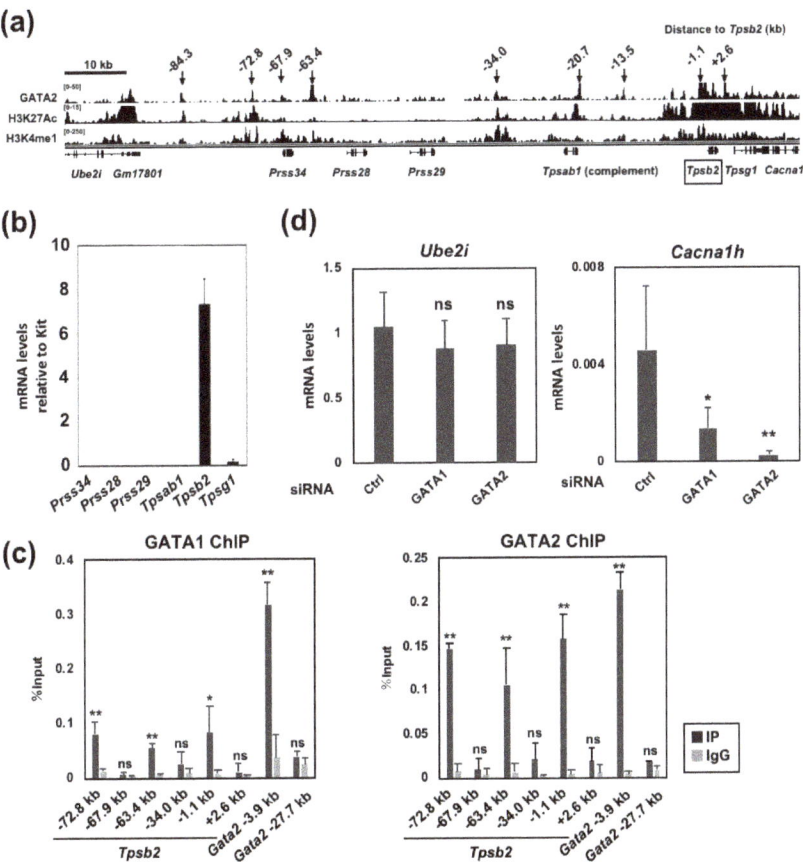

Figure 3. GATA1 and GATA2 bind to multiple regions at the tryptase locus. (**a**) Publicly available ChIP-seq data of the GATA2 binding and the histone modification marks at the tryptase locus in BMMCs [20,21]. The peaks are visualized with the Integrative Genomics Viewer (IGV). (**b**) The results of the qRT-PCR analysis of the genes on mouse chromosome 17A3.3 in BMMCs. The mRNA levels were normalized relative to the level of Kit mRNA. $n = 3$. (**c**) Binding of GATA1 and GATA2 to the tryptase locus was examined by qChIP assays. Chromatin fragments were prepared from wild-type BMMCs. The values of PCR amplicons using immunoprecipitated with an antibody (IP) or the corresponding normal IgG (IgG) relative to those of the input are shown. The regions 3.9 and 27.7 kb upstream of the *Gata2* gene were amplified as positive and negative control regions for GATA2 binding, respectively. In comparison to IgG: *, $p < 0.05$; **, $p < 0.01$; n.s., not significant. $n = 6$. (**d**) The results of qRT-PCR of Ube2i and Cacna1h gene transcript in the BMMCs transfected with the indicated siRNAs. *, $p < 0.05$; **, $p < 0.01$; n.s., not significant. $n = 3$.

To examine whether or not these GATA2 binding regions were also bound by GATA1, qChIP-PCR was performed using either GATA1 or GATA2 antibody (Figure 3C). The −3.9 and −27.7 kb regions of the *Gata2* gene were amplified as positive and negative controls for GATA factor binding, respectively [22]. We found that the −72.8, −63.4 and −1.1 kb regions were bound by GATA2, and their percent input values were similar to that of the *Gata2* −3.9 kb region. GATA1 binding was observed at similar regions, although the percent input values were smaller than that of the *Gata2* −3.9 kb region. The DNA binding of both GATA1 and GATA2 was weak or undetectable at the −67.9, −34.0 and +2.6 kb regions. Although additional peaks of GATA2 binding were observed at −84.3, −20.7 and −13.5 kb in the ChIP-seq data (Figure 3A), the PCR products were not observed despite the use of two different primer sets.

The −72.8 and −1.1 kb regions are localized near the 5′ and 3′ ends of the tryptase gene cluster, respectively (Figure 3A). Both regions are bound by the GATA factors and overlap with the ChIP-seq marks for H3K27Ac and H3K4me1. These observations prompted us to examine whether or not the expression of the genes localized outside of the tryptase gene cluster was also influenced by GATA factors.

Contrary to our hypothesis, the mRNA level of the 5′-neighboring *Ube2i* gene encoding the SUMO-conjugating enzyme UBC9 was not changed in BMMCs treated with either GATA1 or GATA2 siRNA (Figure 3D). In contrast, that of Cacna1h, the 3′ neighboring gene of Tpsg1 encoding a voltage-dependent T-type calcium channel, was significantly decreased in the GATA1 or GATA2 knockdown BMMCs (Figure 3D). These data suggest that the expression of *Cacna1h*, but not *Ube2i*, is regulated by the GATA factors. It is also possible that −72.8 kb region may function as a unidirectional regulatory domain, and the GATA factor binding to this region might affect the expression of downstream (*Tpsb2*, *Tpsg1* and *Cacna1h*), but not upstream (*Ube2i*), genes. Alternatively, although this region is bound by the GATA factors, this region may not have a significant role in gene regulation.

2.4. The GATA2 Binding Activity to the −72.8 kb Region is Reduced by GATA1 Ablation

To further examine the DNA binding specificity of GATA1 and GATA2 to the −72.8 and −1.1 kb regions, we utilized BMMCs prepared from conditional knockout mice of GATA1 (G1KO) and GATA2 (G2KO) and examined whether or not GATA1 and GATA2 affect each other's DNA binding activity to these regions. These mice express *Rosa26CreER^{T2}* gene and their gene recombination is induced by the 4-OHT treatment in BMMCs [17,18]. We previously observed that the Cre-loxP-mediated gene recombination of the GATA1 flox allele takes time, and this is possibly due to the long distance between the two loxP sites (approximately 6.8 kb) [17]. In contrast, the recombination of the GATA2 flox allele, which only excises exon 5 encoding the DNA binding domain, occurs rapidly [18]. The *Kit* −114 kb region was examined as a positive locus for GATA factor binding [17]. The GATA factor binding to the −72.8 and −1.1 kb upstream regions was significantly reduced in the corresponding gene knockout BMMCs, while the residual GATA1 protein might affect the DNA binding activity (Figure 4A,B). Interestingly, the GATA2 binding to the −72.8 and −1.1 kb regions were significantly reduced in the G1KO BMMCs (Figure 4B). In particular, the reduction of GATA2 binding to the −72.8 kb region in the G1KO BMMCs was comparable to that of the G2KO BMMCs. These results indicate that GATA1 is required for the maximal binding activity of GATA2 to the −72.8 and −1.1 kb regions. In contrast to GATA1, GATA2 ablation did not affect the GATA1 binding to the −72.8 kb region (Figure 4A). In contrast, the GATA1 binding activity to the −1.1 kb region was reduced in the G2KO BMMCs, and the percent input value was even less than that in the G1KO BMMCs (Figure 4A). Such cross regulation of the DNA binding activity was not observed at the Kit −114 kb region. (Figure 4A,B).

Taken together, these results indicate that GATA1 and GATA2 affect each other's binding activity to the −72.8 and −1.1 kb regions. In addition, GATA1 might have a critical role in GATA2 binding to the distal −72.8 kb region, whereas GATA2 might be required for GATA1 binding to the proximal −1.1 kb region.

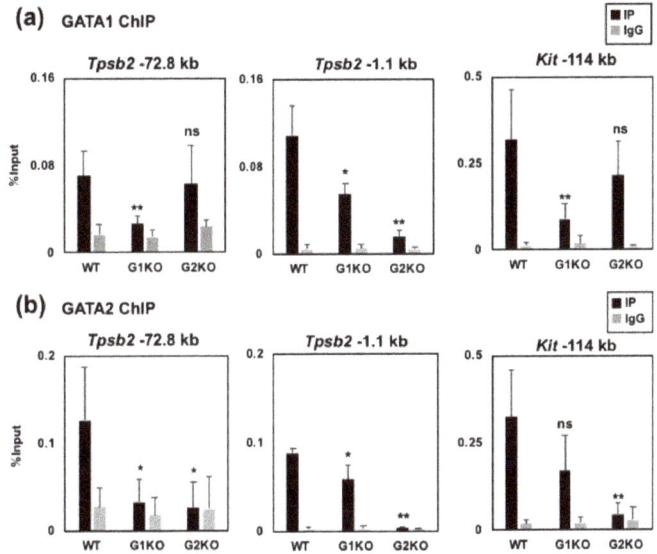

Figure 4. GATA1 and GATA2 affect each other's binding activity to the −72.8 and −1.1 kb regions. (**a**,**b**) Binding of GATA1 (**a**) and GATA2 (**b**) to the −72.8 and −1.1 kb regions was examined by ChIP-qPCR assays. Chromatin fragments were prepared from either wild-type (WT), G1KO, or G2KO BMMCs. The values of PCR amplicons using immunoprecipitated with an antibody (IP) or the corresponding normal IgG (IgG) relative to those of the input are shown. The results were obtained from four independent assays. The region 114 kb upstream of the *Kit* gene was amplified as a positive control region for GATA1 and GATA2 binding. *, $p < 0.05$; **, $p < 0.01$; n.s., not significant. $n = 4$.

2.5. The −72.8 kb Upstream Region of the Tpsb2 Gene is Indispensable for the Expression of the Tpsb2 and Tpsg1 Genes in MEDMC-BRC6 Murine Mast Cells

To determine whether or not the −72.8 kb region contributes to the *Tpsb2* and *Tpsg1* gene expression, this region was deleted using CRISPR/Cas9-mediated genome editing in MEDMC-BRC6 (BRC6) murine mast cells [23]. qRT-PCR analyses showed that transcripts from *Tpsb2* and *Tpsg1* were significantly decreased in the GATA1 or GATA2 knockdown cells (Figure 5A) and increased in the cells transfected with an expression plasmid encoding either GATA1 or GATA2 cDNA (Figure 5B). These results suggest that the expression of these genes was dependent on the GATA factors in BRC6 cells, as observed in BMMCs.

Using CRISPR/Cas9-mediated genome editing, the −72.8 kb region was deleted and replaced with a homologously recombined *PGK-gb2-neo* gene cassette. As a result, we obtained 6 homozygous clones (Δ−72.8 kb) that were used for the qRT-PCR analysis (Figure 5C). The G418 resistant clones in the absence of the −72.8 kb deletion were examined as wild-type controls. The GATA1 and GATA2 mRNA levels were unaffected by the −72.8 kb deletion. Notably, both the *Tpsb2* and *Tpsg1* transcript levels were significantly reduced in the Δ−72.8 kb clones. In contrast, the −72.8 kb deletion did not markedly affect either the *Cpa3* or *Mcpt4* transcript levels, denying any non-specific effects on the mast cell phenotype in the Δ−72.8 kb clones. Interestingly, the transcript level of *Cacna1h*, but not *Ube2i*, was significantly lower in the Δ−72.8 kb clones than in the wild-type clones, as was observed in the GATA factor knockdown BMMCs (Figure 5C). Taken together, these data suggest that the −72.8 kb region is required for the expression of far downstream *Tpsb2*, *Tpsg1* and *Cacna1h* genes, whereas it is dispensable for the upstream *Ube2i* gene expression.

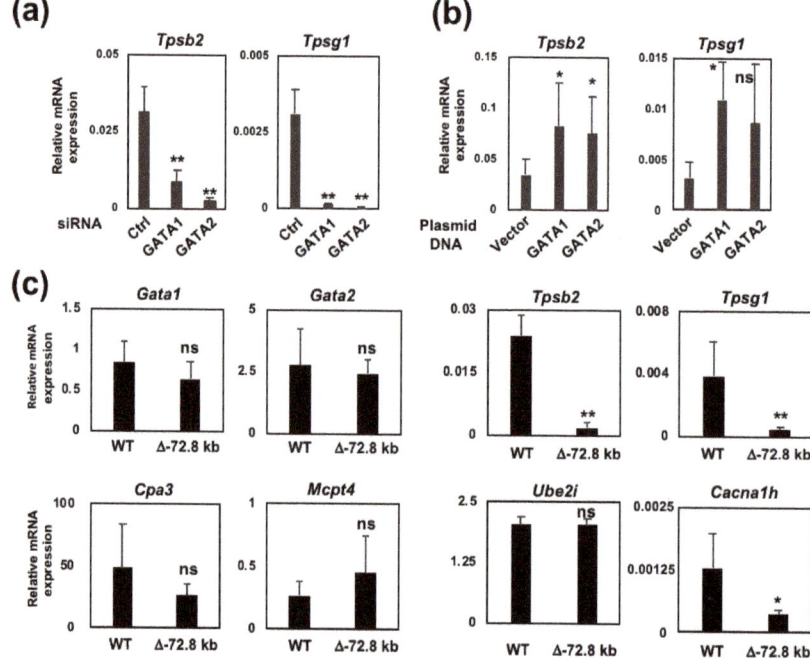

Figure 5. The deletion of the −72.8 kb region reduced the *Tpsb2* and *Tpsg1* gene expression in BRC6 mast cells. (**a,b**) Results of qRT-PCR of the *Tpsb2* and *Tpsg1* gene transcript in BRC6 cells transfected with either control, GATA1 or GATA2 siRNA (**a**) or pEF plasmid DNAs (**b**). In the plasmid transfection, pmaxGFP was co-transfected with pEF plasmid DNAs, and green fluorescent protein (GFP)-positive cells were sorted at 24 h after transfection. (**c**) The results of qRT-PCR of mRNAs transcribed from the indicated genes in genome-edited BRC6 cells. The samples were prepared from undeleted (WT) and homozygous (Δ−72.8 kb) clones. $n = 6$ for each group. *, $p < 0.05$; **, $p < 0.01$; n.s., not significant. $n = 5$.

2.6. GATA1 Regulates the CTCF and Rad21 Binding Activity to the Tryptase Gene Locus

Our data showed that the −72.8 kb region functions as a unidirectional regulatory region for the *Tpsb2* and *Tpsg1* genes, and the GATA2 binding activity to this region is regulated, at least in part, by GATA1. Based on these findings, we surmised that there might be boundary regions that separate the −72.8 kb region and the upstream *Ube2i* gene. Because CTCF is often found in the chromatin domain boundaries [24], we utilized a published ChIP-seq dataset for CTCF binding in BMMCs [20] to visualize the CTCF binding peaks at the tryptase gene locus (Figure 6A). We found three CTCF binding peaks between the −72.8 kb region and the *Ube2i* gene. Additional CTCF binding peaks were observed at −32.4, −2.4 and +7.6 kb upstream of the *Tpsb2* gene.

CTCF often shares DNA binding sites with cohesion, and the CTCF/cohesin complex plays central roles for creating the chromatin boundaries and the loop formation [25]. Our ChIP analysis revealed that the −81.3, −75.9 and −2.4 kb regions (Figure 6A) are bound by both CTCF and the cohesion subunit Rad21 in BMMCs (Figure 6B,C). Surprisingly, the CTCF binding activities at the −81.3, −75.9 and −2.4 kb regions were significantly decreased in the GATA1, but not GATA2, knockout BMMCs (Figure 6B). The Rad21 binding activity to the −81.3 and −75.9 regions was also reduced by GATA1, but not GATA2, ablation, although the reduction at the −2.4 kb region was unaffected in both mice. In summary, these results suggest that GATA1, but not GATA2, can facilitate the CTCF/Rad21 binding to the 5′-boundary regions of the tryptase locus.

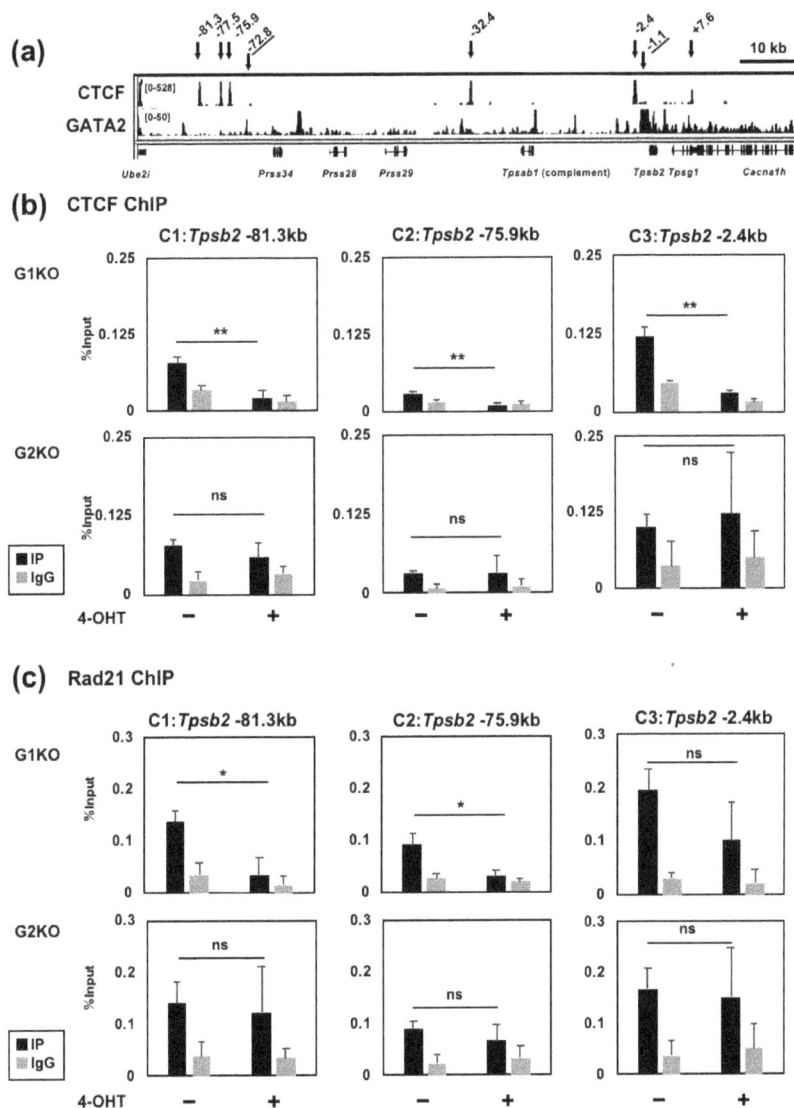

Figure 6. Conditional ablation of GATA1 in BMMCs resulted in a significant reduction in the CTCF binding to the −81.3 and −75.9 kb regions. (**a**) Publicly available ChIP-seq data of the CTCF and GATA2 binding at the tryptase locus in BMMCs. The peaks are visualized with the IGV. (**b**,**c**) Genomic binding of CTCF (**b**) and Rad21 (**c**) to 81.3, 75.9 and 2.4 kb upstream of the *Tpsb2* gene was examined by the ChIP-qPCR assays. Chromatin fragments were prepared from G1KO and G2KO BMMCs cultured either in the presence or absence of 4-OHT. The values of PCR amplicons using immunoprecipitated with an antibody (IP) or the corresponding normal IgG (IgG) relative to those of the input are shown. The results were obtained from four independent assays. *, $p < 0.05$; **, $p < 0.01$; n.s., not significant. $n = 4$.

3. Discussion

In the present study, we investigated the regulation of mouse tryptase gene expression by GATA factors. Our data suggest that the genes encoding mast cell tryptase on mouse chromosome 17A3.3 are coordinately regulated by GATA factors. Within the mouse tryptase gene locus spanning approximately 75 kb, only two genes (*Tpsb2* and *Tpsg1*) were found to be expressed in the BMMCs of C57BL/6 mice. These genes reside next to each other in the 3′-end of the locus. To our surprise, deletion of the −72.8 kb region that resides in the 5′-end of the locus severely affected the expression of *Tpsb2* and *Tpsg1* genes. The −72.8 kb region contains seven classical GATA recognition sequences, (A/T)GATAA, and two of them match the chromatin occupancy sequence for GATA1, (C/G)(A/T)GATAA(G/A/C)(G/A/C), that was reported in previous ChIP-seq studies [26–28]. Of note, deletion of this region affected the expression of the 3′-neighboring *Cacna1h* gene but not the 5′-neighboring *Ube2i* gene. Similar results were also obtained in BMMCs treated with either GATA1 or GATA2 siRNA. The expression of the *Ube2i* gene encoding the SUMO-conjugating enzyme Ubc9 is not mast cell-specific, and its transcript is detected in a variety of tissues [29]. Taken together, these results suggest a possibility that the gene regulatory function of the −72.8 kb region is dependent on the GATA factors and is unidirectional. Further studies that evaluate the expression of other neighboring genes are needed for understanding the function of the −72.8 kb region.

Recently, a chromosome conformation capture (3C) assay and related Hi-C technique reveal that the three-dimensional structure of chromosomes is dynamically regulated, depending on the cell type, stage of development and extracellular condition [30,31]. Eukaryotic chromatin is organized into compartments composed of topologically associating domains (TADs) that are further divided into smaller units termed subTADs [32–35]. TADs and subTADs are critical chromosome structural domains in the regulation of the long-range gene expression. CTCF and cohesion have been shown to play crucial roles in the formation of TADs and subTADs, and their binding sites are often found at the boundary region of TADs [24]. In the mouse tryptase locus, three binding peaks of CTCF residing between the *Ube2i* gene and the −72.8 kb region were found by the ChIP-seq data, and two of them were bound by CTCF and Rad21 in our ChIP analyses. Considering the unidirectional effect of the −72.8 kb region, we speculate that these regions might function as a barrier to prevent the GATA factor-dependent, mast cell-specific gene activation of the *Ube2i* gene. The 3C and Hi-C analyses in combination with deletion of the CTCF or GATA factor binding regions may help clarify the 3D chromosome architecture of the tryptase locus. In addition, whether or not the −72.8 kb region resides in close proximity to the *Tpsb2* and *Tpsg1* promoters due to chromatin looping should be clarified.

Our data indicate that GATA1 plays specific roles that cannot be compensated for by GATA2 in the regulation of mast cell tryptase genes. The ChIP analyses showed that GATA1 ablation significantly reduced the GATA2 binding to the distal −72.8 kb region. Given that deletion of the −72.8 kb region affects the expression of *Tpsb2* and *Tpsg1*, GATA1 might be required for the GATA2-mediated activation of the −72.8 kb region. Notably, ablation of GATA1, but not GATA2, affected the CTCF and Rad21 binding to the −81.3 and −75.9 kb regions. Thus, it is possible that GATA1 facilitates the recruitment of CTCF and cohesin to the 5′-region of the tryptase locus and thereby promotes the formation of active chromatin structure. Interestingly, GATA2 ablation attenuated the GATA1 binding to the proximal −1.1 kb region, whereas the binding to the −72.8 kb was not affected. Thus, GATA2 might have a dominant role in activating the *Tpsb2* and *Tpsg1* promoters.

In erythroid and megakaryocytic cells, the genome-wide DNA binding of GATA1 and GATA2 has been comprehensively studied by ChIP-seq analyses [26–28,36,37]. These studies showed that numerous cell type-specific genes were commonly regulated by both factors. Although these studies defined several unique target genes of either GATA1 or GATA2, the difference between the overlapping and specific target gene regulation has not been clearly defined. GATA1 and its cofactor FOG-1 were shown to be required for looping the β-globin locus control region to the active β-globin promoter [38]. Subsequently, several factors that interact with GATA1, such as Ldb1 [39], BRG1 [40] and SCL/TAL1 [41], have shown to play crucial roles for the chromatin looping formation. These findings suggest that

GATA1 might interact with a specific partner to promote the formation of active chromatin structure in mast cells. Further investigations will be needed in order to define the functional differences between GATA1 and GATA2 in mast cell-specific gene regulation.

An earlier study showed that the expression of tryptase genes in vivo is restricted to a particular cell type or tissue, and each individual gene has a different expression profile [9]. These data seem to be inconsistent with the present data. In this study, we used BMMCs and the mast cell line BRC6, which are not fully differentiated compared to highly differentiated peripheral tissue mast cells. The coordinated gene expression regulation of the entire tryptase locus, that has been shown in this study, might be restricted to immature mast cells. Alternatively, only when the structure of the entire locus is activated can a local gene regulatory system of an individual gene be formed during differentiation. BMMCs can be differentiated to connective tissue-type mast cells by culturing with Swiss 3T3 fibroblasts [42]. This system can be used to determine whether or not the coordinated gene regulation of the tryptase locus is differentiation stage-dependent.

4. Materials and Methods

4.1. Mice

Conditional knockout mice of *Gata1* ($Gata1^{flox/y}$) and *Gata2* ($Gata2^{flox/flox}$) were kindly provided by S. Philipsen (Erasmus MC, Rotterdam, the Netherlands) and S. A. Camper (University of Michigan, Ann Arbor, MI, USA), respectively [43,44]. The knockin mice expressing a 4-hydroxy tamoxifen (4-OHT)-inducible Cre recombinase gene under the control of the Rosa26 promoter (Rosa26CreER^{T2}) were kindly provided by Anton Berns, The Netherlands Cancer Institute. The *Gata1* and *Gata2* knockout phenotype was examined in BMMCs prepared from hemizygous ($Gata1^{-/y}$) and homozygous ($Gata2^{-/-}$) male mice expressing CreER^{T2}. The study was approved by the Animal Experiment Committee of the Takasaki University of Health and Welfare (Kendai1526, 31 Mar 2015, Kendai1601, 1 Apr 2016, Kendai1730, 15 Mar 2017, Kendai1816, 1 Apr 2018 and Kendai1919, 1 Apr 2019). The animal experiments were carried out in accordance with The Guidelines on Animal Experiments in Takasaki University of Health and Welfare, Japanese Government Animal Protection and Management Law (No.105) and Japanese Government Notification on Feeding and Safekeeping of Animals (No.88). The mice were maintained in an animal facility of Takasaki University of Health and Welfare in accordance with institutional guidelines.

4.2. Cell Culture

Bone marrow mononuclear cells isolated from the femurs and tibiae were cultured for two weeks in Roswell Park Memorial Institute (RPMI) 1640 medium supplemented with 10% FBS and penicillin-streptomycin in the presence of 10 ng/mL recombinant murine IL-3 (PeproTech, Rocky Hill, NJ, USA) and subsequently cultured for two weeks with IL-3 and 10 ng/mL recombinant murine stem cell factor (Peprotech). The 293T cells (Thermo Fisher Scientific) were cultured in Dulbecco modified Eagle's medium (DMEM) supplemented with 10% fetal bovine serum (FBS) and penicillin-streptomycin. MEDMC-BRC6 cells [23] were purchased from RIKEN BRC (Tsukuba, Japan) and cultured in Iscove's modified Dulbecco's medium (IMDM; Invitrogen, Thermo Fisher Scientific, Waltham, MA, USA) containing the following: 15% FBS, ITS liquid media supplement (Sigma-Aldrich, St. Louis, MO, USA), 50 mg/mL ascorbic acid (Sigma-Aldrich), 0.45 mM α-monothioglycerol (Sigma-Aldrich), 3 ng/mL IL-3, 30 ng/mL stem cell factor (SCF), 1% penicillin-streptomycin solution and 2 mM L-glutamine (Nacalai Tesque, Kyoto, Japan).

4.3. Transfection of Small Interfering RNA (siRNA) or Plasmid DNA

The siRNA duplexes for mouse GATA1 and GATA2 were purchased from Invitrogen. The control siRNA was purchased from Sigma. In the knockdown experiments, BMMCs (2.0×10^6 cells) were transfected with 200 pmol of siRNA by electroporation using an Amaxa Nucleofector (Lonza, Basel,

Switzerland). Cells were harvested 24 h after transfection and used for the analyses. In the co-expression experiments shown in Figure 2, we generated MITF-A and MITF-MC cDNAs by PCR and cloned them into a bicistronic expression plasmid pIRES2 DsRed-Express2 Vector (Takara Bio USA, Mountain View, CA, USA). BMMCs (2.0×10^6 cells) were transfected with 200 pmol of siRNA and 2.5 μg of plasmid DNA by electroporation, and the cells expressing DsRed were sorted using a FACSJazz cell sorter (BD Biosciences, Franklin Lakes, NJ, USA) at 24 h after transfection. In the plasmid transfection experiments shown in Figure 5B, we used the pEF-BOS [45] expression plasmids GATA1 and GATA2 [46], and pmaxGFP vector (Lonza). pEF plasmids (4 μg; GATA1, GATA2, or empty vector) and 1 μg of pmaxGFP were co-transfected into BRC6 cells by electroporation. At 24 h after transfection, GFP-positive cells were sorted using the cell sorter and used for the analyses.

4.4. Quantitative RT-PCR (qRT-PCR)

Total RNA was isolated from cells using a NucleoSpin RNA II (Macherey-Nagel, Düren, Germany). The reverse transcription reactions were performed using a ReverTra Ace qPCR RT Kit (Toyobo, Osaka, Japan) according to the manufacturer's instructions. Quantitative RT-PCR (qRT-PCR) was performed using the Go Taq qPCR Master Mix (Promega, Madison, WI, USA) and an Mx3000P real-time PCR system (Agilent, Santa Clara, CA, USA), as described previously [47]. The results were normalized to the transcript from the polymerase (RNA) II (DNA directed) polypeptide A (*Polr2a*) gene. The primer sequences used for PCR are shown in Table A1.

4.5. Western Blotting

The whole lysates were prepared as previously described (ref). The samples were resolved by 10% sodium dodecyl sulfate polyacrylamide gel electrophoresis, and the Western blot analyses were performed as described previously [47] using anti-GATA1 (N6; Santa Cruz, Dallas, TX, USA), anti-GATA2 (H-116; Santa Cruz), anti-MCP6 (sc-32474; Santa Cruz), anti-MITF (H-50; Santa Cruz), and anti-lamin B (M-20; Santa Cruz) antibodies.

4.6. Chromatin Immunoprecipitation (ChIP)

A ChIP assay was performed as in a prior report [47] using anti-GATA-1 (N6; Santa Cruz), anti-GATA2 (B9922A; Perseus Proteomics, Tokyo, Japan), anti-CTCF (A300-543A; Bethyl, Montgomery, TX, USA) and anti-Rad21 (Ab992; Abcam, Cambridge, UK) antibodies and normal Rabbit IgG (2729S; Cell Signaling Technology, Danvers, MA, USA) and anti-Rat IgG (sc-2026; Santa Cruz). As described previously, the GATA1 ChIP assay was done using an anti-rat IgG rabbit antibody (Jackson ImmunoResearch, West Grove, PA, USA) as a secondary antibody to precipitate the immune complex [47]. The DNA purified from ChIP samples were amplified was analyzed using an Mx3000P real-time PCR system (Agilent) with the GoTaq qPCR Master Mix (Promega). The primer sequences used are shown in Table A2.

4.7. CRISPR/Cas9 Genome Editing

To delete the −72.8 kb region using the CRISPR/Cas9 system, we used two Cas9 expression plasmids: pSpCas9(BB)-2A-GFP (PX458) and pSpCas9(BB)-2A-Puro (PX459) V2.0. These plasmids were a gift from Feng Zhang (Addgene plasmid #48139 and #48138) [48]. Single-guide RNAs (sgRNAs) targeting the 5' and 3' end of the −72.8 kb region were designed using CRISPRdirect (https://crispr.dbcls.jp). The sgRNA target sequences were synthesized as DNA oligonucleotides, and a pair of annealed oligonucleotides was inserted into either PX458 or PX459 using the golden gate method. To prepare a targeting vector for homologous recombination, the 5' and 3' homology arms were amplified by PCR. The resulting 5' (1.1 kb) and 3' (1 kb) arms and the PGK-gb2-neo template (Gene Bridges, Heidelberg, Germany) were cloned into a pBluescript KS vector (Agilent Technologies). BRC6 cells were co-transfected with 2 μg each of PX458 and PX459 vectors harboring the 5' and 3' gRNAs, respectively, and 1 μg of the targeting plasmid by electroporation using NEPA21 (Nepa Gene,

Chiba, Japan). At 24 h after electroporation, the cells were cultured with 1.0 µg/mL of puromycin for another 24 h, and subsequently, the GFP-positive cells were sorted using a FACSJazz cell sorter into 96-well plates. At 24 h after sorting, G418 was added at a concentration of 1.5 mg/mL, and the cells were cultured for 10 days. The genomic deletion was examined by PCR using genomic DNA isolated with PBND buffer (10 mM Tris-HCl, pH 8.3, 50 mM KCl, 2.5 mM MgCl2, 0.1 mg/mL Gelatin, 0.45% NP-40, 0.45% Tween20 and 20 mg/mL Proteinase K). For homozygous deletion mutants, deletion of the −72.8 kb region was further confirmed by DNA sequencing. The sgRNA target sequences and PCR primers used for the arms are shown in Table A3.

4.8. ChIP-seq Data Processing

The previously described ChIP-seq data sets (GSE48086 and GSE97253) [20,21] were aligned to the mouse genome (mm9 assembly). The data (GATA2, GSM1167578; H3K27Ac, GSM2564722; H3K4me1, GSM2564728; CTCF, GSM1167574) were visualized using the Integrative Genomics Viewer (IGV).

4.9. Statistical Analyses

Comparisons between two groups were made using Student's *t*-test. Data are presented as the means ± standard deviation. For all of the analyses, statistical significance was defined as a *p*-value < 0.05.

Author Contributions: Conceptualization, K.O.; Methodology, K.O. and S.O.; Investigation, K.O. and S.O.; Writing—original draft, K.O.; Writing—review & editing, K.O. and M.Y.; Visualization, K.O. and S.O.; Funding Acquisition, K.O. and S.O.; Resources, S.O., M.Y. and K.O.; Supervision, K.O.

Funding: This work was funded by a Grant-in-Aid for Scientific Research (C) from the Japan Society for the Promotion of Science (grant number 18K06920 to K.O., 17K08643 to S.O.).

Acknowledgments: We thank Yasushi Ishijima, Takuya Ninomiya, Satsuki Hoshikawa, Tatsuya Maruyama, Keiichi Iizuka and Taro Takeuchi for technical assistance.

Conflicts of Interest: The authors declare no conflicts of interest.

Abbreviations

BMMCs	Bone marrow-derived mast cells
ChIP	Chromatin immunoprecipitation
MITF	Microphthalmia-associate transcription factor
RT	Reverse transcription
qPCR	Quantitative polymerase chain reaction
RNA-seq	RNA sequencing
RPKM	reads per kilobase million
ChIP-seq	chromatin immunoprecipitation sequencing
3C	chromosome conformation capture
TAD	topologically associating domains
4-OHT	4-hydroxy tamoxifen
RPMI	Roswell Park Memorial Institute
IMDM	Iscove's modified Dulbecco's medium
FBS	fetal bovine serum
Polr2a	polymerase (RNA) II (DNA directed) polypeptide A
GFP	green fluorescent protein
sgRNA	single-guide RNA
IGV	Integrative Genomics Viewer

Appendix A

Table A1. Primer sequences for qRT-PCR analyses.

Primers for qRT-PCR	Sequences (5′ to 3′)	
	Forward	Reverse
Gata1	CAGAACCGGCCTCTCATCC	TAGTGCATTGGGTGCCTGC
Gata2	GCACCTGTTGTGCAAATTGT	GCCCCTTTCTTGCTCTTCTT
Cebpa	AAAGCCAAGAAGTCGGTGGAC	CTTTATCTCGGCTCTTGCGC
Mitf	GCTGGAGATGCAGGCTAGAG	TGATGATCCGATTCACCAGA
Cpa3	GCTACACATTCAAACTGCCTCCT	GAGAGAGCATCCGTGGCAA
Mcpt4	CATGCTTTGTTGAACCCAAGG	GAAGTGAAAAGCCTGACCTGC
Mcpt8	GTGGGAAATCCCAGTG	GACAACCATACCCCAG
Cma1	CCTGGGTTCCAGCACCAA	GGCGGGAGTGTGGTATGC
Ctsg	GAGTCCAGAAGGGGCTG	GATGGCTCTGAGACAT
Tpsb2	CGACATTGATAATGACGAGCCTC	ACAGGCTGTTTTCCACAATGG
Tpsg1	GGTCACACTGTCTCCCCACT	GCATCCCAGGGTAGAAGTCA
Mitf ex1a	AAGTCGGGGAGGAGTTTCAC	CATCAATTACATCATCCATCTGCATGC
Mitf ex1mc	CGACAAGCTTATGAACCGGCTTTTCCTG	
Mitf ex1e	TCACAGAGGTTAGTAGGTGGATGGG	
Mitf ex1h	GGCGCTTAGATTTGAGATGC	
Mitf ex1m	GAGGACTAAGTGGTCTGCGG	
Mitf ex1b	CCTGAGCTCACCATGTCCAAAC	
Prss34	GCTGATGAAAGTGGTCAAGATCATCCG	AGGAGTGAATGCATCAATATGAGTGGCTG
Prss28	GTACCGTGTTCATGGCCTCT	TGACTTTGGATGCAGTGAGC
Prss29	GTCAAGCTGCCCTCTGAGTC	TGGTTGCCTGCACATAACAT
Tpsab1	ATGACCACCTGATGACTGTGAGCCAG	AGGAACGGAGGTCATCCTGGATGTG
Ube2i	GAGGCTTGTTCAAGCTACGG	GTGATAGCTGGCCTCCAGTC
Cacna1h	CCTTTCTCAGCGTCTCCAAC	GCCACAATGATGTCAACCAG
Polr2a	CTGGACCCTCAAGCCCATACAT	CGTGGCTCATAGGCTGGTGAT

Table A2. Primer sequences for ChIP-qPCR analyses.

Primers		Sequences (5′ to 3′)	
		Forward	Reverse
Tpsb2	−72.8 kb	AACCTTCGACGTGACCTTTG	GGCACAGGATTTGTGAGACC
	−67.9 kb	TCAGTTGGCAGGTTTCTGTG	ACCAGTCAGGGCAAGTTCAC
	−63.4 kb	CTTACTGCTTTGGCCTGGAG	TATGAATTTGGAGGCGATCC
	−34.0 kb	AGCCTCCTAAGGGTCAGAGC	CCGCGATATTATCTGCACCT
	−1.1 kb	GGAGGTCACACTGCAGGATT	AATGGGTAACAGCGTCGTTC
	+2.6 kb	CTTGCCTTCCTTGTCCTCTG	AGAAGAGAGGGAGCCACACA
Gata2	−81.3 kb	GTGAGGCCCATTCAAAAGAA	CTAGGGAACCAGATGCCAAA
	−75.9 kb	GAGGACCCAAGTGAGGTTCA	AGAAGCCCTAGGAGTGAGC
	−2.4 kb	CAGTCCAACTGCACCAACC	CACCCTCAGTTGCCTCCTCA
	−3.9 kb	GAGATGAGCTAATCCCGCTGTA	AAGGCTGTATTTTTCCAGGCC
	−27.7 kb	TGCCATGCCGGATATATTTTG	ACTAGCACGTGTGGCACAGTG
Kit	−114 kb	CGTGCACACAGGTTTGTTTC	TGCTGAGATGTGGCAATAGG

Table A3. Sequences of oligonucleotide used for CRISPR Cas9 genome editing.

Applied Oligonucleotide		Sequences of Oligonucleotide (5′ to 3′)
sgRNAs	5′-fwd	CACCGTCTTACTGTAGATTTAAGC
	5′-rev	AAACGCTTAAATCTACAGTAAGAC
	3′-fwd	CACCGACATTAGAACACTATTAGTA
	3′-rev	AAACTACTAATAGTGTTCTAATGTC
5′ arm	Fwd	TAATGGGCCCACAGGGCCTCATTTTGTAGG
	Rev	ACCGATCGATGCTTAAATCTACAGTAAGAC
3′ arm	Fwd	TATGGGATCCACTACTTTTACACTGCCTCA
	Rev	ACTTGCGGCCGCTACATGTTGGCACAAGCCTG

References

1. Caughey, G.H. Tryptase Genetics and Anaphylaxis. *J. Allergy Clin. Immunol.* **2006**, *117*, 1411–1414. [PubMed]
2. Akin, C.; Soto, D.; Brittain, E.; Chhabra, A.; Schwartz, L.B.; Caughey, G.H.; Metcalfe, D.D. Tryptase Haplotype in Mastocytosis: Relationship to Disease Variant and DiagnostOlic Utility of Total Tryptase Levels. *Clin. Immunol.* **2007**, *123*, 268–271. [CrossRef] [PubMed]
3. Thakurdas, S.M.; Melicoff, E.; Sansores-Garcia, L.; Moreira, D.C.; Petrova, Y.; Stevens, R.L.; Adachi, R. The Mast Cell-Restricted Tryptase mMCP-6 has a Critical Immunoprotective Role in Bacterial Infections. *J. Biol. Chem.* **2007**, *282*, 20809–20815. [CrossRef] [PubMed]
4. Shin, K.; Watts, G.F.; Oettgen, H.C.; Friend, D.S.; Pemberton, A.D.; Gurish, M.F.; Lee, D.M. Mouse Mast Cell Tryptase mMCP-6 is a Critical Link between Adaptive and Innate Immunity in the Chronic Phase of Trichinella Spiralis Infection. *J. Immunol.* **2008**, *180*, 4885–4891. [CrossRef] [PubMed]
5. Trivedi, N.N.; Tamraz, B.; Chu, C.; Kwok, P.Y.; Caughey, G.H. Human Subjects are Protected from Mast Cell Tryptase Deficiency Despite Frequent Inheritance of Loss-of-Function Mutations. *J. Allergy Clin. Immunol.* **2009**, *124*, 1099–1105.e4. [CrossRef]
6. Trivedi, N.N.; Caughey, G.H. Mast Cell Peptidases: Chameleons of Innate Immunity and Host Defense. *Am. J. Respir. Cell Mol. Biol.* **2010**, *42*, 257–267. [CrossRef] [PubMed]
7. Reimer, J.M.; Samollow, P.B.; Hellman, L. High Degree of Conservation of the Multigene Tryptase Locus Over the Past 150-200 Million Years of Mammalian Evolution. *Immunogenetics* **2010**, *62*, 369–382. [CrossRef]
8. Hunt, J.E.; Stevens, R.L.; Austen, K.F.; Zhang, J.; Xia, Z.; Ghildyal, N. Natural Disruption of the Mouse Mast Cell Protease 7 Gene in the C57BL/6 Mouse. *J. Biol. Chem.* **1996**, *271*, 2851–2855. [CrossRef]
9. Wong, G.W.; Yasuda, S.; Morokawa, N.; Li, L.; Stevens, R.L. Mouse Chromosome 17A3.3 Contains 13 Genes that Encode Functional Tryptic-Like Serine Proteases with Distinct Tissue and Cell Expression Patterns. *J. Biol. Chem.* **2004**, *279*, 2438–2452. [CrossRef]
10. Lyons, J.J.; Yu, X.; Hughes, J.D.; Le, Q.T.; Jamil, A.; Bai, Y.; Ho, N.; Zhao, M.; Liu, Y.; O'Connell, M.P.; et al. Elevated Basal Serum Tryptase Identifies a Multisystem Disorder Associated with Increased TPSAB1 Copy Number. *Nat. Genet.* **2016**, *48*, 1564–1569. [CrossRef]
11. Cildir, G.; Pant, H.; Lopez, A.F.; Tergaonkar, V. The Transcriptional Program, Functional Heterogeneity, and Clinical Targeting of Mast Cells. *J. Exp. Med.* **2017**, *214*, 2491–2506. [CrossRef] [PubMed]
12. Morii, E.; Tsujimura, T.; Jippo, T.; Hashimoto, K.; Takebayashi, K.; Tsujino, K.; Nomura, S.; Yamamoto, M.; Kitamura, Y. Regulation of Mouse Mast Cell Protease 6 Gene Expression by Transcription Factor Encoded by the Mi Locus. *Blood* **1996**, *88*, 2488–2494. [PubMed]
13. Ogihara, H.; Kanno, T.; Morii, E.; Kim, D.K.; Lee, Y.M.; Sato, M.; Kim, W.Y.; Nomura, S.; Ito, Y.; Kitamura, Y. Synergy of PEBP2/CBF with Mi Transcription Factor (MITF) for Transactivation of Mouse Mast Cell Protease 6 Gene. *Oncogene* **1999**, *18*, 4632–4639. [CrossRef] [PubMed]
14. Ogihara, H.; Morii, E.; Kim, D.K.; Oboki, K.; Kitamura, Y. Inhibitory Effect of the Transcription Factor Encoded by the Mutant Mi Microphthalmia Allele on Transactivation of Mouse Mast Cell Protease 7 Gene. *Blood* **2001**, *97*, 645–651. [CrossRef] [PubMed]

15. Morii, E.; Ogihara, H.; Oboki, K.; Kataoka, T.R.; Jippo, T.; Kitamura, Y. Effect of MITF on Transcription of Transmembrane Tryptase Gene in Cultured Mast Cells of Mice. *Biochem. Biophys. Res. Commun.* **2001**, *289*, 1243–1246. [CrossRef] [PubMed]
16. Hu Frisk, J.M.; Kjellen, L.; Kaler, S.G.; Pejler, G.; Ohrvik, H. Copper Regulates Maturation and Expression of an MITF:Tryptase Axis in Mast Cells. *J. Immunol.* **2017**, *199*, 4132–4141. [CrossRef] [PubMed]
17. Ohneda, K.; Moriguchi, T.; Ohmori, S.; Ishijima, Y.; Satoh, H.; Philipsen, S.; Yamamoto, M. Transcription Factor GATA1 is Dispensable for Mast Cell Differentiation in Adult Mice. *Mol. Cell. Biol.* **2014**, *34*, 1812–1826. [CrossRef] [PubMed]
18. Ohmori, S.; Moriguchi, T.; Noguchi, Y.; Ikeda, M.; Kobayashi, K.; Tomaru, N.; Ishijima, Y.; Ohneda, O.; Yamamoto, M.; Ohneda, K. GATA2 is Critical for the Maintenance of Cellular Identity in Differentiated Mast Cells Derived from Mouse Bone Marrow. *Blood* **2015**, *125*, 3306–3315. [CrossRef] [PubMed]
19. Takemoto, C.M.; Yoon, Y.J.; Fisher, D.E. The Identification and Functional Characterization of a Novel Mast Cell Isoform of the Microphthalmia-Associated Transcription Factor. *J. Biol. Chem.* **2002**, *277*, 30244–30252. [CrossRef]
20. Calero-Nieto, F.J.; Ng, F.S.; Wilson, N.K.; Hannah, R.; Moignard, V.; Leal-Cervantes, A.I.; Jimenez-Madrid, I.; Diamanti, E.; Wernisch, L.; Gottgens, B. Key Regulators Control Distinct Transcriptional Programmes in Blood Progenitor and Mast Cells. *EMBO J.* **2014**, *33*, 1212–1226. [CrossRef]
21. Li, Y.; Liu, B.; Harmacek, L.; Long, Z.; Liang, J.; Lukin, K.; Leach, S.M.; O'Connor, B.; Gerber, A.N.; Hagman, J.; et al. The Transcription Factors GATA2 and Microphthalmia-Associated Transcription Factor Regulate Hdc Gene Expression in Mast Cells and are Required for IgE/mast Cell-Mediated Anaphylaxis. *J. Allergy Clin. Immunol.* **2018**, *142*, 1173–1184. [CrossRef] [PubMed]
22. Ohmori, S.; Takai, J.; Ishijima, Y.; Suzuki, M.; Moriguchi, T.; Philipsen, S.; Yamamoto, M.; Ohneda, K. Regulation of GATA Factor Expression is Distinct between Erythroid and Mast Cell Lineages. *Mol. Cell. Biol.* **2012**, *32*, 4742–4755. [CrossRef] [PubMed]
23. Hiroyama, T.; Miharada, K.; Sudo, K.; Danjo, I.; Aoki, N.; Nakamura, Y. Establishment of Mouse Embryonic Stem Cell-Derived Erythroid Progenitor Cell Lines Able to Produce Functional Red Blood Cells. *PLoS ONE* **2008**, *3*, e1544. [CrossRef] [PubMed]
24. Ghirlando, R.; Felsenfeld, G. CTCF: Making the Right Connections. *Genes Dev.* **2016**, *30*, 881–891. [CrossRef] [PubMed]
25. Zhu, Z.; Wang, X. Roles of Cohesin in Chromosome Architecture and Gene Expression. *Semin. Cell Dev. Biol.* **2019**, *90*, 187–193. [CrossRef] [PubMed]
26. Fujiwara, T.; O'Geen, H.; Keles, S.; Blahnik, K.; Linnemann, A.K.; Kang, Y.A.; Choi, K.; Farnham, P.J.; Bresnick, E.H. Discovering Hematopoietic Mechanisms through Genome-Wide Analysis of GATA Factor Chromatin Occupancy. *Mol. Cell* **2009**, *36*, 667–681. [CrossRef] [PubMed]
27. Yu, M.; Riva, L.; Xie, H.; Schindler, Y.; Moran, T.B.; Cheng, Y.; Yu, D.; Hardison, R.; Weiss, M.J.; Orkin, S.H.; et al. Insights into GATA-1-Mediated Gene Activation Versus Repression Via Genome-Wide Chromatin Occupancy Analysis. *Mol. Cell* **2009**, *36*, 682–695. [CrossRef]
28. Soler, E.; Andrieu-Soler, C.; de Boer, E.; Bryne, J.C.; Thongjuea, S.; Stadhouders, R.; Palstra, R.J.; Stevens, M.; Kockx, C.; van Ijcken, W.; et al. The Genome-Wide Dynamics of the Binding of Ldb1 Complexes during Erythroid Differentiation. *Genes Dev.* **2010**, *24*, 277–289. [CrossRef]
29. Yue, F.; Cheng, Y.; Breschi, A.; Vierstra, J.; Wu, W.; Ryba, T.; Sandstrom, R.; Ma, Z.; Davis, C.; Pope, B.D.; et al. A Comparative Encyclopedia of DNA Elements in the Mouse Genome. *Nature* **2014**, *515*, 355–364. [CrossRef]
30. Robson, M.I.; Ringel, A.R.; Mundlos, S. Regulatory Landscaping: How Enhancer-Promoter Communication is Sculpted in 3D. *Mol. Cell* **2019**, *74*, 1110–1122. [CrossRef]
31. Zheng, H.; Xie, W. The Role of 3D Genome Organization in Development and Cell Differentiation. *Nat. Rev. Mol. Cell Biol.* **2019**, *20*, 535–550. [CrossRef] [PubMed]
32. Nora, E.P.; Lajoie, B.R.; Schulz, E.G.; Giorgetti, L.; Okamoto, I.; Servant, N.; Piolot, T.; van Berkum, N.L.; Meisig, J.; Sedat, J.; et al. Spatial Partitioning of the Regulatory Landscape of the X-Inactivation Centre. *Nature* **2012**, *485*, 381–385. [CrossRef] [PubMed]
33. Dixon, J.R.; Selvaraj, S.; Yue, F.; Kim, A.; Li, Y.; Shen, Y.; Hu, M.; Liu, J.S.; Ren, B. Topological Domains in Mammalian Genomes Identified by Analysis of Chromatin Interactions. *Nature* **2012**, *485*, 376–380. [CrossRef] [PubMed]

34. Phillips-Cremins, J.E.; Sauria, M.E.; Sanyal, A.; Gerasimova, T.I.; Lajoie, B.R.; Bell, J.S.; Ong, C.T.; Hookway, T.A.; Guo, C.; Sun, Y.; et al. Architectural Protein Subclasses Shape 3D Organization of Genomes during Lineage Commitment. *Cell* **2013**, *153*, 1281–1295. [CrossRef] [PubMed]
35. Catarino, R.R.; Stark, A. Assessing Sufficiency and Necessity of Enhancer Activities for Gene Expression and the Mechanisms of Transcription Activation. *Genes Dev.* **2018**, *32*, 202–223. [CrossRef] [PubMed]
36. Dore, L.C.; Chlon, T.M.; Brown, C.D.; White, K.P.; Crispino, J.D. Chromatin Occupancy Analysis Reveals Genome-Wide GATA Factor Switching during Hematopoiesis. *Blood* **2012**, *119*, 3724–3733. [CrossRef]
37. Papadopoulos, G.L.; Karkoulia, E.; Tsamardinos, I.; Porcher, C.; Ragoussis, J.; Bungert, J.; Strouboulis, J. GATA-1 Genome-Wide Occupancy Associates with Distinct Epigenetic Profiles in Mouse Fetal Liver Erythropoiesis. *Nucleic Acids Res.* **2013**, *41*, 4938–4948. [CrossRef] [PubMed]
38. Vakoc, C.R.; Letting, D.L.; Gheldof, N.; Sawado, T.; Bender, M.A.; Groudine, M.; Weiss, M.J.; Dekker, J.; Blobel, G.A. Proximity among Distant Regulatory Elements at the Beta-Globin Locus Requires GATA-1 and FOG-1. *Mol. Cell* **2005**, *17*, 453–462. [CrossRef]
39. Lee, J.; Krivega, I.; Dale, R.K.; Dean, A. The LDB1 Complex Co-Opts CTCF for Erythroid Lineage-Specific Long-Range Enhancer Interactions. *Cell Rep.* **2017**, *19*, 2490–2502. [CrossRef]
40. Kim, S.I.; Bultman, S.J.; Kiefer, C.M.; Dean, A.; Bresnick, E.H. BRG1 Requirement for Long-Range Interaction of a Locus Control Region with a Downstream Promoter. *Proc. Natl. Acad. Sci. USA* **2009**, *106*, 2259–2264. [CrossRef]
41. Yun, W.J.; Kim, Y.W.; Kang, Y.; Lee, J.; Dean, A.; Kim, A. The Hematopoietic Regulator TAL1 is Required for Chromatin Looping between the Beta-Globin LCR and Human Gamma-Globin Genes to Activate Transcription. *Nucleic Acids Res.* **2014**, *42*, 4283–4293. [CrossRef] [PubMed]
42. Takano, H.; Nakazawa, S.; Okuno, Y.; Shirata, N.; Tsuchiya, S.; Kainoh, T.; Takamatsu, S.; Furuta, K.; Taketomi, Y.; Naito, Y.; et al. Establishment of the Culture Model System that Reflects the Process of Terminal Differentiation of Connective Tissue-Type Mast Cells. *FEBS Lett.* **2008**, *582*, 1444–1450. [CrossRef] [PubMed]
43. Gutiérrez, L.; Tsukamoto, S.; Suzuki, M.; Yamamoto-Mukai, H.; Yamamoto, M.; Philipsen, S.; Ohneda, K. Ablation of Gata1 in Adult Mice Results in Aplastic Crisis, Revealing its Essential Role in Steady-State and Stress Erythropoiesis. *Blood* **2008**, *111*, 4375–4385. [CrossRef] [PubMed]
44. Charles, M.A.; Saunders, T.L.; Wood, W.M.; Owens, K.; Parlow, A.F.; Camper, S.A.; Ridgway, E.C.; Gordon, D.F. Pituitary-Specific Gata2 Knockout: Effects on Gonadotrope and Thyrotrope Function. *Mol. Endocrinol.* **2006**, *20*, 1366–1377. [CrossRef] [PubMed]
45. Mizushima, S.; Nagata, S. PEF-BOS, a Powerful Mammalian Expression Vector. *Nucleic Acids Res.* **1990**, *18*, 5322. [CrossRef]
46. Shimizu, R.; Takahashi, S.; Ohneda, K.; Engel, J.D.; Yamamoto, M. In Vivo Requirements for GATA-1 Functional Domains during Primitive and Definitive Erythropoiesis. *EMBO J.* **2001**, *20*, 5250–5260. [CrossRef] [PubMed]
47. Ishijima, Y.; Ohmori, S.; Uenishi, A.; Ohneda, K. GATA Transcription Factors are Involved in IgE-Dependent Mast Cell Degranulation by Enhancing the Expression of Phospholipase C-gamma1. *Genes Cells* **2012**, *17*, 285–301. [CrossRef]
48. Ran, F.A.; Hsu, P.D.; Wright, J.; Agarwala, V.; Scott, D.A.; Zhang, F. Genome Engineering using the CRISPR-Cas9 System. *Nat. Protoc.* **2013**, *8*, 2281–2308. [CrossRef]

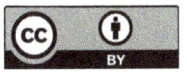

© 2019 by the authors. Licensee MDPI, Basel, Switzerland. This article is an open access article distributed under the terms and conditions of the Creative Commons Attribution (CC BY) license (http://creativecommons.org/licenses/by/4.0/).

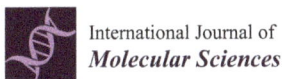

Article

Identification of 5-Hydroxymethylfurfural (5-HMF) as an Active Component Citrus Jabara That Suppresses FcεRI-Mediated Mast Cell Activation

Ryota Uchida [1], Michiko Kato [1], Yuka Hattori [2], Hiroko Kikuchi [3], Emi Watanabe [3], Katsuumi Kobayashi [3] and Keigo Nishida [1,2,*]

[1] Laboratory of Immune Regulation, Graduate School of Pharmaceutical Sciences, Suzuka University of Medical Science, 3500-3 Minamitamagaki, Suzuka Mie 513-8607, Japan; mumyojoyani@gmail.com (R.U.); m-kato@suzuka-u.ac.jp (M.K.)
[2] Laboratory of Immune Regulation, Faculty of Pharmaceutical Sciences, Suzuka University of Medical Science, 3500-3 Minamitamagaki-cho, Suzuka Mie 513-8670, Japan; pp13078@st.suzuka-u.ac.jp
[3] Development Planning Department, Nisshin Honey Co.,LTD, 3133-1 Maki Anpachi-cho, Anpachi-gun, Gifu 503-0125, Japan; hiroko.kikuchi@nisshin-honey.co.jp (H.K.); emi.watanabe@nisshin-honey.co.jp (E.W.); katsuumi.kobayashi@nisshin-honey.co.jp (K.K.)
* Correspondence: knishida@suzuka-u.ac.jp; Tel.: +81-59-340-0577; Fax: +81-59-368-1271

Received: 23 March 2020; Accepted: 31 March 2020; Published: 2 April 2020

Abstract: Jabara (*Citrus jabara* Hort. ex Y. Tanaka) is a type of citrus fruit known for its beneficial effect against seasonal allergies. Jabara is rich in the antioxidant narirutin whose anti-allergy effect has been demonstrated. One of the disadvantages in consuming Jabara is its bitter flavor. Therefore, we fermented the fruit to reduce the bitterness and make Jabara easy to consume. Here, we examined whether fermentation alters the anti-allergic property of Jabara. Suppression of degranulation and cytokine production was observed in mast cells treated with fermented Jabara and the effect was dependent on the length of fermentation. We also showed that 5-hydroxymethylfurfural (5-HMF) increases as fermentation progresses and was identified as an active component of fermented Jabara, which inhibited mast cell degranulation. Mast cells treated with 5-HMF also exhibited reduced degranulation and cytokine production. In addition, we showed that the expression levels of phospho-PLCγ1 and phospho-ERK1/2 were markedly reduced upon FcεRI stimulation. These results indicate that 5-HMF is one of the active components of fermented Jabara that is involved in the inhibition of mast cell activation.

Keywords: mast cells; allergy; degranulation; cytokine; *Citrus jabara*; fermentation; 5-HMF

1. Introduction

Millions of people who react to airborne allergens such as pollens suffer from symptoms including rhinitis, atopic dermatitis, and asthma, which could reduce the patients' quality of life. These allergic symptoms are induced by the activation of inflammatory cells such as mast cells [1–3].

Mast cells express Fc epsilon receptor (FcεRI), which can bind to immunoglobulin E (IgE). Stimulation of IgE-sensitized mast cells with a specific antigen results in a cascade of events leading to the secretion and production of proinflammatory molecules such as histamine, lipid mediators and cytokines [4,5]. These secreted molecules play critical roles in the inflammatory reactions in patients with allergic diseases. Allergic symptoms can impair the patients' quality of life by causing chronic fatigue, cognitive impairment, and many other symptoms associated with the condition. While there are many anti-allergy medications on the market, more effective and safer drugs are still being sought. Use of natural products for the prevention and treatment of allergic diseases is an attractive and advantageous option in that they have fewer side effects.

Citrus jabara is a cultivar of citrus native to Kitayama village in Wakayama prefecture, Japan. Jabara has gained much attention in recent years for its effect on alleviating seasonal allergy symptoms [6]. Jabara has been found to be particularly rich in the dietary flavonoid narirutin (naringenin-7-O-β-D-rutinoside) commonly found in citrus that is reported to possess anti-allergic property. The anti-allergic property of narirutin has been shown in both in vitro and in vivo studies using a mouse model of atopic dermatitis and airway inflammation [7–9]. However, it is still unknown whether Jabara contains other active compounds that have anti-allergic activity.

While the consumption of Jabara has been shown to be effective in alleviating allergic symptoms in patients suffering from seasonal allergy, its use as a health food has some restrictions due to its flavor, especially the bitterness of the peel where narirutin is primarily present. To overcome this disadvantage, we reduced the bitterness of the fruit by processing it with our proprietary procedure that incorporates self-fermentation and maturation. However, it is unknown whether Jabara's chemical composition changes and its anti-allergic effects are affected by fermentation.

In this study, we investigated the effect of fermented Jabara extract on allergic responses by examining in vitro anti-allergic activity using mouse mast cells. We identified 5-hydroxymethylfurfural (5-HMF) as an active compound that inhibits FcεRI-mediated degranulation and cytokine production in mouse mast cells.

2. Results

2.1. Fermented Jabara Suppressed Mast Cell Activation

We first examined the effect of fermented Jabara on the activation of mast cells by measuring the release of the mast cell degranulation marker β-hexosaminidase. Antigen-dependent degranulation of mast cells was significantly suppressed by pretreating the cells with four-week fermented Jabara as well as flesh and peel of raw Jabara (Figure 1A). Next, we measured the concentration of cytokines in the culture supernatant of mast cells by ELISA (Figure 1B,C). Cytokine production was suppressed by pretreating mast cells with fermented Jabara. In addition, no significant change in the cell viability was observed after 6-h exposure to Jabara extracts (Figure S1). These data suggest that inhibition of mast cell degranulation and cytokine production induced by antigen stimulation is not due to cytotoxic effect of Jabara extracts.

We then examined whether the length of fermentation influences the effectiveness of inhibition of degranulation. As shown in Figure 2, the inhibitory effect of Jabara increased as the length of fermentation increased. Degranulation was significantly inhibited when cells were treated with Jabara fermented for 12 weeks.

2.2. 5-HMF is the Active Component in Fermented Jabara that Inhibits Mast Cell Activation

To identify the active component of fermented Jabara that exerts inhibitory effect against mast cell degranulation, we fractionated the extract of fermented Jabara by HPLC and examined the inhibitory effect of each fraction on degranulation. The chromatogram of the fermented sample showed two major peaks at 3.7 min (peak *a*) and 9.85 min (peak *b*) (Figure 3A). The retention time of peak *b* in the fermented sample as well as the single peak in the unfermented sample corresponded to the retention time of the narirutin standard (data not shown). The 3.7 min peak appeared in the fermented sample (Figure 3A) but not in the unfermented sample (Figure 3B), suggesting that this compound is produced by fermentation. In addition, the amount of this compound increased as the fermentation progressed.

We then analyzed the fraction containing the compound in peak *a* for its effect on mast cell degranulation. As shown in Figure 3C, the compound in peak *a* exerted similar inhibitory effect on degranulation as the compound in peak *b* (Narirutin).

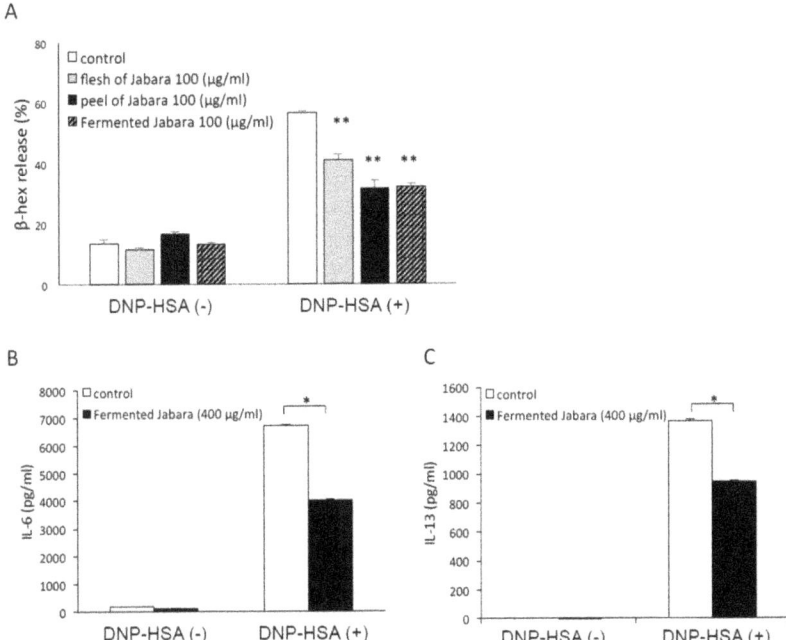

Figure 1. (**A**) Inhibitory effect of DMSO extract of flesh and peel of raw Jabara, as well as the extract of fermented Jabara (four weeks) on β-hexosaminidase (β-hex) release from mast cells. IgE-sensitized mast cells (1.0×10^5 cells/well) were preincubated with each extract at 37 °C for 15 min prior to 30 min stimulation with DNP-HSA. Data represent one of at least three trials that showed similar results. Data are presented as mean (SD). **$p < 0.01$, two-tailed Student's t-test. (**B**,**C**) Inhibitory effect of DMSO extract of fermented Jabara on cytokine production in mast cells. Mast cells were stimulated with 10 ng/mL DNP-HSA for 6 h with or without the addition of fermented Jabara. IL-6 (**B**) and IL-13 (**C**) production were measured by ELISA. Data represent one of at least three trials that showed similar results. Data are presented as mean (SD). *$p < 0.05$, two-tailed Student's t-test.

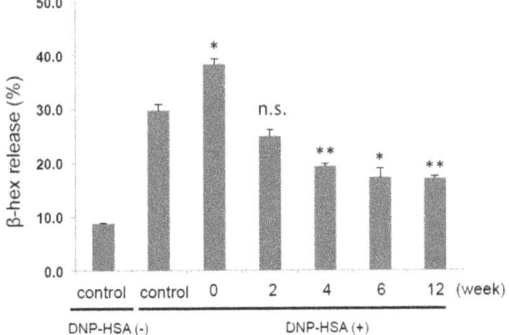

Figure 2. Inhibitory effect of DMSO extract from fermented Jabara on β-hex release from mast cells. IgE-sensitized mast cells (1.0×10^5 cells/well) were preincubated with each extract (200 μg/mL) at 37 °C for 15 min prior to 30 min stimulation with DNP-HSA. Results represent one trial. At least three additional trials show similar results. Data are presented as mean + SD. *$p < 0.05$, **$p < 0.01$, two-tailed Student's **t**-test. n.s., not significant.

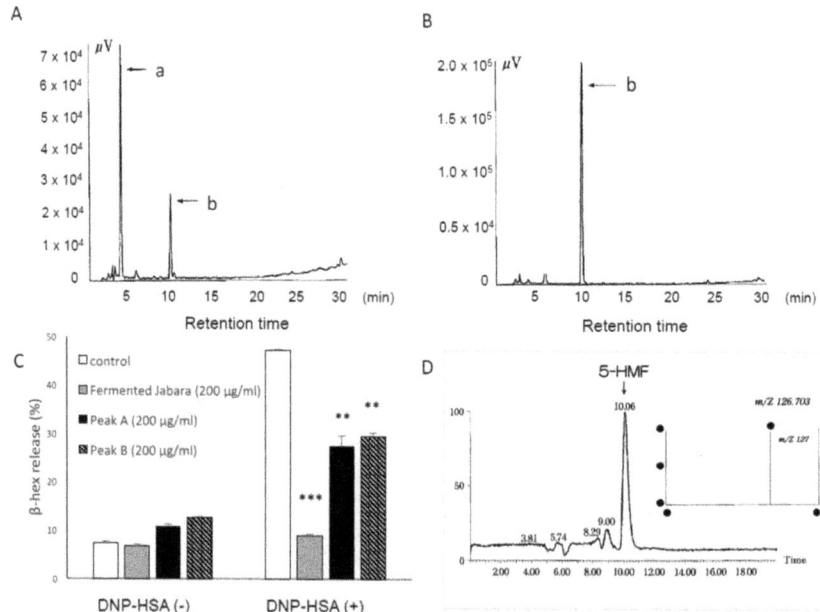

Figure 3. HPLC chromatograms of extracts (DMSO: MeOH = 1:1) of fermented Jabara (**A**) and flesh of Jabara (**B**). Column: ODS-HG-5 (φ4.6 × 250 mm, 5 μm) NOMURA CHEMICAL; flow rate, 1.0 mL/min; detected with UV at 285 nm. (**C**) Inhibitory effect of the compounds in peak a and b extracted from fermented Jabara on β-hex release from mast cells. IgE-sensitized mast cells (1.0 × 10^5 cells/well) were preincubated with each extract at 37 °C for 15 min prior to 30 min stimulation with DNP-HSA. Data represent one of at least three trials that showed similar results. Data are presented as mean (SD). **$p < 0.01$, ***$p < 0.001$, one-way ANOVA with Tukey–Kramer multiple comparison test. (**D**) LC-MS analysis of peak a revealed its molecular weight.

Peak a was identified as 5-hydroxymethylfurfural (5-HMF) on the basis of ^{1}H NMR, ^{13}C NMR LC-MS, and HPLC. The ^{13}C NMR spectrum of the compound recovered from peak a revealed six signals, indicating the presence of six (or a multiple of six) carbon atoms. When these signals were compared to the reference signals from the Aldrich Spectral Library, they corresponded with the NMR profile of 5-HMF This compound was further analyzed by LC-MS, and the MS spectrum showed the ion peak at m/z 126, which matched that of 5-HMF (Figure 3D, right). The compound from peak a also eluted at the same retention time as the 5-HMF standard. Based on these analyses, we identified this compound as 5-HMF.

2.3. 5-HMF Increased as Fermentation Progressed

HPLC analysis showed that unfermented Jabara is rich in narirutin while 5-HMF was barely detectable. As fermentation progressed, the amount of 5-HMF increased with a concomitant decrease of narirutin. After 4–6 weeks of fermentation, the amount of 5-HMF equaled or exceeded the amount of narirutin (Figure 4A).

The effect of 5-HMF on degranulation was examined using various concentrations of 5-HMF standard and Jabara fermented for four weeks. As shown in Figure 4B, β-hexosaminidase release was suppressed by 5-HMF in a concentration-dependent manner. Fermented Jabara suppressed β-hexosaminidase release to the basal level, suggesting that the anti-degranulation effect of Jabara becomes more potent as fermentation time increases. In addition, no significant change in the cell viability was observed after 6-h exposure to various doses of 5-HMF (Figure S1). These data suggested that inhibition of mast cell degranulation induced by antigen stimulation is not due to cytotoxic effect of 5-HMF.

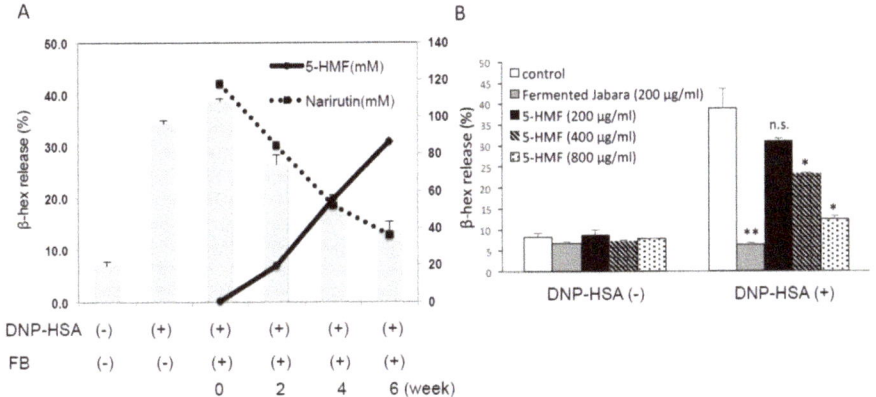

Figure 4. (**A**) Inhibitory effect of the DMSO extract of fermented Jabara (FB) on β-hex release from mast cells. IgE-sensitized mast cells (1.0×10^5 cells / well) were preincubated with each extract (200 ug/mL) at 37 °C for 15 min prior to 30 min stimulation with DNP-HSA. Data are presented as mean (SD). Solid and dashed lines: Amount of 5-HMF (mM) and Narirutin (mM) in Jabara, respectively, determined on different days of fermentation by HPLC analysis. (**B**) Inhibitory effect of 5-HMF on β-hex release from mast cells. IgE-sensitized mast cells (1.0×10^5 cells/well) were preincubated with each extract at 37 °C for 15 min prior to 30 min stimulation with DNP-HSA. Results represent one trial. At least three additional trials show similar results. Data are presented as mean (SD). *$p < 0.05$, **$p < 0.01$, two-tailed Student's *t*-test. n.s., not significant.

2.4. Effect of 5-HMF on the Expression of Proinflammatory Cytokine

Next, we examined whether 5-HMF inhibits cytokine production. The effect of 5-HMF on the expression of the proinflammatory cytokine IL-6 in FcεRI-induced mast cells was assessed by ELISA. When cells were pretreated with 5-HMF, the expression level of IL-6 was significantly decreased in a concentration-dependent manner as compared with the untreated group (Figure 5). Next, we analyzed the mRNA levels of cytokines by quantitative PCR. Antigen stimulation of mast cells led to an increase in the *Il6* mRNA level (Figure 5B), and treating these cells with 5-HMF decreased the *Il6* mRNA level in a dose-dependent manner (Figure 5B). These results indicate that 5-HMF is capable of suppressing the induction and production of proinflammatory cytokines.

2.5. The effect of 5-HMF on the PLCγ and MAPK Signaling Pathways

To gain some insight into the molecular mechanisms involved in the suppression on FcεRI-stimulated mast cell activation by 5-HMF, we examined the MAPK signaling pathway, which is known to regulate the expression of proinflammatory genes in response to FcεRI stimulation [10]. We hypothesized that 5-HMF downregulates cytokine expression by suppressing the activation of MAPK signaling, and analyzed the phosphorylation status of PLCγ and ERK1/2 by Western blot analysis. The expression levels of unphosphorylated PLCγ1 and ERK1/2 were comparable among all treatment groups. In addition, phosphorylated proteins were marginally expressed in the negative control group (no 5-HMF pretreatment, no stimulation) but were highly expressed in cells stimulated with DNP-HSA. Phosphorylation of both PLCγ1 and ERK1/2 was completely suppressed by treating mast cells with 800 μg/mL 5-HMF (Figure 6). Thus, our results support the idea that 5-HMF inhibits the expression of cytokine expression by suppressing the MAPK signaling pathways.

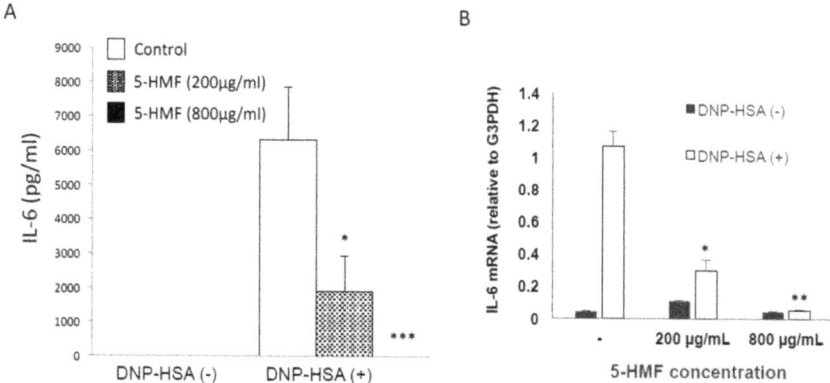

Figure 5. Inhibitory effect of 5-HMF on cytokine production and gene induction in mast cells. (**A**) Mast cells were stimulated with 10 ng/mL DNP-HSA for 6 h and 5-HMF was added at the time of stimulation. IL-6 production was then measured by ELISA. Data are from a representative of at least three trials that showed similar results. Data are presented as mean (SD). *$p < 0.05$, ***$p < 0.001$, two-tailed Student's t-test. (**B**) Expression of IL-6 mRNA relative to G3PDH mRNA. Mast cells were stimulated with 10 ng/mL DNP-HSA for 1 h in the presence of 200 or 800 µg/mL 5-HMF. A representative of three experiments is shown. Error bars represent standard deviation among duplicate samples. *$p < 0.05$, **$p < 0.01$, two-tailed Student's t-test.

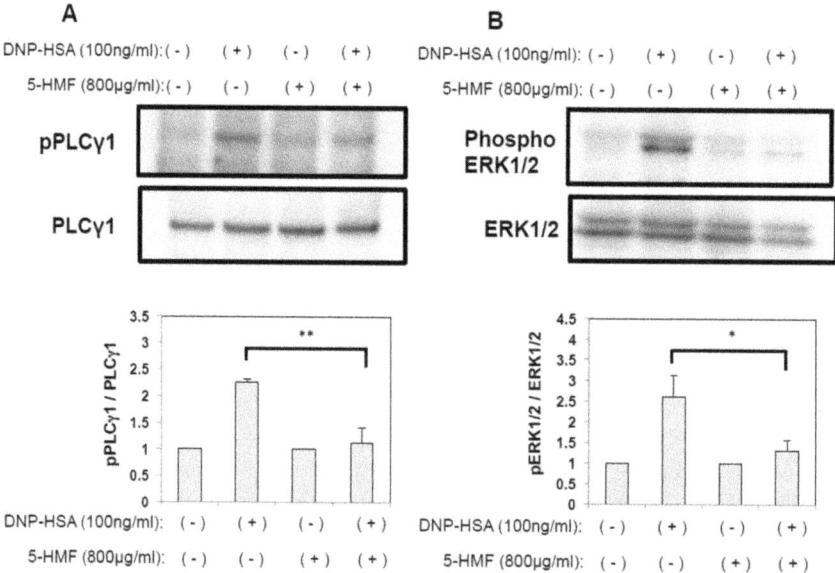

Figure 6. (**A**) Inhibition of PLCγ1 phosphorylation in mast cells treated with 5-HMF. After stimulation with DNP-HSA, mast cells were lysed and the cytosol fraction was immunoblotted with anti-phospho-PLCγ1 (Top). Data were normalized to the expression levels of non-phosphorylated PLCγ1 (Bottom). (**B**) Inhibition ERK1/2 phosphorylation in mast cells treated with 5-HMF. After stimulation with DNP-HSA, mast cells were lysed and the cytosol fraction was immunoblotted with anti-phospho-ERK1/2 (Top). Data were normalized to the expression levels of non-phosphorylated ERK1/2 (Bottom). Data are presented as mean (SD). *$p < 0.05$, **$p < 0.01$, two-tailed Student's t-test.

3. Discussion

This study examined the anti-allergic effect of citrus Jabara that was fermented in order to reduce bitterness. We showed that β-hexosaminidase release was significantly decreased in mast cells treated with fermented Jabara, and the effect was enhanced as the fermentation period increased.

Currently, the flavonoid narirutin is believed to be the major contributor of anti-allergic effect in Jabara. It has been shown that narirutin inhibits histamine release from rat peritoneal mast cells in vitro and exerts an inhibitory effect on allergic skin reactions in a murine model of atopic dermatitis [8]. Interestingly, the amount of narirutin abundant in raw Jabara fruit decreased as fermentation progressed, while the amount of 5-HMF, which is barely present in raw fruit, increased. We also observed that the extract of freeze-dried unfermented Jabara, which is expected to be rich in narirutin (Figure 2), did not inhibit mast cell degranulation. Since the HPLC-purified compound *b* (narirutin) suppressed degranulation (Figure 3C), we considered the possibility that there is an unidentified factor in the freeze-dried peel that interferes with the effect of narirutin.

Our data indicate that the fermentation process, during which narirutin is decreased, does not affect the anti-allergic effect of Jabara. We also observed that the amount of 5-HMF and the anti-degranulation effect increased proportionately to the length of fermentation, which led us to further investigate 5-HMF as the major anti-allergic/anti-inflammatory agent in fermented Jabara.

5-HMF is an organic compound generated by sugar reduction through the Maillard reaction [11–13]; therefore, it is normally present in heat-processed foods such as honey, dried fruits, and fruit juices [14–16]. The anti-inflammatory and anti-allergic effects of 5-HMF have been reported in several recent studies [17–21]. For example, it has been reported that *Lycium chinense*, commonly called wolfberry, contains large amount of 5-HMF and that the fruit extract inhibits degranulation of rat basophilic leukemia (RBL) cells [17]. In addition, Kong et al. showed that lipopolysaccharide (LPS)-stimulated production of pro-inflammatory cytokines was suppressed in RAW 264.7 cells pretreated with 5-HMF [21].

With regards to the mechanism underlying the anti-inflammatory activities of 5-HMF, little has been understood. Yamada et al. described that 5-HMF inhibits the release of chemical mediators by suppressing Ca^{2+} signaling in basophils though its detailed mechanism is unclear [17].

Calcium signaling is critical for the activation of mast cells. In mast cells, tyrosine kinase Syk is recruited by aggregated FcεRI and phosphorylates phospholipase Cγ (PLCγ), leading to the generation of inositol 1, 4, 5-triphosphate (IP_3). IP_3 causes Ca^{2+} release from intracellular Ca^{2+} stores and activates Ca^{2+} influx via Ca^{2+} release-activated Ca^{2+} channels (CRAC) to replenish Ca^{2+} stores [22–25]. Therefore, it can be said that an increase in the intracellular Ca^{2+} is a necessary and sufficient stimulus to trigger degranulation in mast cells. We investigated whether the mechanism by which 5-HMF inhibits degranulation in mast cells involves the suppression of calcium signaling. We found that 5-HMF pretreatment inhibited FcεRI-mediated phosphorylation of PLCγ1 in DNP-HSA-stimulated BMMC. This observation suggests that 5-HMF suppresses calcium influx by modulating PLCγ phosphorylation and it agrees with previous reports that 5-HMF suppresses the elevation of intracellular Ca^{2+} concentration [17,26]. Thus, our study suggests that 5-HMF may prevent mast cell degranulation by regulating intracellular Ca^{2+} flux, but how 5-HMF might inhibit PLCγ1 phosphorylation is unclear and is a subject of further investigation.

We also showed that FcεRI-mediated cytokine production is inhibited by 5-HMF. When mast cells are activated via FcεRI, production of pro-inflammatory cytokines such as IL-6 occurs via the MAPK signaling pathway [27]. The main components of the MAPK signaling cascades include ERK1/2, SAPK/JNK, and p38 protein kinases, which are involved in number of physiological processes such as cell proliferation, differentiation, and inflammatory responses [28,29]. We observed that 5-HMF clearly inhibited FcεRI-mediated phosphorylation of ERK1/2, suggesting that 5-HMF could disturb FcεRI-activated MAPK signaling pathway (Figure 6B). Collectively, our data provide further insights into the mechanism(s) controlling mast cell activation by 5-HMF that was previously unknown.

In conclusion, our findings suggest that the anti-allergic effect of Jabara is enhanced by fermentation, during which 5-HMF is produced. Further studies including in vivo experiments are required, but 5-HMF has potential to be useful for controlling allergy symptoms. We consider fermentation as a useful and effective way to produce 5-HMF as well as to improve the taste for consumption.

4. Materials and Methods

4.1. Fermentation of Jabara

Raw Jabara peel was aged in a fermenter for 4–12 weeks at a temperature of 70 °C and a humidity of 75% or higher with no additives or water added.

4.2. Reagents and Antibodies

Narirutin (141-09301) and 5-HMF (AC121460010) were purchased from FUJIFILM (Tokyo, Japan) and Thermo Fisher Scientific (Waltham, MA, USA), respectively. The following antibodies were commercially obtained: anti-phospho PLCγ1 (Tyr783), anti- PLCγ1 (Cell Signaling, Farmingdale, NY, USA), anti-phospho ERK1/2 (V803A), and anti-ERK1/2 (V114A) (Promega, Madison, WI, USA).

4.3. Mice

C57BL/6J and BALB/c mice were obtained from Japan SLC (Hamamatsu, Japan). The mice were maintained under specific pathogen-free conditions and were analyzed between 8 and 12 weeks of age for all studies performed. We obtained approval from the animal research committee at Suzuka University of Medical Science for all animal experiments performed (approved #75).

4.4. Cell Culture

Bone marrow-derived mast cells (BMMC) were prepared as described previously [30]. Briefly, 8-week-old C57BL6J mice were sacrificed and their bone marrow cells were cultured in RPMI 1640 supplemented with 10% heat-inactivated FBS, 10 mU/mL penicillin, 0.1 mg/mL streptomycin, and IL-3 in a 5% CO_2 and 95% humidified atmosphere at 37 °C. After 4–5 weeks of culture, cell-surface expression of FcεRI and c-Kit was confirmed by FACSCalibur (BD Biosciences, San Diego, CA, USA).

4.5. BMMC Degranulation Assay

BMMC degranulation assay was performed as previously described [31]. Cells were sensitized with 0.5 μg/mL IgE for 12 h at 37 °C. After sensitization, the cells were washed twice with Tyrode's buffer (10 mM HEPES pH 7.4, 130 mM NaCl, 5 mM KCl, 1.4 mM $CaCl_2$, 1 mM $MgCl_2$, and 5.6 mM glucose), and then suspended in the same buffer and stimulated with polyvalent dinitrophenyl-human serum albumin (DNP-HSA, Biosearch Technologies, Hoddesdon, UK) for 30 min at 37 °C. To measure β-hexosaminidase activity, 50 μL of supernatant or cell lysate was transferred in duplicates into a 96-well plate and 100 μL of 1.3 mg/mL p-nitrophenyl-N-acetyl-D-glucosaminide (in 0.1 M citrate, pH 4.5) was added to each well. The plate was then incubated for color development for 50 min at 37 °C. The enzyme reaction was stopped by adding 150 μL of 0.2 M glycine-NaOH (pH 10.2) followed by the measurement of absorbance at 405 nm. Tyrode's buffer containing 1% Triton X-100 was used to lyse cells. The percentage of released β-hexosaminidase was calculated using the following formula:

$$\text{Degranulation (\%)} = (\text{OD supernatant}) / (\text{OD supernatant} + \text{OD lysate}) \times 100 \qquad (1)$$

4.6. Measurement of Cytokines

Mast cells (0.5×10^5 cells) were treated with Jabara extracts or 5-HMF for 6 h. IL-6 and IL-13 in the cell culture supernatants were measured with an ELISA kit (BD Biosciences, San Diego, CA, USA for IL-6; Thermo Fisher Scientific for IL-13).

4.7. Extraction from Fermented Jabara

Fermented of Jabara was pulverized and lyophilized for powder preparations. Before adding to the cultured mast cells, the entire fraction was dissolved in DMSO.

4.8. Identification of the Active Component from Fermented Jabara

The active fraction of fermented Jabara was subjected to Cosmosil $5C_{18}$-MS-II (φ4.6 mm × 150 mm, MeOH:H_2O = 3:7) to yield two fractions (Fr. A and B). All fractions were tested for β- hexosaminidase release assay from mast cells. The chemical structure of the main active compound was identified based on HPLC-MS analysis and NMR analysis.

4.9. Cell lysates and Immunoblotting

Cell lysates and immunoblotting were performed as previously described [32]. BMMCs were harvested, lysed in lysis buffer (20 mM Tris-HCl pH 7.4, 150 mM NaCl, 1% NP-40, and proteinase inhibitor cocktail (Roche, Basel, Swizerland) for 30 min at 4 °C, and spun at 12,000× g at 4 °C for 30 min. The eluted and reduced samples were resolved by SDS-PAGE using a 5-20% gradient polyacrylamide gel (Wako Pure Chemical, Osaka Japan) and transferred to a PVDF membrane (Immobilon-P, Millipore, Billeria, MA, USA). For immunoblotting, the membranes were incubated with primary antibodies for 1 h at room temperature, and then incubated with HRP-conjugated anti-mouse (Thermo Fisher Scientific) or anti-rabbit (Thermo Fisher Scientific) antibody for 1 h at room temperature. After extensive washing of the membranes, immunoreactive proteins were visualized using the Western Lightning-ECL system (GE Healthcare Life Sciences, Buckinghamshire, England) according to the manufacturer's recommendation. The PVDF membranes were exposed to Fuji RX film (Fujifilm). Densitometric analysis was performed using a LAS-4000 fluorescence image analyzer (Fujifilm, Tokyo, Japan).

4.10. Real-time PCR Analysis

Cells were homogenized with Sepasol RNAI (Nacalai Tesque, Kyoto, Japan), and total RNA was isolated following the manufacturer's instructions. For standard RT-PCR, cDNA was synthesized from 1 µg of total RNA with reverse transcriptase (ReverTra Ace; TOYOBO, Osaka, Japan) and 500 ng of oligo (dT) primer (Life Technologies, Grand Island, NY, USA) for 30 min at 42 °C. A portion of the cDNA was used for real-time PCR. The relative expression of *Il-6* gene was determined compared to a reference gene *g3pdh* using the SYBR® Green reagent (TaKaRa Bio inc., Kusatsu, Japan). Primers used in these experiments were purchased from TaKaRa, and the sequences were as follows: IL-6: forward primer, 5'- GAGGATACCACTCCCAACAGACC-3' and reverse primer, 5'- AAGTGCATCATCGTTGTTCATACA-3'; G3PDH: forward primer, 5'- TTCACCACCATGGAG AAGGCCG-3' and reverse primer, 5'- GGCATGGACTGTGGTCATGA-3'.

4.11. Cell Viability

BMMC was diluted to 1×10^6 cells/mL in RPMI-1640 medium and 200 µL cell suspension was added to duplicate wells in a 96-well plate. 5-HMF was added to the final concentration of 200, 400 or 800 µg/mL in each well. Jabara extract was added to the final concentration of 400 µg/mL. The plate was incubated at 37 °C, and a 1:1 dilution of cell suspension and trypan blue (0.5%) was prepared at each timepoint. Cell viability was measured using an automated cell counter (TC20, Bio-Rad, Hercules, CA, USA).

4.12. Statistical Analysis

All data were statistically analyzed using Dunnett's test or Student's two-tailed t test with IBM SPSS Statistics software (version 24). Data were considered statistically significant when the *p* value was less than 0.05.

Supplementary Materials: Supplementary materials can be found at http://www.mdpi.com/1422-0067/21/7/2472/s1.

Author Contributions: Conceptualization, M.K., K.K., and K.N.; Data curation, R.U., M.K., Y.H., H.K., and E.W.; Formal analysis, R.U., M.K., Y.H., H.K., E.W., and K.N.; Funding acquisition, K.N.; Investigation, R.U., M.K., E.W., and K.N.; Methodology, H.K., E.W., and K.K.; Resources, H.K., E.W., and K.K.; Supervision, K.N.; Writing—original draft, M.K. and K.N.; and Writing—review and editing, M.K., H.K., E.W., and K.K. All authors have read and agreed to the published version of the manuscript.

Funding: This work was supported in part by Grants-in-Aid for Scientific Research (KAKENHI #16K15152) (K.N.).

Conflicts of Interest: The authors declare no conflict of interest.

References

1. Kawakami, T.; Ando, T.; Kimura, M.; Wilson, B.S.; Kawakami, Y. Mast cells in atopic dermatitis. *Curr. Opin. Immunol.* **2009**, *21*, 666–678. [CrossRef] [PubMed]
2. Galli, S.J.; Tsai, M. IgE and mast cells in allergic disease. *Nat. Med.* **2012**, *18*, 693–704. [CrossRef] [PubMed]
3. Dema, B.; Suzuki, R.; Rivera, J. Rethinking the role of immunoglobulin E and its high-affinity receptor: New insights into allergy and beyond. *Int. Arch. Allergy Immunol.* **2014**, *164*, 271–279. [CrossRef] [PubMed]
4. Galli, S.J.; Nakae, S.; Tsai, M. Mast cells in the development of adaptive immune responses. *Nat. Immunol.* **2005**, *6*, 135–142. [CrossRef] [PubMed]
5. Mukai, K.; Tsai, M.; Saito, H.; Galli, S.J. Mast cells as sources of cytokines, chemokines, and growth factors. *Immunol. Rev.* **2018**, *282*, 121–150. [CrossRef]
6. Minatoguchi, S.; Ohno, Y.; Funaguchi, N.; Baila, B.; Nagashima, K.; Fujiwara, H. Effect of "Jabara" juice on symptoms and QOL in patients cedar pollinosis. *Clin. Immunol. Allergol.* **2008**, *50*, 360–364.
7. Kubo, M.; Matsuda, H.; Tomohiro, N.; Harima, S. History and therapeutic evaluation of Citrus hassaku HORT. Tanaka. *Yakushigaku Zasshi* **2004**, *39*, 363–364.
8. Funaguchi, N.; Ohno, Y.; La, B.L.; Asai, T.; Yuhgetsu, H.; Sawada, M.; Takemura, G.; Minatoguchi, S.; Fujiwara, T.; Fujiwara, H. Narirutin inhibits airway inflammation in an allergic mouse model. *Clin. Exp. Pharmacol. Physiol.* **2007**, *34*, 766–770. [CrossRef]
9. Murata, K.; Takano, S.; Masuda, M.; Iinuma, M.; Matsuda, H. Anti-degranulating activity in rat basophil leukemia RBL-2H3 cells of flavanone glycosides and their aglycones in citrus fruits. *J. Nat. Med.* **2013**, *67*, 643–646. [CrossRef]
10. Gonzalez-Espinosa, C.; Odom, S.; Olivera, A.; Hobson, J.P.; Martinez, M.E.; Oliveira-Dos-Santos, A.; Barra, L.; Spiegel, S.; Penninger, J.M.; Rivera, J. Preferential signaling and induction of allergy-promoting lymphokines upon weak stimulation of the high affinity IgE receptor on mast cells. *J. Exp. Med.* **2003**, *197*, 1453–1465. [CrossRef]
11. Jeuring, H.J.; Kuppers, F.J. High performance liquid chromatography of furfural and hydroxymethylfurfural in spirits and honey. *J. Assoc. Off. Anal. Chem.* **1980**, *63*, 1215–1218. [CrossRef] [PubMed]
12. Janzowski, C.; Glaab, V.; Samimi, E.; Schlatter, J.; Eisenbrand, G. 5-Hydroxymethylfurfural: Assessment of mutagenicity, DNA-damaging potential and reactivity towards cellular glutathione. *Food Chem. Toxicol.* **2000**, *38*, 801–809. [CrossRef]
13. Antal, M.J., Jr.; Mok, W.S.; Richards, G.N. Mechanism of formation of 5-(hydroxymethyl)-2-furaldehyde from D-fructose an sucrose. *Carbohydr. Res.* **1990**, *199*, 91–109. [CrossRef]
14. Lo Coco, F.; Novelli, V.; Valentini, C.; Ceccon, L. High-performance liquid chromatographic determination of 2-furaldehyde and 5-hydroxymethyl-2-furaldehyde in fruit juices. *J. Chromatogr. Sci.* **1997**, *35*, 578–583. [CrossRef]
15. Shapla, U.M.; Solayman, M.; Alam, N.; Khalil, M.I.; Gan, S.H. 5-Hydroxymethylfurfural (HMF) levels in honey and other food products: Effects on bees and human health. *Chem. Cent. J.* **2018**, *12*, 35. [CrossRef]
16. Murkovic, M.; Pichler, N. Analysis of 5-hydroxymethylfurfural in coffee, dried fruits and urine. *Mol. Nutr. Food Res.* **2006**, *50*, 842–846. [CrossRef]
17. Yamada, P.; Nemoto, M.; Shigemori, H.; Yokota, S.; Isoda, H. Isolation of 5-(hydroxymethyl)furfural from Lycium chinense and its inhibitory effect on the chemical mediator release by basophilic cells. *Planta Med.* **2011**, *77*, 434–440. [CrossRef]

18. Alizadeh, M.; Khodaei, H.; Mesgari Abbasi, M.; Saleh-Ghadimi, S. Assessing the effect of 5-hydroxymethylfurfural on selected components of immune responses in mice immunised with ovalbumin. *J. Sci. Food Agric.* **2017**, *97*, 3979–3984. [CrossRef]
19. Ziadlou, R.; Barbero, A.; Stoddart, M.J.; Wirth, M.; Li, Z.; Martin, I.; Wang, X.L.; Qin, L.; Alini, M.; Grad, S. Regulation of Inflammatory Response in Human Osteoarthritic Chondrocytes by Novel Herbal Small Molecules. *Int. J. Mol. Sci.* **2019**, *20*, 5745. [CrossRef]
20. Kong, F.; Fan, C.; Yang, Y.; Lee, B.H.; Wei, K. 5-hydroxymethylfurfural-embedded poly (vinyl alcohol)/sodium alginate hybrid hydrogels accelerate wound healing. *Int. J. Biol. Macromol.* **2019**, *138*, 933–949. [CrossRef]
21. Kong, F.; Lee, B.H.; Wei, K. 5-Hydroxymethylfurfural Mitigates Lipopolysaccharide-Stimulated Inflammation via Suppression of MAPK, NF-kappaB and mTOR Activation in RAW 264.7 Cells. *Molecules* **2019**, *24*, 275. [CrossRef] [PubMed]
22. Baba, Y.; Nishida, K.; Fujii, Y.; Hirano, T.; Hikida, M.; Kurosaki, T. Essential function for the calcium sensor STIM1 in mast cell activation and anaphylactic responses. *Nat. Immunol.* **2008**, *9*, 81–88. [CrossRef] [PubMed]
23. Wen, R.; Jou, S.T.; Chen, Y.; Hoffmeyer, A.; Wang, D. Phospholipase C gamma 2 is essential for specific functions of Fc epsilon R and Fc gamma R. *J. Immunol.* **2002**, *169*, 6743–6752. [CrossRef] [PubMed]
24. Turner, H.; Kinet, J.P. Signalling through the high-affinity IgE receptor Fc epsilonRI. *Nature* **1999**, *402* (Suppl. 6760), B24–B30. [CrossRef] [PubMed]
25. Vig, M.; Kinet, J.P. Calcium signaling in immune cells. *Nat. Immunol.* **2009**, *10*, 21–27. [CrossRef]
26. Wolkart, G.; Schrammel, A.; Koyani, C.N.; Scherubel, S.; Zorn-Pauly, K.; Malle, E.; Pelzmann, B.; Andra, M.; Ortner, A.; Mayer, B. Cardioprotective effects of 5-hydroxymethylfurfural mediated by inhibition of L-type Ca(2+) currents. *Br. J. Pharmacol.* **2017**, *174*, 3640–3653. [CrossRef]
27. Gibbs, B.F.; Grabbe, J. Inhibitors of PI 3-kinase and MEK kinase differentially affect mediator secretion from immunologically activated human basophils. *J. Leukoc. Biol.* **1999**, *65*, 883–890. [CrossRef]
28. Karin, M. Signal transduction from the cell surface to the nucleus through the phosphorylation of transcription factors. *Curr. Opin. Cell Biol.* **1994**, *6*, 415–424. [CrossRef]
29. Davis, R.J. Transcriptional regulation by MAP kinases. *Mol. Reprod. Dev.* **1995**, *42*, 459–467. [CrossRef]
30. Nishida, K.; Hasegawa, A.; Yamasaki, S.; Uchida, R.; Ohashi, W.; Kurashima, Y.; Kunisawa, J.; Kimura, S.; Iwanaga, T.; Watarai, H.; et al. Mast cells play role in wound healing through the ZnT2/GPR39/IL-6 axis. *Sci. Rep.* **2019**, *9*, 10842. [CrossRef]
31. Uchida, R.; Egawa, T.; Fujita, Y.; Furuta, K.; Taguchi, H.; Tanaka, S.; Nishida, K. Identification of the minimal region of peptide derived from ADP-ribosylation factor1 (ARF1) that inhibits IgE-mediated mast cell activation. *Mol. Immunol.* **2019**, *105*, 32–37. [CrossRef] [PubMed]
32. Uchida, R.; Xiang, H.; Arai, H.; Kitamura, H.; Nishida, K. L-Type Calcium Channel-Mediated Zinc Wave Is Involved in the Regulation of IL-6 by Stimulating Non-IgE with LPS and IL-33 in Mast Cells and Dendritic Cells. *Biol. Pharm. Bull.* **2019**, *42*, 87–93. [CrossRef] [PubMed]

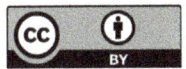

© 2020 by the authors. Licensee MDPI, Basel, Switzerland. This article is an open access article distributed under the terms and conditions of the Creative Commons Attribution (CC BY) license (http://creativecommons.org/licenses/by/4.0/).

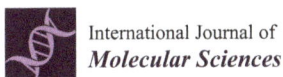

Review

Killer Immunoglobulin-Like Receptor 2DL4 (CD158d) Regulates Human Mast Cells both Positively and Negatively: Possible Roles in Pregnancy and Cancer Metastasis

Tatsuki R. Kataoka *, Chiyuki Ueshima, Masahiro Hirata, Sachiko Minamiguchi and Hironori Haga

Department of Diagnostic Pathology, Kyoto University Hospital, Kyoto 606-8507, Japan; ueshima@kuhp.kyoto-u.ac.jp (C.U.); hiratama@kuhp.kyoto-u.ac.jp (M.H.); minami@kuhp.kyoto-u.ac.jp (S.M.); haga@kuhp.kyoto-u.ac.jp (H.H.)
* Correspondence: trkata@kuhp.kyoto-u.ac.jp; Tel: +81-75-751-3491; Fax: +81-75-751-3499

Received: 25 December 2019; Accepted: 30 January 2020; Published: 31 January 2020

Abstract: Killer immunoglobulin-like receptor (KIR) 2DL4 (CD158d) was previously thought to be a human NK cell-specific protein. Mast cells are involved in allergic reactions via their KIT-mediated and FcεRI-mediated responses. We recently detected the expression of KIR2DL4 in human cultured mast cells established from peripheral blood of healthy volunteers (PB-mast), in the human mast cell line LAD2, and in human tissue mast cells. Agonistic antibodies against KIR2DL4 negatively regulate the KIT-mediated and FcεRI-mediated responses of PB-mast and LAD2 cells. In addition, agonistic antibodies and human leukocyte antigen (HLA)-G, a natural ligand for KIR2DL4, induce the secretion of leukemia inhibitory factor and serine proteases from human mast cells, which have been implicated in pregnancy establishment and cancer metastasis. Therefore, KIR2DL4 stimulation with agonistic antibodies and recombinant HLA-G protein may enhance both processes, in addition to suppressing mast-cell-mediated allergic reactions.

Keywords: allergic reaction; CD158d; FcεRI; KIR2DL4; KIT; mast cell; pregnancy

1. Introduction

Mast cells were first described by Paul Ehrlich in 1878 [1]. Mast cells originate from hematopoietic precursors, and mature in almost all tissues [2,3]. The cells are characterized by their intracellular granules, containing heparin, histamine, serotonin, β-hexosaminidase, prostaglandins (for example in human mast cells, prostaglandin D_2), growth factors (for example in human mast cells, basic fibroblast growth factor (FGF)/FGF-2, granulocyte macrophage colony-stimulating factor (GM-CSF), nerve growth factor (NGF), vascular endothelial growth factor (VEGF), and stem cell factor (SCF)/KIT ligand/mast cell growth factor), cytokines (for example in human mast cells, tumor necrosis factor (TNF)-α, transforming growth factor (TGF)-β, interleukin (IL)-1β, IL-3, IL-4, IL-5, IL-6, IL-10, IL-11, IL-12, IL-13, IL-16, and interferon (IFN)-γ), chemokines (for example in human mast cells, CC chemokine legend (CCL) 1, CCL2, CCL3, CCL4, CCL5, CCL7, CCL8, CCL11,CCL17, CCL20, CCL22, CXC chemokine legend (CXCL) 2, CXCL8, and CXCL10), and serine proteases (for example in human mast cells, tryptases, chymases, carboxypeptidase A3, granzyme B (GrB), and matrix metalloproteases (MMPs)) [4–6]. Mast cells play important roles in both innate and adaptive immune responses by secreting these mediators [4–6]. Studies using mast cell-deficient mice, such as Kit[W/Wv] mice and Kit[Wsh/Wsh] mice, revealed that mast cells protect against parasitic infections including *Strongyloides ratti* and *Strongyloides brasiliensis* [7,8], as well as the venoms of honeybees or vipers [9]. Mast cells are categorized by the contents of granules. More specifically, human mast cells can be classified into MCT (tryptase-positive and chymase-negative), MCTC (tryptase-positive and chymase-positive), and MCC (tryptase-negative and chymase-positive), while mouse mast cells can be classified into MMC (mucosal type mast cells, which are tryptase-positive and chymase-negative) and CTMC (connective tissue type mast cells, which are tryptase-positive and chymase-positive) [4–6]. Mast cells distribute almost all tissues [4–6]. MCT or MMC are mainly located in the mucosa of gastrointestinal systems and airways, while MCTC or CTMC are primarily found in the connective tissue like dermis and soft tissues [4–6]. Activated gastrointestinal mast cells increase fluid secretion, smooth muscle contraction, peristalsis, and diarrhea. Moreover, activated mast cell in the airways induce airway constriction, increased mucous production, edema, and cough. Activated skin mast cells induce urticaria and angioedema. Thus, mast cells are considered to be as a major effector cell type in allergic diseases including food allergy, asthma, atopic rhinitis, atopic dermatitis, and anaphylaxis [10]. In addition, the roles and functions of mast cells have been focused in autoimmune diseases (Crohn diseases, celiac disease, irritable bowel syndrome, etc.) [11] and cardiovascular diseases (atherosclerosis, etc.) [12]. Mast cell activation and their functions are regulated by cell surface receptors, among which the high-affinity receptor for IgE (FcεRI) and KIT (CD117/SCF receptor) have been studied extensively [13,14].

FcεRI expressed on mast cells consists of four subunits: an IgE-binding α chain, a β chain, and two disulfide-bonded γ chains (FcεRIγ) that are the main signal transducers. Among these chains, the β chain plays key roles by amplifying the expression and signaling of FcεRI, and the followed allergic reactions via its immunoreceptor tyrosine-based activation motifs (ITAMs) [15]. When a multivalent antigen-IgE complex binds to FcεRI on the cell surface, FcεRI become aggregated or crosslinked, resulting in degranulation and cytokine secretion from the mast cells. KIT is a Type III receptor tyrosine kinase, consisting of an extracellular domain, a juxtamembrane domain, and two tyrosine-kinase domains (TKDs). The TKDs contain a phosphotransferase domain and an ATP binding site. The ligand for KIT, SCF, induces the development, proliferation, maturation, and survival of mast cells. In addition, KIT signaling stimulates cytokine and chemokine release, and augments FcεRI-mediated responses. The regulation of FcεRI and KIT should be a promising strategy to control mast cell-mediated allergic reactions [13,14].

Gain-of-function mutations in *KIT* genes, among which D816V is most common, cause the dysregulated cell growth and subsequent clonal accumulation of mast cells in various tissues, a condition referred as mastocytosis [16]. Mastocytosis had been categorized into cutaneous mastocytosis (urticaria pigmentosa) and systemic mastocytosis according to the distribution of neoplastic mast cells, and has been recently recategorized into indolent systemic mastocytosis (ISM), systemic mastocytosis with an associated clonal hematologic non-MC-lineage disease (SM-AHNMD), aggressive systemic mastocytosis (ASM), and mast cell leukemia (MCL) according to the clinical parameters [16]. Patients with mastocytosis often experience mast cell mediator-related symptoms including anaphylaxis, in addition to tissue damage caused by neoplastic mast cell infiltration [17]. To alleviate these symptoms, the numbers of neoplastic mast cells should be reduced in the patients. The regulation on mutated KIT signal pathways should also be a promising approach to control the numbers of neoplastic mast cells. Gain-of-function type KIT mutations are observed in other malignancies, such as gastrointestinal stromal tumor (GIST), seminoma, and acute myelogenous leukemia (AML), though the mutated sites are varied among these malignancies [18].

2. Inhibitory Receptors

KIT-mediated and FcεRI-mediated responses can be modulated by other receptors expressed on the surface of mast cells, including FcγRIIb, Siglecs, mast cell function-associated antigen, signal regulatory protein α, and leukocyte Ig-like receptor B4 (formerly gp49B1), paired Ig-like receptor-B, myeloid-associated immunoglobulin-like receptor I, CD200 receptor, CD300a, CD300f, Allergin-1, 2B4, CD72, programmed death-1 (PD-1), NKp46, carcinoembryonic antigen-related cell adhesion molecule 1, signaling lymphocytic activation molecule family member 8, and killer immunoglobulin-like receptor (KIR) 2DL4 [19–31]. These include inhibitory receptors characterized by immunoreceptor tyrosine-based inhibitory motifs (ITIMs) within their cytosolic domains (Figure 1) [32]. ITIMs comprise the homology sequence (I/V/L/S)xYxx(L/V) (x; any residue). When the receptors are stimulated, their tyrosine residues become phosphorylated following the activation of receptor or Src family tyrosine kinases. This is followed by the recruitment and activation of non-receptor protein phosphatases, such as Src homology 2 domain-containing tyrosine phosphatase (SHP)-1, SHP-2, and Src homology 2 domain-containing inositol 5-phosphatase (SHIP) 1. SHP-1 and SHP-2 dephosphorylate tyrosine-containing signaling molecules, thus reversing the action of tyrosine kinases. SHIP1 dephosphorylates phosphatidylinositol 3,4,5 trisphosphate at the 3′ position, thereby terminating phosphatidylinositol 3-kinase (PI3K)-driven signaling pathways [32].

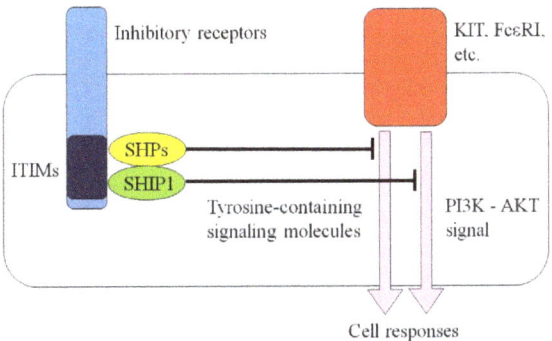

Figure 1. Inhibitory receptor. ITIM: immunoreceptor tyrosine-based inhibitory motif; PI3K: phosphatidylinositol 3-kinase; SHIP: Src homology 2 domain-containing inositol 5-phosphatase; SHP: Src homology 2 domain-containing tyrosine phosphatase.

Several inhibitory receptors on T and natural killer (NK) cells are classified as immune checkpoint proteins. The discovery of inhibitors against such immune checkpoint proteins, including anti-PD-1 antibodies (nivolumab, pembrolizumab, and cemiplimab), anti-cytotoxic T lymphocyte-associated antigen-4 (CTLA-4) antibody (ipilimumab), anti-lymphocyte activation gene-3 (LAG-3) antibody, anti-T cell immunoglobulin and mucin-domain containing-3 (TIM-3) antibody, anti-T cell immunoglobulin ITIM domain (TIGIT) antibody, anti-V-domain Ig suppressor of T cell activation (VISTA) antibody, and anti-killer immunoglobulin-like receptor (KIR2D) antibody (lirilumab), represents a breakthrough in the field of tumor immunotherapy [33,34]. Anti-PD-L1 (ligand for PD-1) antibody (atezolizumab, avelumab, and durvalumab) and anti-CD200 (ligand for CD200 receptor) antibody (samalitumab) target the ligands for inhibitory receptors on these cells [33,35]. The above-mentioned antibodies interfere with the inhibition of cytotoxic activities of T and NK cells against tumor cells, therefore, they are regarded as "inhibitors" for inhibitory receptors. Gemtuzumab is an antibody against CD33, a member of inhibitory receptors, utilized for the treatment on hematopoietic malignancies [36]. This antibody binds to tumor cells without inducing activation of CD33. To our knowledge, the agonistic antibodies against inhibitory receptors have not been therapeutically utilized.

3. KIR2DL4, a Member of the KIR Family

KIRs are human-specific transmembrane proteins which modulate the functions of human NK cells, and some of them are members of inhibitory receptors [37]. NK cells can kill major histocompatibility (MHC) class I-negative tumor cells but cannot kill MHC class I-positive tumor cells. To explain this observation, the missing self-hypothesis had been proposed. This hypothesis predicted that NK cells express MHC class I-receptors, transducing inhibitory signals. KIRs had been identified as such receptors (at the time, KIRs termed killer "inhibitory" receptors). Then, it revealed that the at least 14 KIR genes have been identified in the human genome and are clustered on chromosome 19q13.4 (then, KIRs are called killer "immunoglobulin-like" receptors) [37]. The number and combination of

KIR genes in the genome varies within the human population. Additionally, the expression of each KIR is regulated at the transcriptional level by DNA methylation. Therefore, KIR protein expression repertoires are varied within the human population. The KIR nomenclature reflects the structure of the proteins: the first two characters correspond to the number of the extracellular domains (2D and 3D), and the third digit corresponds to the length of the cytoplasmic tail (L or S). KIRs with a long cytoplasmic domain (L) contain ITIMs (KIR-L), while those with a short cytoplasmic domain (S) lack ITIMs (KIR-S) [37]. Therefore, KIR-Ls are categorized into the inhibitory receptors, and expected to transduce inhibitory signals to NK cells.

Unlike other KIR members, KIR2DL4 is constitutively expressed in all NK cells on the transcriptional level [38]. Human leukocyte antigen (HLA)-G has been identified as the ligand for KIR2DL4 [38,39]. HLA-G is a non-classical HLA class I molecule, and composed of four membrane-bound (HLA-G1, -G2, -G3, and -G4) and three soluble (HLA-G5, -G6, and -G7) isoforms [39]. These isoforms are generated by alternative splicing of HLA-G mRNA. In addition to KIR2DL4, CD85j/immunoglobulin-like transcript 2 (ILT2), CD85d/ILT4, CD8, and CD160 have also been reported to bind HLA-G [39]. CD85j is expressed by monocytes, B cells, dendritic cells (DCs), myeloid derived suppressive cells (MDSCs), NK cells, and T cells. CD85d is expressed by DCs, monocytes, neutrophils, and MDSCs. KIR2DL4 contains two extracellular domains and a long cytoplasmic domain, therefore has been classified as a KIR-L [37]. The ITIM of KIR2DL4 protein has been shown to interact with SHP-1 and SHP-2, like other inhibitory receptors, and the followed inhibition of CD16/FcγRIIIa signaling in human NK cells [40]. CD16 mediates antibody-dependent cell-mediated cytotoxicity, therefore KIR2DL4-mediated CD16 inhibition is in line with the missing self-hypothesis. In contrast to such inhibitory activity, KIR2DL4 stimulation induces weak cytotoxicity and the secretions of IFN-γ, TNF-α, IL-1α, IL-1β, IL-6, and IL-8 from human NK cells, mediated by activating signals via FcεRIγ independent of the presence of ITIM [41–44]. These responses could potentially enhance tumor and virus elimination, although their physiological roles have not been established. Soluble HLA-G has been shown to induce similar cytokine secretions [44]. It is thought that soluble HLA-G binds to KIR2DL4 in endosomes and activates DNA-PKcs (DNA-dependent protein kinase, catalytic subunit)–AKT–NF-κB signals [44,45]. The expression and function of KIR2DL4 in other immune cells remains poorly understood.

4. KIR2DL4 Expression in Human Mast Cells

Similar to NK cells, mast cells secrete the Th1 cytokine IFN-γ [46,47] and show cytotoxic activity by producing GrB [48,49]. Therefore, we hypothesized and explored the expression of KIR2DL4 in human mast cells.

We detected the expression of KIR2DL4 in human cultured mast cells established from the peripheral blood of healthy volunteers (PB-mast) [50], in a human mast cell line LAD2 expressing normal KIT and normal FcεRI [51], and in human tissue mast cells [30]. We could not detect the expression of other HLA-G receptors, such as CD85j, CD85d, CD8, and CD160, in these cultured mast cells. In contrast, we observed that the KIR2DL4 protein expression was lacking in the human neoplastic mast cell line HMC1.2 expressing mutated KIT and deficient in FcεRI expression [52], and that nine of 15 cutaneous mastocytosis samples were KIR2DL4-negative [30]. These observations suggest that a lack of KIR2DL4 protein expression could serve as a diagnostic marker of neoplastic changes in mast cells, as is the case that lack of or decreased expression of KIR2DL4 is detected in neoplastic NK cells, NK cell lymphoma [53,54].

5. Possible Regulation by KIR2DL4 Stimulation on Mast Cell-Associated Allergic Reactions and Mastocytosis

Both PB-mast and LAD2 cells have been used to examine the role of KIR2DL4 in FcεRI-mediated and/or KIT-mediated reactions of human mast cells. Treatment of PB-mast and LAD2 cells with two agonistic antibodies against KIR2DL4 suppressed FcεRI-mediated degranulation and KIT-mediated growth of these cells [30]. These results suggested that KIR2DL4 stimulation is expected to suppress mast cell-mediated allergic reactions. In addition, administration of the same antibodies induced the secretion of the serine protease, GrB [30]. The inhibitory effects on FcεRI-mediated and KIT-mediated responses, as well as the GrB secretion, were abrogated when a SHP-2 inhibitor was used [30], suggesting that the KIR2DL4-mediated responses were SHP-2-dependent [30]. SHP-2 regulates cell functions both positively and negatively; SHP-2 enhances cell functions by activating Grb2-associated binder family member (Gab) 2–mitogen-activated protein kinase (MAPK) signal pathways, and suppresses cell functions by dephosphorylating phopho-proteins that are involved in various other signal pathways [55]. In human mast cells, KIR2DL4-induced suppression of FcεRI-mediated and KIT-mediated responses would be mediated by the dephosphorylating activity of SHP-2, and at the same time KIR2DL4-induced GrB secretion would be mediated by the Gab2–MAPK signal pathway. We observed that KIR2DL4-induced GrB secretion was c-Jun N-terminal kinase (JNK)-dependent in human mast cells [30], therefore KIR2DL4–SHP-2–Gab2–JNK signaling would exist in human mast cells.

As mentioned above, interference with the KIT-mediated and FcεRI-mediated signal pathways has been proposed as a potential strategy to control mast cell-mediated allergic reactions [13,14], highlighting the importance of KIR2DL4 as a target for allergic diseases. In other words, the agonistic antibodies against KIR2DL4 would be useful for allergy therapy, similar to the anti-IgE antibody omalizumab clinically utilized to neutralize IgE in blood, and eliminate of FcεRI-mediated function and control mast cell-mediated allergic reactions [56]. Imatinib is known to inhibit KIT signal pathways, and the efficacy of this drug is shown in patients with severe refractory asthma, one of the mast cell-mediated allergic diseases [57]. KIR2DL4 can inhibit both KIT-mediated and FcεRI-mediated signal pathways, therefore the agonistic antibodies against KIR2DL4 could potentially exert synergistic effects in combination with omalizumab and imatinib.

Some human mastocytosis (six of 15 cutaneous mastocytosis cases) expressed KIR2DL4 protein, however, whether KIR2DL4 stimulation suppresses the growth of KIT-mutated neoplastic mast cells in vitro has not been determined. It is believed that KIR2DL4 may inhibit the growth of KIT-mutated neoplastic mast cells. This hypothesis is supported by the fact that PD-1-mediated SHP-2 activation could inhibit the growth of KIT-mutated neoplastic mast cells [26]. Moreover, avapritinib is a recently identified KIT D816V inhibitor and shown to be useful for mastocytosis treatment [58]. Another KIT inhibitor imatinib is ineffective on KIT D816V observing almost all mastocytosis [59] but is effective on KIT mutations in GISTs [60]. Resistance to this drug, mainly caused by the second mutation in KIT gene, is a problem arising during imatinib therapy on GISTs [60]. KIR2DL4-targeted therapy might be useful, especially when a second mutation in the *KIT* gene is caused during avapritinib-utilized mastocytosis therapy.

6. Involvement of KIR2DL4 on Human Mast Cells in the Establishment of Pregnancy

The natural ligand of KIR2DL4 is HLA-G, as mentioned above [38,39]. The HLA-G expression was physiologically restricted in trophoblasts, cornea, thymic medulla, and islets of pancreas [39]. HLA-G is involved in tumor progression, viral infection, organ transplantation, autoimmune and inflammatory diseases [39]. Furthermore, soluble HLA-G levels have been associated with allergen-specific IgE levels in the serum of patients with allergic rhinitis [61]. Herein, we then focused on the interaction of human mast cells expressing KIR2DL4 with HLA-G-positive trophoblasts during pregnancy establishment and with HLA-G-positive cancer cells during cancer progression.

Interactions between KIR2DL4 and HLA-G have been investigated in the context of decidual NK cell-trophoblast interactions during the establishment of pregnancy [62]. The reduced expression of KIR2DL4 protein in decidual NK cells was observed in some women with recurrent spontaneous abortion [63]. KIR2DL4 is expressed on human decidual NK cells, and suppresses the cytotoxic activity against the HLA-G-expressing fetuses [62,63]. Therefore, the reduced KIR2DL4 expression levels on decidual NK cells have been thought to increase the susceptibility of NK cell-mediated cytotoxic activity and the following recurrent spontaneous abortion [63]. Regulatory T cells (Tregs) have also been also implicated in the establishment of pregnancy [64]. Reduced numbers of decidual Tregs were observed in some women with recurrent spontaneous abortion [65–67]. Decidual Tregs is necessary for the tolerance toward semi-allogenic fetuses [65–67]. Thus, the studies on the roles of decidual immune cells have been focused on the suppression of semi-allogenic fetus rejections in the establishment of pregnancy. Additionally, recent studies show that decidual immune cells are necessary for angiogenesis in the establishment of pregnancy [68]. For example, decidual NK cells secrete angiogenic factors, such as VEGF, angiopoietin-2, placental growth factor (PlGF), and chymase [69,70]. Decidual NK cells are thought to secrete these factors, induce angiogenesis and spiral artery remodeling. Recently, a new subset of decidual NK cells, pregnancy trained decidual NK cells (PTdNKs) has been characterized as an enhancer of proper placentation, which increases the secretion of VEGF which supporting angiogenesis [71].

Another immunocompetent cell, mast cell, is also distributed to the uterus [72]. Mast cells are identified in the endometrium throughout the menstrual cycle, and the activation of mast cells are observed prior to menstruation [72]. Nevertheless, mast cells had been thought to be indispensable for pregnancy; mast-cell-deficient $Kit^{W/Wv}$ and $Kit^{Wsh/Wsh}$ mice are infertile, though blastocyst transfer can archive implantation and live births in both mice [73,74]. Moreover, mast cell transfer to uterus could improve the success ratio of establishment of pregnancy in $Kit^{Wsh/Wsh}$ mice [75]. Mast cell chymase was subsequently shown to be important for angiogenesis in the decidual tissues of mice and humans, as is the case of NK cell-derived chymase [65]. In addition, mast cells produce other angiogenic molecules such as VEGF, bFGF, heparin, histamine, SCF, as mentioned above [4–6]. Transfer of Tregs into abortion-prone mice promoted the expansion of uterine mast cells and the angiogenesis, resulting in the improvement of the success ratio of establishment of pregnancy [76].

We observed that mast cells in the decidual tissues of parous women expressed KIR2DL4 [31]. In contrast, the numbers of decidual mast cells and KIR2DL4 expression was significantly reduced in infertile women long-term treated with corticosteroids for autoimmune diseases, liver transplantation, or kidney transplantation [31]. The numbers of NK cells and Tregs in decidual tissues were not significantly different among the infertile women long-term treated with corticosteroids, infertile women of uncertain etiology, and the parous women, as is not the case of mouse experiments. We suspected that KIR2DL4 on decidual mast cells seemed to be involved in the establishment of pregnancy. To elucidate the importance of the interaction between KIR2DL4 on mast cells and HLA-G on trophoblasts, we co-cultured a HLA-G-positive human trophoblast cell line HTR-8/SVneo cells [77] with a human mast cell LAD2. The co-culture showed enhanced migration and tube formation of HTR-8/SVneo in the KIR2DL4-HLA-G interaction-dependent manner [31]. When KIR2DL4 was stimulated, LAD2 cells secreted leukemia growth factor (LIF) and a serine protease MMP-9 [31]. LIF is a member of the IL-6 family of cytokines [78]. LIF receptor consists of gp130 and LIF receptor β subunit, and transduces the Janus kinase (JAK)–signal transducer and activator of transcription (STAT) signaling pathway [78]. LIF-knockout female mice are infertile due to embryo implantation failure [78]. LIF is highly expressed in the endometrial glands, as well as decidual NK and mast cells [31,78]. LIF enhances the invasion and differentiation of trophoblasts, resulting in the implantation of fetuses [78]. LIF also enhances tumor progression by promoting cell cycle progression and invasive activity of tumor cells via STAT3 activation, as is the case of other IL-6 family of cytokines [79]. Similarly, KIR2DL4-induced LIF secretion by LAD2 enhanced the migration of HTR-8/SVneo via STAT3 activation. Serine proteases, including MMP-9, induce the degradation of protease-activated receptors [80], which subsequently decreases in the secretion of soluble fms-like tyrosine kinase-1 (sFlt-1), an inhibitor of VEGF, from trophoblasts [81]. KIR2DL4-induced MMP-9 secretion from LAD2 decreased the secretion of sFlt-1 from HTR-8/SVneo, and the followed increase of tube formation by HTR-8/SVneo. Thus, mast cell deficiency in decidual tissues leads to pregnancy and parturition disorder, and KIR2DL4 downregulation is associated with infertility, suggesting that selective KIR2DL4-induced production of LIF and MMP-9 by mast cells that may illustrate the critical context-specific role of mast cells in pregnancy.

7. Involvement of KIR2DL4 on Human Mast Cells in Tumor Progression

HLA-G is expressed in various tumors, as mentioned above [38,39]. The expression of HLA-G in neoplasms was first identified in choriocarcinomas, neoplastic trophoblastic cells [82], and secondly identified in malignant melanoma [83]. HLA-G expression has also been reported in lung cancer, oral and nasopharyngeal squamous cell carcinoma, esophageal cancer, gastric cancer, colorectal cancer, hepatocellular carcinoma, pancreatic cancer, uterine cancer (cervical cancer and endometrial cancer), ovarian cancer, glioblastoma, malignant lymphoma, and so on. Additionally, HLA-G expression levels have been associated with advanced tumor stage, metastasis status and poor diagnosis in various tumors [84]. This is partially explained by the fact that HLA-G is thought to suppress the cytotoxic activity of human NK cells against HLA-G-positive tumor cells via KIR2DL4 or other receptors, such as CD85j, CD85d, CD8, and CD160 [84]. Therefore, HLA-G could be a target for immune checkpoint therapy, though the HLA-G-targeted drugs have not been therapeutically utilized to our knowledge. Breast cancer cells also express HLA-G, and HLA-G expression in breast cancers is associated with poor prognosis [85–88].

A role for mast cells in tumor progression has been under discussion [89,90]. When mast cells were first described by Paul Ehrlich, he reported mast cells distributed around skin cancers and pointed out the association between mast cell and tumorigenesis [1]. Experimental tumorigenesis after subcutaneous treatment with 3-methylcholanthrene revealed that the tumor incidence in mast cell-deficient $KIT^{W/Wv}$ mice was increased compared to that in control mice, therefore mast cells had been thought to be involved in tumor suppression [91]. This finding could be attributed to the fact that mast cells produce anti-tumor mediators, such as granzyme B, reactive oxygen species, and Th1 cytokines, including TNF-α and IFN-γ [46–49]. Mast-cell-produced IL-9 were shown to inhibit tumor cell engraftment [92]. Mast cells are a major source of histamine, and histamine was shown to inhibit tumor growth by promoting the development of monocyte-derived DCs [93]. The combined deficiency in mast cell chymase, tryptase, and carboxypeptidase A3 was associated with reduced invariant NKT cells and increased melanoma dissemination [94]. Contrary to these reports on suppressive roles of mast cells in tumor progression, there are reports on enhancing roles of mast cells. The association between mast cells and tumor angiogenesis has been focused in this area. Mast cells produce angiogenetic mediators, such as VEGF, bFGF, heparin, histamine, SCF, IL-8, NGF, TNF-α, tryptase, in forming tumor vessels and the followed invasion or metastasis of cancers [87,88,93]. Mast cells produce Th2 cytokines which contributes to M2 (pro-tumor) polarization of tumor-associated macrophages, and the cells produce TNF-α and IL-10 which promote the Treg-mediated immune tolerance and immune tolerance against tumors [4–6]. Mast cells produce TGF-β, CXCL8, and TNF-α, promoting epithelial-to-mesenchymal transition in tumor invasion and metastasis [94–96]. Mast-cell-produced histamine was shown to inhibit hypoxia inducible factor-1 alpha expression and the followed growth suppression in melanoma [97]. Mast cells producing serine proteases such as tryptase and MMPs [4–6] degrade the extracellular matrix to increase the angiogenesis, resulting in metastasis [98]. The association between infiltrating mast cells and tumor angiogenesis has clinically been shown in pulmonary carcinoma, gastric carcinoma, colorectal carcinoma, endometrial carcinoma, cervix carcinoma, prostatic carcinoma, skin tumors including basal cell carcinoma and melanomas, lymphomas, multiple myeloma, myelodysplastic syndrome, and leukemia [89,90]. Thus, mast cells play dual roles in tumor progression, and the classification into anti-tumorigenic MC1 and pro-tumorigenic MC2 mast cell types have been advocated recently [90]. In breast cancer cells, mast cell infiltration is also related to increased angiogenesis and poor prognosis [99,100]. We examined the association between HLA-G, its receptor KIR2DL4, mast cells, and breast cancer progression.

Using clinical samples, we have shown that HLA-G-positive breast cancer cells interact directly with KIR2DL4-positive tissue mast cells immunohistochemically [30]. The interaction is associated with lymph node metastasis and lymphovascular invasion [30]. Thus, KIR2DL4 on mast cells seems to be involved in cancer progression. To elucidate the importance of the interaction between KIR2DL4 on mast cells and HLA-G on cancer cells, we co-cultured the HLA-G-positive human breast cancer cell line

MCF-7 cells [101] with the human mast cell LAD2. The co-culture showed enhanced invasion of MCF-7 in a KIR2DL4–HLA-G interaction-dependent manner [30]. MMP-9 secreted from KIR2DL4-stimulated LAD2 cells were found to be involved in this process [30]. Thus, human mast cells are associated with an invasive phenotype of HLA-G-positive breast cancers.

8. KIR2DL4 as a Potent Therapeutic Target

KIR2DL4 can be activated by recombinant HLA-G or by agonistic antibodies, such as clone 181,703 and clone 33. The ability of these molecules to enhance the establishment of pregnancy suggests their therapeutic use in the treatment of infertility, in addition to allergic diseases and mastocytosis. KIR2DL4 is expressed by human NK cells, and KIR2DL4-targeted drugs are expected to enhance NK activity and to induce IFN-γ secretion [46–49]. Therefore, KIR2DL4-targeted drugs might enhance NK activity and the following enhancing defensive effects against virus infections. However, KIR2DL4-targeted drugs might enhance HLA-G-positive cancer progression, and patients treated with KIR2DL4 stimulants should first be carefully screened for the presence of malignancy. Additionally, KIR2DL4 expression has been detected in dendritic cells [102]. KIR2DL4-targeting therapies may exert undesirable effects by modulating the function of these cells.

The IL-33/ST2 signal pathway and Mas-related G protein-coupled receptor X2 also play important roles in mast cell biology [14], and the effects of KIR2DL4 on the function of these receptors should be elucidated before KIR2DL4-targeting therapies can enter into clinical practice.

9. Conclusions

KIR2DL4, a member of the KIR family, is expressed by human mast cells. It positively and negatively regulates the functions of human mast cells such that its stimulation may suppress mast cell-mediated allergic reactions and enhance the establishment of pregnancy (Figure 2).

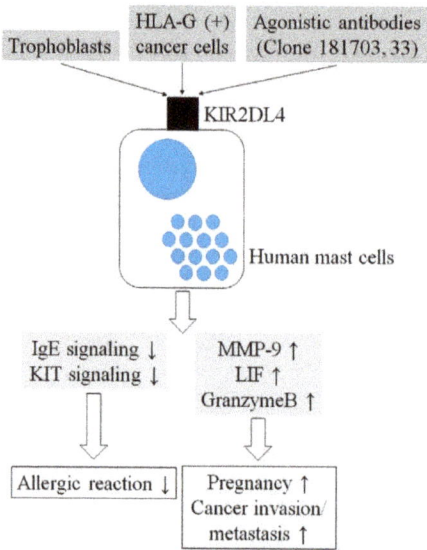

Figure 2. The current model. HLA: human leukocyte antigen; KIR: killer immunoglobulin-like receptor; LIF: Leukemia inhibitory factor; MMP: matrix metalloprotease.

Funding: This research was funded by grants from JSPS KAKENHI (23590437, 15K08362, 16K19080, 18K07014, and 19K16556). The authors thank K. Ijiri (Department of Diagnostic Pathology, Kyoto University Hospital, Kyoto, Japan) for her secretarial assistance.

Conflicts of Interest: The authors declare no conflict of interest.

Abbreviations

AML	acute myelogenous leukemia
ASM	aggressive systemic mastocytosis
CTLA-4	cytotoxic T lymphocyte-associated antigen-4
DC	dendritic cell
DNA-PKcs	DNA-dependent protein kinase, catalytic subunit
FcεRIγ	Fc receptor γ chain
FGF	fibroblast growth factor
Gab	Grb2-associated binder family member (Gab)
GIST	gastrointestinal stromal tumor
GM-CSF	granulocyte macrophage colony-stimulating factor
GrB	granzyme B
HLA	human leukocyte antigen
IFN	interferon
IL	interleukin
ILT	immunoglobulin-like transcript
ISM	indolent systemic mastocytosis
ITAM	immunoreceptor tyrosine-based activation motifs
ITIM	immunoreceptor tyrosine-based inhibitory motif
JAK	Janus kinase
JNK	c-Jun N-terminal kinase
KIR	killer immunoglobulin-like receptor
LAG-3	lymphocyte activation gene-3
LIF	leukemia growth factor
MAPK	mitogen-activated protein kinase
MCL	mast cell leukemia
MDSC	myeloid derived suppressive cell
MHC	major histocompatibility
MMP	matrix metalloprotease
NK	natural killer
NGF	nerve growth factor
PB-mast	human cultured mast cells established from peripheral blood derived from healthy volunteers
PD	programmed death
PI3K	phosphatidylinositol 3-kinase
PlGF	placental growth factor
PTdNK	pregnancy trained decidual NK cell
SCF	stem cell factor
sFlt-1	soluble fms-like tyrosine kinase-1
SHIP	Src homology 2 domain-containing inositol 5-phosphatase
SHP	Src homology 2 domain-containing tyrosine phosphatase
SM-AHNMD	systemic mastocytosis with an associated clonal hematologic non-MC-lineage disease
STAT	signal transducer and activator of transcription
TGF	transforming growth factor
TIGIT	T cell immunoglobulin ITIM domain
TIM-3	T cell immunoglobulin and mucin-domain containing-3
TKD	tyrosine-kinase domain
TNF	tumor necrosis factor
Treg	regulatory T cell
VEGF	vascular endothelial growth factor
VISTA	V-domain Ig suppressor of T cell activation

References

1. Crivellato, E.; Beltrami, C.; Mallardi, F.; Ribatti, D. Paul Ehrlich's doctoral thesis: A milestone in the study of mast cells. *Br. J. Haematol.* **2003**, *123*, 19–21. [PubMed]
2. Kitamura, Y.; Matsuda, H.; Hatanaka, K. Clonal nature of mast-cell clusters formed in W/Wv mice after bone marrow transplantation. *Nature* **1979**, *281*, 154–155. [CrossRef] [PubMed]
3. Nakano, T.; Sonoda, T.; Hayashi, C.; Yamatodani, A.; Kanayama, Y.; Yamamura, T.; Asai, H.; Yonezawa, T.; Kitamura, Y.; Galli, S.J. Fate of bone marrow-derived cultured mast cells after intracutaneous, intraperitoneal, and intravenous transfer into genetically mast cell-deficient W/Wv mice. Evidence that cultured mast cells can give rise to both connective tissue type and mucosal mast cells. *J. Exp. Med.* **1985**, *162*, 1025–1043. [PubMed]
4. Mukai, K.; Tsai, M.; Saito, H.; Galli, S.J. Mast cells as sources of cytokines, chemokines, and growth factors. *Immunol. Rev.* **2018**, *282*, 121–150. [CrossRef] [PubMed]
5. Espinosa, E.; Valitutti, S. New roles and controls of mast cells. *Curr. Opin. Immunol.* **2018**, *50*, 39–47. [CrossRef]
6. Dudeck, A.; Köberle, M.; Goldmann, O.; Meyer, N.; Dudeck, J.; Lemmens, S.; Rohde, M.; Roldán, N.G.; Dietze-Schwonberg, K.; Orinska, Z.; et al. Mast cells as protectors of health. *J. Allergy Clin. Immunol.* **2019**, *144(4S)*, S4–S18. [CrossRef]
7. Reitz, M.; Brunn, M.L.; Rodewald, H.R.; Feyerabend, T.B.; Roers, A.; Dudeck, A.; Voehringer, D.; Jonsson, F.; Kuhl, A.A.; Breloer, M. Mucosal mast cells are indispensable for the timely termination of *Strongyloides ratti* infection. *Mucosal. Immunol.* **2017**, *10*, 481–492. [CrossRef]
8. Mukai, K.; Karasuyama, H.; Kabashima, K.; Kubo, M.; Galli, S.J. Differences in the Importance of Mast Cells, Basophils, IgE, and IgG versus That of CD4(+) T Cells and ILC2 Cells in Primary and Secondary Immunity to *Strongyloides venezuelensis*. *Infect. Immun.* **2017**, *85*, e00053-17. [CrossRef]
9. Galli, S.J.; Starkl, P.; Marichal, T.; Tsai, M. Mast Cells and IgE can Enhance Survival During Innate and Acquired Host Responses to Venoms. *Trans. Am. Clin. Climatol. Assoc.* **2017**, *128*, 193–221.
10. Kubo, M. Mast cells and basophils in allergic inflammation. *Curr. Opin. Immunol.* **2018**, *54*, 74–79. [CrossRef]
11. Bischoff, S.C. Mast cells in gastrointestinal disorders. *Eur. J. Pharmacol.* **2016**, *778*, 139–145. [CrossRef] [PubMed]
12. Hermans, M.; Lennep, J.R.V.; van Daele, P.; Bot, I. Mast Cells in Cardiovascular Disease: From Bench to Bedside. *Int. J. Mol. Sci.* **2019**, *20*, 3395. [CrossRef] [PubMed]
13. Draber, P.; Halova, I.; Polakovicova, I.; Kawakami, T. Signal transduction and chemotaxis in mast cells. *Eur. J. Pharmacol.* **2016**, *778*, 11–23. [CrossRef] [PubMed]
14. Olivera, A.; Beaven, M.A.; Metcalfe, D.D. Mast cells signal their importance in health and disease. *J. Allergy Clin. Immunol.* **2018**, *142*, 381–393. [CrossRef] [PubMed]
15. Ra, C.; Nunomura, S.; Okayama, Y. Fine-Tuning of Mast Cell Activation by FcεRIβ Chain. *Front. Immunol.* **2012**, *3*, 112. [CrossRef]
16. Valent, P.; Akin, C.; Hartmann, K.; Nilsson, G.; Reiter, A.; Hermine, O.; Sotlar, K.; Sperr, W.R.; Escribano, L.; George, T.I.; et al. Advances in the Classification and Treatment of Mastocytosis: Current Status and Outlook toward the Future. *Cancer Res.* **2017**, *77*, 1261–1270. [CrossRef]
17. Castells, M.; Butterfield, J. Mast Cell Activation Syndrome and Mastocytosis: Initial Treatment Options and Long-Term Management. *J. Allergy Clin. Immunol. Pract.* **2019**, *7*, 1097–1106. [CrossRef]
18. Heinrich, M.C.; Blanke, C.D.; Druker, B.J.; Corless, C.L. Inhibition of KIT tyrosine kinase activity: A novel molecular approach to the treatment of KIT-positive malignancies. *J. Clin. Oncol.* **2002**, *20*, 1692–1703. [CrossRef]
19. Bulfone-Paus, S.; Nilsson, G.; Draber, P.; Blank, U.; Levi-Schaffer, F. Positive and Negative Signals in Mast Cell Activation. *Trends Immunol.* **2017**, *38*, 657–667. [CrossRef]
20. Hitomi, K.; Tahara-Hanaoka, S.; Someya, S.; Fujiki, A.; Tada, H.; Sugiyama, T.; Shibayama, S.; Shibuya, K.; Shibuya, A. An immunoglobulin-like receptor, Allergin-1, inhibits immunoglobulin E-mediated immediate hypersensitivity reactions. *Nat. Immunol.* **2010**, *11*, 601–607. [CrossRef]
21. Izawa, K.; Yamanishi, Y.; Maehara, A.; Takahashi, M.; Isobe, M.; Ito, S.; Kaitani, A.; Matsukawa, T.; Matsuoka, T.; Nakahara, F.; et al. The receptor LMIR3 negatively regulates mast cell activation and allergic responses by binding to extracellular ceramide. *Immunity* **2012**, *37*, 827–839. [CrossRef] [PubMed]

22. Mizrahi, S.; Gibbs, B.F.; Karra, L.; Ben-Zimra, M.; Levi-Schaffer, F. Siglec-7 is an inhibitory receptor on human mast cells and basophils. *J. Allergy Clin. Immunol.* **2014**, *134*, 230–233. [CrossRef] [PubMed]
23. Elishmereni, M.; Fyhrquist, N.; Singh Gangwar, R.; Lehtimäki, S.; Alenius, H.; Levi-Schaffer, F. Complex 2B4 regulation of mast cells and eosinophils in murine allergic inflammation. *J. Investig. Dermatol.* **2014**, *134*, 2928–2937. [CrossRef] [PubMed]
24. Yu, Y.; Blokhuis, B.R.J.; Diks, M.A.P.; Keshavarzian, A.; Garssen, J.; Redegeld, F.A. Functional Inhibitory Siglec-6 Is Upregulated in Human Colorectal Cancer-Associated Mast Cells. *Front. Immunol.* **2018**, *9*, 2138. [CrossRef] [PubMed]
25. Kataoka, T.R.; Kumanogoh, A.; Bandara, G.; Metcalfe, D.D.; Gilfillan, A.M. CD72 negatively regulates KIT-mediated responses in human mast cells. *J. Immunol.* **2010**, *184*, 2468–2475. [CrossRef] [PubMed]
26. Kataoka, T.R.; Fujimoto, M.; Moriyoshi, K.; Koyanagi, I.; Ueshima, C.; Kono, F.; Tsuruyama, T.; Okayama, Y.; Ra, C.; Haga, H. PD-1 Regulates the Growth of Human Mastocytosis Cells. *Allergol. Int.* **2013**, *62*, 99–104. [CrossRef]
27. Ueshima, C.; Kataoka, T.R.; Hirata, M.; Koyanagi, I.; Honda, T.; Tsuruyama, T.; Okayama, Y.; Seiyama, A.; Haga, H. NKp46 regulates the production of serine proteases and IL-22 in human mast cells in urticaria pigmentosa. *Exp. Dermatol.* **2015**, *24*, 675–679. [CrossRef]
28. Ueshima, C.; Kataoka, T.R.; Takei, Y.; Hirata, M.; Sugimoto, A.; Hirokawa, M.; Okayama, Y.; Blumberg, R.S.; Haga, H. CEACAM1 long isoform has opposite effects on the growth of human mastocytosis and medullary thyroid carcinoma cells. *Cancer Med.* **2017**, *6*, 845–856. [CrossRef]
29. Sugimoto, A.; Kataoka, T.R.; Ueshima, C.; Takei, Y.; Kitamura, K.; Hirata, M.; Nomura, T.; Haga, H. SLAM family member 8 is involved in oncogenic KIT-mediated signalling in human mastocytosis. *Exp. Dermatol.* **2018**, *27*, 641–646. [CrossRef]
30. Ueshima, C.; Kataoka, T.R.; Hirata, M.; Furuhata, A.; Suzuki, E.; Toi, M.; Tsuruyama, T.; Okayama, Y.; Haga, H. The Killer Cell Ig-like Receptor 2DL4 Expression in Human Mast Cells and Its Potential Role in Breast Cancer Invasion. *Cancer Immunol. Res.* **2015**, *3*, 871–880. [CrossRef]
31. Ueshima, C.; Kataoka, T.R.; Hirata, M.; Sugimoto, A.; Iemura, Y.; Minamiguchi, S.; Nomura, T.; Haga, H. Possible Involvement of Human Mast Cells in the Establishment of Pregnancy via Killer Cell Ig-Like Receptor 2DL. *Am. J. Pathol.* **2018**, *188*, 1497–1508.
32. Unkeless, J.C.; Jin, J. Inhibitory receptors, ITIM sequences and phosphatases. *Curr. Opin. Immunol.* **1997**, *9*, 338–343. [CrossRef]
33. Qin, S.; Xu, L.; Yi, M.; Yu, S.; Wu, K.; Luo, S. Novel immune checkpoint targets: Moving beyond PD-1 and CTLA-4. *Mol. Cancer* **2019**, *18*, 155. [CrossRef] [PubMed]
34. Terszowski, G.; Klein, C.; Schmied, L.; Stern, M. How to outsmart NK cell tolerance. *Oncoimmunology* **2015**, *4*, e1016708. [CrossRef] [PubMed]
35. Mahadevan, D.; Lanasa, M.C.; Farber, C.; Pandey, M.; Whelden, M.; Faas, S.J.; Ulery, T.; Kukreja, A.; Li, L.; Bedrosian, C.L.; et al. Phase I study of samalizumab in chronic lymphocytic leukemia and multiple myeloma: Blockade of the immune checkpoint CD200. *J. Immunother. Cancer* **2019**, *7*, 227. [CrossRef] [PubMed]
36. Morsink, L.M.; Walter, R.B. Novel monoclonal antibody-based therapies for acute myeloid leukemia. *Best Pract. Res. Clin. Haematol.* **2019**, *32*, 116–126. [CrossRef]
37. Kumar, S. Natural killer cell cytotoxicity and its regulation by inhibitory receptors. *Immunology* **2018**, *154*, 383–393. [CrossRef]
38. Rajagopalan, S.; Long, E.O. A human histocompatibility leukocyte antigen (HLA)-G-specific receptor expressed on all natural killer cells. *J. Exp. Med.* **1999**, *189*, 1093–1100. [CrossRef]
39. Fainardi, E.; Castellazzi, M.; Stignani, M.; Morandi, F.; Sana, G.; Gonzalez, R.; Pistoia, V.; Baricordi, O.R.; Sokal, E.; Peña, J. Emerging topics and new perspectives on HLA-G. *Cell. Mol. Life Sci.* **2011**, *68*, 433–451. [CrossRef]
40. Faure, M.; Long, E.O. KIR2DL4 (CD158d), an NK cell-activating receptor with inhibitory potential. *J. Immunol.* **2002**, *168*, 6208–6214. [CrossRef]
41. Kikuchi-Maki, A.; Yusa, S.; Catina, T.L.; Campbell, K.S. KIR2DL4 is an IL-2-regulated NK cell receptor that exhibits limited expression in humans but triggers strong IFN-γ production. *J. Immunol.* **2003**, *171*, 3415–3425. [CrossRef] [PubMed]

42. Kikuchi-Maki, A.; Catina, T.L.; Campbell, K.S. Cutting edge: KIR2DL4 transduces signals into human NK cells through association with the Fc receptor γ protein. *J. Immunol.* **2005**, *174*, 3859–3863. [CrossRef] [PubMed]
43. Miah, S.M.; Hughes, T.L.; Campbell, K.S. KIR2DL4 differentially signals downstream functions in human NK cells through distinct structural modules. *J. Immunol.* **2008**, *180*, 2922–2932. [CrossRef] [PubMed]
44. Rajagopalan, S.; Bryceson, Y.T.; Kuppusamy, S.P.; Geraghty, D.E.; van der Meer, A.; Joosten, I.; Long, E.O. Activation of NK cells by an endocytosed receptor for soluble HLA-G. *PLoS Biol.* **2006**, *4*, e9. [CrossRef]
45. Rajagopalan, S. Endosomal signaling and a novel pathway defined by the natural killer receptor KIR2DL4 (CD158d). *Traffic* **2010**, *11*, 1381–1390. [CrossRef]
46. Gupta, A.A.; Leal-Berumen, I.; Croitoru, K.; Marshall, J.S. Rat peritoneal mast cells produce IFN-γ following IL-12 treatment but not in response to IgE-mediated activation. *J. Immunol.* **1996**, *157*, 2123–2128.
47. Kataoka, T.R.; Komazawa, N.; Morii, E.; Oboki, K.; Nakano, T. Involvement of connective tissue-type mast cells in Th1 immune responses via Stat4 expression. *Blood* **2005**, *105*, 1016–1020. [CrossRef]
48. Kataoka, T.R.; Morii, E.; Oboki, K.; Kitamura, Y. Strain-dependent inhibitory effect of mutant mi-MITF on cytotoxic activities of cultured mast cells and natural killer cells of mice. *Lab. Investig.* **2004**, *84*, 376–384. [CrossRef]
49. Ito, A.; Morii, E.; Kim, D.K.; Kataoka, T.R.; Jippo, T.; Maeyama, K.; Nojima, H.; Kitamura, Y. Inhibitory effect of the transcription factor encoded by the mi mutant allele in cultured mast cells of mice. *Blood* **1999**, *93*, 1189–1196. [CrossRef]
50. Kirshenbaum, A.S.; Goff, J.P.; Semere, T.; Foster, B.; Scott, L.M.; Metcalfe, D.D. Demonstration that human mast cells arise from a progenitor cell population that is CD34(+), c-kit(+), and expresses aminopeptidase N (CD13). *Blood* **1999**, *94*, 2333–2342. [CrossRef]
51. Kirshenbaum, A.S.; Akin, C.; Wu, Y.; Rottem, M.; Goff, J.P.; Beaven, M.A.; Rao, V.K.; Metcalfe, D.D. Characterization of novel stem cell factor responsive human mast cell lines LAD 1 and 2 established from a patient with mast cell sarcoma/leukemia; activation following aggregation of FcεRI or FcγRI. *Leuk. Res.* **2003**, *27*, 677–682. [CrossRef]
52. Butterfield, J.H.; Weiler, D.; Dewald, G.; Gleich, G.J. Establishment of an immature mast cell line from a patient with mast cell leukemia. *Leuk. Res.* **1988**, *12*, 345–355. [CrossRef]
53. Maki, G.; Klingemann, H.G.; Martinson, J.A.; Tam, Y.K. Factors regulating the cytotoxic activity of the human natural killer cell line, NK-92. *J. Hematother. Stem Cell Res.* **2001**, *10*, 369–383. [CrossRef] [PubMed]
54. Küçük, C.; Hu, X.; Gong, Q.; Jiang, B.; Cornish, A.; Gaulard, P.; McKeithan, T.; Chan, W.C. Diagnostic and Biological Significance of KIR Expression Profile Determined by RNA-Seq in Natural Killer/T-Cell Lymphoma. *Am. J. Pathol.* **2016**, *186*, 1435–1441. [CrossRef]
55. Stein-Gerlach, M.; Wallasch, C.; Ullrich, A. SHP-2, SH2-containing protein tyrosine phosphatase-2. *Int. J. Biochem. Cell. Biol.* **1998**, *30*, 559–566. [CrossRef]
56. Kawakami, T.; Blank, U. From IgE to Omalizumab. *J. Immunol.* **2016**, *197*, 4187–4192. [CrossRef]
57. Cahill, KN.; Katz, H.R.; Cui, J.; Lai, J.; Kazani, S.; Crosby-Thompson, A.; Garofalo, D.; Castro, M.; Jarjour, N.; DiMango, E.; et al. KIT Inhibition by Imatinib in Patients with Severe Refractory Asthma. *N. Engl. J. Med.* **2017**, *376*, 1911–1920. [CrossRef]
58. Lübke, J.; Naumann, N.; Kluger, S.; Schwaab, J.; Metzgeroth, G.; Evans, E.; Gardino, A.K.; Lengauer, C.; Hofmann, W.K.; Fabarius, A.; et al. Inhibitory effects of midostaurin and avapritinib on myeloid progenitors derived from patients with KIT D816V positive advanced systemic mastocytosis. *Leukemia* **2019**, *33*, 1195–1205. [CrossRef]
59. Frost, M.J.; Ferrao, P.T.; Hughes, T.P.; Ashman, L.K. Juxtamembrane mutant V560GKit is more sensitive to Imatinib (STI571) compared with wild-type c-kit whereas the kinase domain mutant D816VKit is resistant. *Mol. Cancer Ther.* **2002**, *1*, 1115–1124.
60. Serrano, C.; George, S.; Valverde, C.; Olivares, D.; García-Valverde, A.; Suárez, C.; Morales-Barrera, R.; Carles, J. Novel Insights into the Treatment of Imatinib-Resistant Gastrointestinal Stromal Tumors. *Target. Oncol.* **2017**, *12*, 277–288. [CrossRef]
61. Murdaca, G.; Contini, P.; Negrini, S.; Ciprandi, G.; Puppo, F. Immunoregulatory Role of HLA-G in Allergic Diseases. *J. Immunol. Res.* **2016**, *2016*, 6865758. [CrossRef] [PubMed]
62. Ferreira, L.M.R.; Meissner, T.B.; Tilburgs, T.; Strominger, J.L. HLA-G: At the interface of maternal-fetal tolerance. *Trends Immunol.* **2017**, *38*, 272–286. [CrossRef]

63. Yan, W.H.; Lin, A.; Chen, B.G.; Zhou, M.Y.; Dai, M.Z.; Chen, X.J.; Gan, L.H.; Zhu, M.; Shi, W.W.; Li, B.L. Possible roles of KIR2DL4 expression on uNK cells in human pregnancy. *Am. J. Reprod. Immunol.* **2007**, *57*, 233–242. [CrossRef]
64. Tsuda, S.; Nakashima, A.; Shima, T.; Saito, S. New Paradigm in the Role of Regulatory T Cells During Pregnancy. *Front. Immunol.* **2019**, *10*, 573. [CrossRef] [PubMed]
65. Sasaki, Y.; Sakai, M.; Miyazaki, S.; Higuma, S.; Shiozaki, A.; Saito, S. Decidual and peripheral blood CD4+CD25+ regulatory T cells in early pregnancy subjects and spontaneous abortion cases. *Mol. Hum. Reprod.* **2004**, *10*, 347–353. [CrossRef] [PubMed]
66. Yang, H.; Qiu, L.; Chen, G.; Ye, Z.; Lu, C.; Lin, Q. Proportional change of CD4+CD25+ regulatory T cells in decidua and peripheral blood in unexplained recurrent spontaneous abortion patients. *Fertil. Steril.* **2008**, *89*, 656–661. [CrossRef]
67. Mei, S.; Tan, J.; Chen, H.; Chen, Y.; Zhang, J. Changes of CD4+CD25high regulatory T cells and FOXP3 expression in unexplained recurrent spontaneous abortion patients. *Fertil. Steril.* **2010**, *94*, 2244–2247. [CrossRef]
68. Pollheimer, J.; Vondra, S.; Baltayeva, J.; Beristain, A.G.; Knöfler, M. Regulation of Placental Extravillous Trophoblasts by the Maternal Uterine Environment. *Front. Immunol.* **2018**, *9*, 2597. [CrossRef]
69. Lash, G.E.; Schiessl, B.; Kirkley, M.; Innes, B.A.; Cooper, A.; Searle, R.F.; Robson, S.C.; Bulmer, J.N. Expression of angiogenic growth factors by uterine natural killer cells during early pregnancy. *J. Leukoc. Biol.* **2006**, *80*, 572–580. [CrossRef]
70. Meyer, N.; Woidacki, K.; Knöfler, M.; Meinhardt, G.; Nowak, D.; Velicky, P.; Pollheimer, J.; Zenclussen, A.C. Chymase-producing cells of the innate immune system are required for decidual vascular remodeling and fetal growth. *Sci. Rep.* **2017**, *7*, 45106. [CrossRef]
71. Gamliel, M.; Goldman-Wohl, D.; Isaacson, B.; Gur, C.; Stein, N.; Yamin, R.; Berger, M.; Grunewald, M.; Keshet, E.; Rais, Y.; et al. Trained Memory of Human Uterine NK Cells Enhances Their Function in Subsequent Pregnancies. *Immunity* **2018**, *48*, 951–962. [CrossRef] [PubMed]
72. Lee, S.K.; Kim, C.J.; Kim, D.-J.; Kang, J.-H. Immune Cells in the Female Reproductive Tract. *Immune Netw.* **2015**, *15*, 16–26. [CrossRef] [PubMed]
73. Wordinger, R.J.; Jackson, F.L.; Morrill, A. Implantation, deciduoma formation and live births in mast cell-deficient mice (W/Wv). *J. Reprod. Fertil.* **1986**, *77*, 471–476. [CrossRef] [PubMed]
74. Menzies, F.M.; Higgins, C.A.; Shepherd, M.C.; Nibbs, R.J.; Nelson, S.M. Mast cells reside in myometrium and cervix, but are dispensable in mice for successful pregnancy and labor. *Immunol. Cell. Biol.* **2012**, *90*, 321–329. [CrossRef]
75. Woidacki, K.; Popovic, M.; Metz, M.; Schumacher, A.; Linzke, N.; Teles, A.; Poirier, F.; Fest, S.; Jensen, F.; Rabinovich, G.A.; et al. Mast cells rescue implantation defects caused by c-kit deficiency. *Cell Death Dis.* **2013**, *4*, e462. [CrossRef]
76. Woidacki, K.; Meyer, N.; Schumacher, A.; Goldschmidt, A.; Maurer, M.; Zenclussen, A.C. Transfer of regulatory T cells into abortion-prone mice promotes the expansion of uterine mast cells and normalizes early pregnancy angiogenesis. *Sci. Rep.* **2015**, *5*, 13938. [CrossRef]
77. Graham, C.H.; Hawley, T.S.; Hawley, R.G.; MacDougall, J.R.; Kerbel, R.S.; Khoo, N.; Lala, P.K. Establishment and characterization of first trimester human trophoblast cells with extended lifespan. *Exp. Cell. Res.* **1993**, *206*, 204–211. [CrossRef]
78. Nicola, N.A.; Babon, J.J. Leukemia inhibitory factor (LIF). *Cytokine Growth Factor Rev.* **2015**, *26*, 533–544. [CrossRef]
79. Jones, S.A.; Jenkins, B.J. Recent insights into targeting the IL-6 cytokine family in inflammatory diseases and cancer. *Nat. Rev. Immunol.* **2018**, *18*, 773–789. [CrossRef]
80. Zhao, Y.; Koga, K.; Osuga, Y.; Nagai, M.; Izumi, G.; Takamura, M.; Harada, M.; Hirota, Y.; Yoshino, O.; Taketani, Y. Thrombin enhances soluble Fms-like tyrosine kinase 1 expression in trophoblasts; possible involvement in the pathogenesis of preeclampsia. *Fertil. Steril.* **2012**, *98*, 917–921. [CrossRef]
81. Huang, Q.T.; Chen, J.H.; Hang, L.L.; Liu, S.S.; Zhong, M. Activation of PAR-1/NADPH oxidase/ROS signaling pathways is crucial for the thrombin-induced sFlt-1 production in extravillous trophoblasts: Possible involvement in the pathogenesis of preeclampsia. *Cell. Physiol. Biochem.* **2015**, *35*, 1654–1662. [CrossRef] [PubMed]

82. Ellis, S.A.; Palmer, M.S.; McMichael, A.J. Human trophoblast and the choriocarcinoma cell line BeWo express a truncated HLA Class I molecule. *J. Immunol.* **1990**, *144*, 731–735. [PubMed]
83. Paul, P.; Cabestre, F.A.; Le Gal, F.A.; Khalil-Daher, I.; Le Danff, C.; Schmid, M.; Mercier, S.; Avril, M.F.; Dausset, J.; Guillet, J.G.; et al. Heterogeneity of HLA-G gene transcription and protein expression in malignant melanoma biopsies. *Cancer Res.* **1999**, *59*, 1954–1960. [PubMed]
84. Lin, A.; Yan, W.H. Heterogeneity of HLA-G Expression in Cancers: Facing the Challenges. *Front. Immunol.* **2018**, *9*, 2164. [CrossRef]
85. He, X.; Dong, D.D.; Yie, S.M.; Yang, H.; Cao, M.; Ye, S.R.; Li, K.; Liu, J.; Chen, J. HLA-G expression in human breast cancer: Implications for diagnosis and prognosis, and effect on allocytotoxic lymphocyte response after hormone treatment in vitro. *Ann. Surg. Oncol.* **2010**, *17*, 1459–1469. [CrossRef]
86. Chen, H.X.; Lin, A.; Shen, C.J.; Zhen, R.; Chen, B.G.; Zhang, X.; Cao, F.L.; Zhang, J.G.; Yan, W.H. Upregulation of human leukocyte antigen-G expression and its clinical significance in ductal breast cancer. *Hum. Immunol.* **2010**, *71*, 892–898. [CrossRef]
87. De Kruijf, E.M.; Sajet, A.; van Nes, J.G.; Natanov, R.; Putter, H.; Smit, V.T.; Liefers, G.J.; van den Elsen, P.J.; van de Velde, C.J.; Kuppen, P.J. HLA-E and HLA-G expression in classical HLA class I-negative tumors is of prognostic value for clinical outcome of early breast cancer patients. *J. Immunol.* **2010**, *185*, 7452–7459. [CrossRef]
88. Engels, C.C.; Fontein, D.B.; Kuppen, P.J.; de Kruijf, E.M.; Smit, V.T.; Nortier, J.W.; Liefers, G.J.; van de Velde, C.J.; Bastiaannet, E. Immunological subtypes in breast cancer are prognostic for invasive ductal but not for invasive lobular breast carcinoma. *Br. J. Cancer* **2014**, *111*, 532–538. [CrossRef]
89. Ribatti, D.; Tamma, R.; Crivellato, E. The dual role of mast cells in tumor fate. *Cancer Lett.* **2018**, *433*, 252–258. [CrossRef]
90. Varricchi, G.; de Paulis, A.; Marone, G.; Galli, S.J. Future Needs in Mast Cell Biology. *Int. J. Mol. Sci.* **2019**, *20*, 4397. [CrossRef]
91. Tanooka, H.; Kitamura, Y.; Sado, T.; Tanaka, K.; Nagase, M.; Kondo, S. Evidence for involvement of mast cells in tumor suppression in mice. *J. Natl. Cancer Inst.* **1982**, *69*, 1305–1309. [PubMed]
92. Abdul-Wahid, A.; Cydzik, M.; Prodeus, A.; Alwash, M.; Stanojcic, M.; Thompson, M.; Huang, E.H.; Shively, J.E.; Gray-Owen, S.D.; Gariépy, J. Induction of antigen-specific TH 9 immunity accompanied by mast cell activation blocks tumor cell engraftment. *Int. J. Cancer* **2016**, *139*, 841–853. [CrossRef] [PubMed]
93. Martner, A.; Wiktorin, H.G.; Lenox, B.; Ewald Sander, F.; Aydin, E.; Aurelius, J.; Thoren, F.B.; Stahlberg, A.; Hermodsson, S.; Hellstrand, K. Histamine promotes the development of monocyte-derived dendritic cells and reduces tumor growth by targeting the myeloid NADPH oxidase. *J. Immunol.* **2015**, *194*, 5014–5021. [CrossRef] [PubMed]
94. Grujic, M.; Paivandy, A.; Gustafson, A.M.; Thomsen, A.R.; Ohrvik, H.; Pejler, G. The combined action of mast cell chymase, tryptase and carboxypeptidase A3 protects against melanoma colonization of the lung. *Oncotarget* **2017**, *8*, 25066–25079. [CrossRef] [PubMed]
95. De Palma, M.; Biziato, D.; Petrova, T.V. Microenvironmental regulation of tumour angiogenesis. *Nat. Rev. Cancer* **2017**, *17*, 457–474. [CrossRef]
96. Montfort, A.; Colacios, C.; Levade, T.; Andrieu-Abadie, N.; Meyer, N.; Segui, B. The TNF Paradox in Cancer Progression and Immunotherapy. *Front. Immunol.* **2019**, *10*, 1818. [CrossRef]
97. Jeong, H.J.; Oh, H.A.; Nam, S.Y.; Han, N.R.; Kim, Y.S.; Kim, J.H.; Lee, S.J.; Kim, M.H.; Moon, P.D.; Kim, H.M.; et al. The critical role of mast cell-derived hypoxia-inducible factor-1α in human and mice melanoma growth. *Int. J. Cancer* **2013**, *132*, 2492–2501. [CrossRef]
98. Blair, R.J.; Meng, H.; Marchese, M.J.; Ren, S.; Schwartz, L.B.; Tonnesen, M.G.; Gruber, B.L. Human mast cells stimulate vascular tube formation. Tryptase is a novel, potent angiogenic factor. *J. Clin. Investig.* **1997**, *99*, 2691–2700. [CrossRef]
99. Aponte-López, A.; Fuentes-Pananá, E.M.; Cortes-Muñoz, D.; Muñoz-Cruz, S. Mast Cell, the Neglected Member of the Tumor Microenvironment: Role in Breast Cancer. *J. Immunol. Res.* **2018**, *2018*, 2584243. [CrossRef]
100. Reddy, S.M.; Reuben, A.; Barua, S.; Jiang, H.; Zhang, S.; Wang, L.; Gopalakrishnan, V.; Hudgens, C.W.; Tetzlaff, M.T.; Reuben, J.M.; et al. Poor Response to Neoadjuvant Chemotherapy Correlates with Mast Cell Infiltration in Inflammatory Breast Cancer. *Cancer Immunol. Res.* **2019**, *7*, 1025–1035. [CrossRef]

101. Pangault, C.; Amiot, L.; Caulet-Maugendre, S.; Brasseur, F.; Burtin, F.; Guilloux, V.; Drenou, B.; Fauchet, R.; Onno, M. HLA-G protein expression is not induced during malignant transformation. *Tissue Antigens* **1999**, *53*(4 Pt. 1), 335–346. [CrossRef]
102. Takei, Y.; Ueshima, C.; Kataoka, T.R.; Hirata, M.; Sugimoto, A.; Rokutan-Kurata, M.; Moriyoshi, K.; Ono, K.; Murakami, I.; Iwamoto, S.; et al. Killer cell immunoglobulin-like receptor 2DL4 is expressed in and suppresses the cell growth of Langerhans cell histiocytosis. *Oncotarget* **2017**, *8*, 36964–36972. [CrossRef] [PubMed]

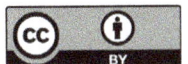 © 2020 by the authors. Licensee MDPI, Basel, Switzerland. This article is an open access article distributed under the terms and conditions of the Creative Commons Attribution (CC BY) license (http://creativecommons.org/licenses/by/4.0/).

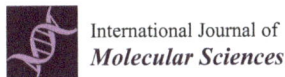

Review

Beyond IgE: Alternative Mast Cell Activation Across Different Disease States

David O. Lyons and Nicholas A. Pullen *

School of Biological Sciences, University of Northern Colorado, Greeley, CO 80639, USA; david.lyons@unco.edu
* Correspondence: nicholas.pullen@unco.edu; Tel.: +1-(970)-351-1843

Received: 9 February 2020; Accepted: 21 February 2020; Published: 22 February 2020

Abstract: Mast cells are often regarded through the lens of IgE-dependent reactions as a cell specialized only for anti-parasitic and type I hypersensitive responses. However, recently many researchers have begun to appreciate the expansive repertoire of stimuli that mast cells can respond to. After the characterization of the interleukin (IL)-33/suppression of tumorigenicity 2 (ST2) axis of mast cell activation—a pathway that is independent of the adaptive immune system—researchers are revisiting other stimuli to induce mast cell activation and/or subsequent degranulation independent of IgE. This discovery also underscores that mast cells act as important mediators in maintaining body wide homeostasis, especially through barrier defense, and can thus be the source of disease as well. Particularly in the gut, inflammatory bowel diseases (Crohn's disease, ulcerative colitis, etc.) are characterized with enhanced mast cell activity in the context of autoimmune disease. Mast cells show phenotypic differences based on tissue residency, which could manifest as different receptor expression profiles, allowing for unique mast cell responses (both IgE and non-IgE mediated) across varying tissues as well. This variety in receptor expression suggests mast cells respond differently, such as in the gut where immunosuppressive IL-10 stimulates the development of food allergy or in the lungs where transforming growth factor-β1 (TGF-β1) can enhance mast cell IL-6 production. Such differences in receptor expression illustrate the truly diverse effector capabilities of mast cells, and careful consideration must be given toward the phenotype of mast cells observed in vitro. Given mast cells' ubiquitous tissue presence and their capability to respond to a broad spectrum of non-IgE stimuli, it is expected that mast cells may also contribute to the progression of autoimmune disorders and other disease states such as metastatic cancer through promoting chronic inflammation in the local tissue microenvironment and ultimately polarizing toward a unique T_h17 immune response. Furthermore, these interconnected, atypical activation pathways may crosstalk with IgE-mediated signaling differently across disorders such as parasitism, food allergies, and autoimmune disorders of the gut. In this review, we summarize recent research into familiar and novel pathways of mast cells activation and draw connections to clinical human disease.

Keywords: mast cell; innate immunity; NLRP3; MRGPRX2; inflammatory bowel disease; cancer; food allergy; trained immunity; TGF-β1; IL-10

1. Introduction

Mast cells (MCs) are innate immune cells of the myeloid lineage that are popularly associated with allergic, asthmatic, and anti-worm responses. In the past, research predominantly focused on the IgE-mediated activation of MCs; this mode of activation is dependent on the adaptive immune system to supply antigen-specific IgE to sensitize MCs. Recently, researchers began to focus on characterization of novel MC activation paradigms that are not only independent of IgE-mediated crosslinking but also express unique cytokine secretion profiles. Perhaps the most heavily discussed pathway is mediated through interleukin (IL)-33/suppression of tumorigenicity 2 (ST2) signaling. IL-33-mediated signaling is capable of inducing cytokine expression by MCs, which can also produce IL-33 during IgE-mediated activation but not IL-33-mediated activation [1]. Signaling through this alarmin also synergizes with IgE-mediated responses by increasing MC abundance and enhancing their activation [2]. Not only can MCs respond differently depending on the stimulus, there are also notable differences across MCs based on their tissue residency. Like macrophages, prenatal MCs come from the yolk sac in the developing embryo and are gradually replaced with definitive MCs as the organism matures [3]. These MCs are also phenotypically distinct from one another. In an adult, MC heterogeneity comes from their tissue residence. Although all MCs are capable of producing common T_h2 cytokines such as IL-4, 5, and 13, their toll-like receptor (TLR) expression and ability to produce renin give those tissue-specific MCs the capability to modulate inflammatory responses and remodel the surrounding ECM [4]. These unique expression patterns manifest differently, and tissue-specific MCs may promote pathologies in a manner unique to their tissue residence. Lung MCs were found to promote bleomycin-induced pulmonary fibrosis through histamine and renin production which promoted wound repair mechanisms and transforming growth factor-$\beta1$ (TGF-$\beta1$) secretion [5]. Specifically, in the intestines, these mucosal MCs (MMCs) express cysteinyl leukotrienes compared to connective tissue MCs (CTMCs). In addition to this, the expression of P2X7 is present in both intestinal and lung MCs. Both subtypes of MCs also have high TLR expression, further suggesting the MCs in these tissues are predisposed for inflammatory responses [4]. Because of the diversity in MC receptor expression across different tissue types, understanding the microenvironment in which pathology is occurring will lend itself toward developing specific and targeted therapies. Furthermore, the different receptor expression patterns observed across tissue-resident MCs suggest that MCs are specialized for their tissue niche. Across multiple diseases, the phenotypic and morphological changes to the tissue microenvironment may include tissue-resident MCs and thus MCs could be a source of pathology as a result of disrupted homeostatic activity. MCs are experts at initiating and driving inflammation, and their dysregulated activity exacerbates inflammatory conditions in the tissue. Here, we review emerging alternative paradigms for MC activation and discuss their relevance to major gut-related disease states. The possible issue of trained immunity and the paradoxical roles of classical immunosuppressive cytokines are specifically reviewed to stimulate further consideration of these topics specific to MCs.

2. Alternative Activation Paradigms

Across all the following inflammatory disorders, MCs are major promoters of pathology and the extent of their activation in these disorders is directly dependent on both the MC's tissue origin as well as the initiating stimulus. Interestingly, MC activation in the context of these diseases is not solely FcεRI mediated; MCs play a pathological role in an antigen-independent, adaptive immune-independent manner. MCs deserve careful consideration in these gut inflammatory disorders as they are major gut homeostatic mediators. Through IgE signaling, MCs are potent sentinels poised to mitigate helminth threats and unfortunately also drive some allergies. However, we will discuss how they are directly involved in coordinating immune responses and inflammation through their ability to detect and respond to other, non-allergenic stimuli. We open this discussion with a review of such non IgE-mediated signals.

For example, MCs are not only capable of secreting histamine, but they also possess cell-surface histamine receptors, allowing for potential paracrine and autocrine MC signaling in response to histamine release. The expression of the four identified histamine receptors (H1-4R) is specialized for interacting with other cell types and the expression of these receptors on MCs is dependent on the tissue localization of the MC. Human skin MCs were found to express H2R and H4R, and furthermore, these are primarily responsible for mediating the gut immune-microenvironment and signaling with other immune cells, respectively [6,7]. The H1 receptor, which has also been studied for its role in allergic responses, was weakly expressed in normal skin human MCs but was more highly expressed in HMC-1 cells, possibly due to constitutively active c-kit expression in the cell line; this receptor is not hypothesized to be involved in direct signaling in response to histamine [6]. Taken together, the H2 and H4 receptors appear to act as a means of negative feedback on MC degranulation. Expression of these histamine receptors on other cell types suggests MCs can directly signal to other cell types through histamine release. The H3 receptor is a pre-synaptic receptor on neurons which inhibits neurotransmitter and histamine release [8]. These interactions connect the nervous system with the innate immune system; MC-neuronal signaling is largely mediated through substance P (SP) which is released by neurons in response to MC-produced histamine and tryptase; other neuropeptides such as vasoactive intestinal polypeptide can also induce MC degranulation [9–11]. In disease states where nervous function may be altered, improper MC-neuronal signaling may induce chronic inflammation without a means for drawing back the inflammatory cell signaling.

Purinergic receptors have also been implicated in mediating MC activation. P2X4 stimulation enhanced prostaglandin E-stimulated degranulation through an alternative mechanism [12]. This enhanced stimulation could be the result of activation of the NLR family pyrin domain containing 3 (NLRP3) inflammasome acting synergistically with typical MC activation paradigms [13].

An emerging unique MC receptor is a GPCR named MAS-related G protein coupled receptor X-2 (MRGPRX2). This membrane and intracellular GPCR is responsible for MC innate immunity and wound healing as well as neurogenic inflammation, pain, and itch. Activation of this receptor results in MC degranulation and is important in mobilizing the adaptive immune system in tissues [14]. Signaling through MRGPRX2 is capable of inducing activation and degranulation of MCs in an IgE-independent manner [15]. MCs are present throughout the body and have also been identified near nerve endings across the skin, gut, and airways [9,16]. Comparable to IgE-mediated T_h2 signaling, this paradigm can potentiate a MC-dependent positive feedback loop, perpetuating pathologic inflammation in the tissue through exuberant MC activation and cytokine secretion in conjunction with SP release from neurons. SP binds to the neurokinin-1 receptor (NK-1R) and therapeutic inhibition of the receptor reduces symptoms of chemotherapy-induced nausea but strangely does not affect inflammation [17,18]. SP activation on MCs, however, is not mediated through NK-1R but instead through MRGPRX2 in humans or Mrgprb2 in mice [19,20]. Although the mechanism behind this signaling is not yet understood, the ability of MCs to interact with the nervous system suggests their importance in diseases where excessive neuronal activity is present. Such a receptor is not only capable of initiating an inflammatory response without the adaptive immune system, but its ability to mediate MC-neuronal interactions and its relatively exclusive MC expression makes it an attractive target for MC-directed immunotherapeutics. Specific antagonism of the MRGPRX2 receptor is sufficient in inhibiting IgE-independent degranulation and could be used to lessen some drug-induced allergic reactions [21].

The 8-oxoguanine DNA glycosylase 1 (OGG1) is involved in base excision repair (BER) in response to DNA damage, specifically oxidative stress-induced 8-oxoguanine lesions on DNA. These bases excised during OGG1-mediated BER are capable of forming a complex with cytoplasmic OGG1 in the cytosol, changing the conformation of OGG1 and inducing gene expression changes in the MC. These changes promote pro-inflammatory and pro-degranulation gene expression in [22,23]. Interestingly, multiple challenges with 8-oxoguanine resulted in a significant fold-change increase in MC-degranulation-associated genes—these lesions are related to oxidative stress, suggesting inflammasome related signaling may be mediating this effect by priming the MC for enhanced activation through NLRP3 activity; reactive oxygen species (ROS)-induced stress in the gut would likely promote OGG1 activity and could act as a means for promoting a trained immune response.

In addition to these alternative activation paradigms that result in MC cytokine secretion, and sometimes degranulation, we and others hypothesize that MCs possess a form of potentiation unique from adaptive immune system memory. This concept, also known as immune training or trained immunity, has been well described in macrophages but the significance of this training in other myeloid cells, specifically in MCs, has yet to be clearly described. Trained immunity allows for innate immune cells to adapt their response to a broad variety of stimuli, which can protect against future insults; this potentiation manifests as changes in gene expression and epigenetic changes such as histone methylation/acetylation [24]. This response is mediated through detection of pathogen and damage-associated molecular pattern molecules (PAMPs and DAMPs) via pattern recognition receptors (PRRs), namely extracellular TLRs and intracellular NOD-like receptors (NLRs) [13]. The binding of ligands to these PRRs initiates a signaling cascade resulting in inflammasome priming or activation upon re-exposure. There are several inflammasome sensors, each with unique stimuli and diseases associated with their dysfunction. However, most researchers select the NLRP3 inflammasome for study due to its ability to respond to the largest variety of stimuli as well as its two-step activation process [25]. Full activation of the NLRP3 inflammasome induces caspase-1 activity, which cleaves pro-IL-1β and pro-IL-18 to yield biologically active forms. Release of these active cytokines (through secretion or release from damaged cells) results in inflammation and immune cell activity [13]. MCs are not only capable of producing active IL-1β but stimulation with IL-1β is sufficient in inducing histamine release and degranulation from MCs, suggesting MCs can initiate and perpetuate this pyroptotic process in tissues [13,26]. This interaction is also implicated as a potential positive feedback loop for MCs, as histamine can then promote *IL-1* gene expression and synthesis [27]. In the gut, NLRP3 is key in maintaining intestinal homeostasis; NLRP3-deficient mice were more susceptible to ulcerative colitis and displayed reduced IL-1β, IL-10, and TGF-β [28]. The NLRP3 inflammasome is a robust sensor of extracellular threats and is a potent regulator of innate immune responses throughout the body; its role in stimulating trained immunity in myeloid cells highlights the long-term protective effects to a broad variety of pathogens.

In sum, MCs are capable responders to broad immunogenic stimuli. Their response is MC specific and tissue specific; disease states in which these signaling pathways are disrupted demonstrate the unique pathogenic roles MCs can have in the etiology and progression of several inflammatory diseases (see Figure 1). Both the mechanisms of disease and the cellular environment of the affected tissue determine the nature of inflammation. For the remainder of this review, we focus on recent findings in inflammatory bowel diseases, food allergy, cancer, autoimmunity, and autoinflammation, and then we close with special attention to novel effects of IL-10 and TGF-β1.

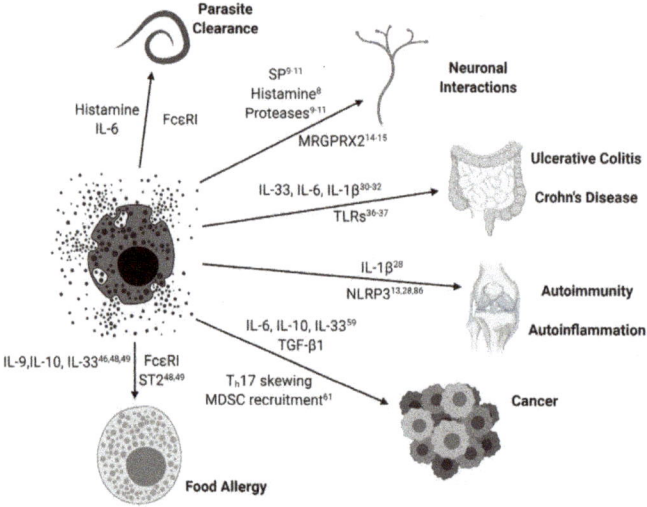

Figure 1. Mast cell activation paradigms. Mast cells and their simplified interactions with clinical diseases are represented with arrowed connections. Relevant MC-mediated soluble factors and associated signaling pathways are represented for each disease state. Subscripts correspond to relevant references from this review.

3. Ulcerative Colitis/Crohn's Disease/Inflammatory Bowel Disease

MCs are pivotal in maintaining gut mucosal homeostasis; inflammatory bowel diseases (IBDs) likely present with defects to MC-related biology. Ulcerative colitis (UC) and Crohn's disease are the major types of IBDs that arise from chronic inflammation against harmless microbiota; the etiology stems from both genetic and environmental factors [29]. Errors in autophagic responses and polymorphisms, which result in the overproduction of IL-1β and IL-6, have been identified as drivers of chronic inflammation in these diseases; innate immune markers such as *NOD2* and mucin genes are also mutated [30–32].

TLR signaling is required in maintaining gut homeostasis and is also important in the clearance of pathogens [33]. Interestingly, MCs in the small intestine weakly express TLR whilst MCs in the colon express high levels of TLR 2 and 4 [4]. The differential expression of TLR could explain why the pathology of ulcerative colitis is limited to colonic tissues compared to more widespread inflammatory bowel disorders such as Crohn's disease; differential TLR expression could also be explained by the bacterial burden experienced in the small intestines versus the colon [34]. Although the activation of TLRs does not directly induce broad degranulation, ligand binding does lead to cytokine and leukotriene secretion, which promote local inflammation and immune cell recruitment. This change to the surrounding tissue microenvironment likely alters MC activation and response to stimuli such as FcεRI, IL-33, or SP [35]. Across both diseases, innate immunity of the gut is disturbed differently. TLR3 (constitutively expressed in healthy epithelial cells) is down regulated in Crohn's disease but not UC. However, TLR4 (normally low expression in healthy tissue; receptor for LPS) is highly upregulated across both diseases [36]. In addition to aberrant TLR signaling and expression, NLRP3-related proteins NOD1 and NOD2 were also found to be suppressively mutated in 15–20% of patients with IBDs [37]. The pathogenesis of these diseases arises from a failure of the immune system to quell inflammatory responses leading to excessive, uncontrolled inflammation.

Patients with IBDs exhibit upregulated NK-1R and SP and severity of disease in patients with UC was correlated to levels of SP; rectal SP levels were only increased in patients with UC and not Crohn's disease and is correlated to a shift in the tissue microenvironment to favor SP production [38,39]. In addition, MCs harboring missense mutations in MRGPRX2 are unable to respond to SP-mediated degranulation—Ca^{2+} mobilization is impacted in this context, which could be the mechanism behind suppression of MCs [40].

Specifically regarding MC activity, patients with UC were found to have greatly enhanced IL-33 expression, and IL-33 producing myofibroblasts were a primary source of IL-33 in these ulcerative lesions and synergized with TGF-β to induce further myofibroblast differentiation; such cells were nearly absent in patients with Crohn's disease [41]. These IL-33 producing cells in an inflamed gut likely promote MC activation; the protective benefits of this inflammation are likely not present in this disease state and instead exacerbate the inflammatory environment. Beyond the body's own cells, parasites are capable of mediating the inflammatory responses in the gut. Helminth infestation is inversely correlated with IBDs and clinical treatment using a helminth benefits patients with UC due to the parasite's capability of inducing a T_h2 response [42,43]. Patients with UC or Crohn's disease have higher histamine levels as well as increased H4R expression; MC-produced histamine likely exacerbates the inflammation whilst promoting neutrophilic recruitment and further inflammation [44]. Indeed, these inflammatory bowel diseases are multifaceted and arise as a result of a combination of biological errors and mutations regarding inflammation.

MCs appear to play a greater role in the pathogenesis of UC by promoting a pro-inflammatory microenvironment, mediated by IL-33 and SP-producing cells in the gut. Both diseases present with autoinflammation. However, MCs play a direct role in UC as both signals directly induce MC activation and subsequent TNF-α production in a synergistic manner [45]. Therapies targeting MCs will likely prove more effective in managing the symptoms of UC than Crohn's disease. However, MCs play a pro-inflammatory role in both diseases.

4. Food Allergy

In the context of common food allergies, MCs are essential in the development of allergic responses. This is a case where a typically suppressive cytokine, IL-10, was shown to be necessary for priming mast cells against consumed food antigens (murine oral OVA model); IL-10 was sufficient to enhance IgE-mediated mast cell activation as well [46]. This unexpected response by MCs to IL-10 could be the result of an evolutionary adaptation in response to immunosuppression by parasites—as parasites evolved the ability to suppress anti-worm responses in the gut, perhaps MCs adapted by paradoxically activating in response to select immunosuppressive cytokines. Despite the immunosuppressive nature of parasites, some parasites instead induce an allergic response which can lead to the development of food allergies. Tick bites promote strong allergic responses to the antigen secreted by the tick; the lone star tick induces an allergy to red meat (Alpha-gal syndrome), which behaves like a typical type I hypersensitivity response. IgE production in response to this insult is reliant on TLR stimulation on B-cells through MyD88 [47]. CTMCs in the skin may facilitate the development of such a hypersensitive response through a distinct mechanism rather than typical IgE-mediated food allergy.

IL-33 is also implicated in the development of food allergies. In addition to its direct effects in enhancing IgE-mediated activity, IL-33 promotes oral OVA-mediated anaphylaxis through enhancing MC activity in mice. ST2-deficient mice displayed reduced anaphylaxis. However, the full effect could be reconstituted using WT bone marrow-derived MCs [48]. IL-9 is also implicated in the development of food allergy as well as parasite protection. IL-33 promotes IL-9 and IL-13 production from a unique subpopulation of MMCs; intestinal expression of IL-9 and IL-13 was also increased in atopic patients [49]. These IL-9 producing MMCs were also found to express MC enzymes tryptase and chymase at increased levels compared to healthy patients.

Large extracellular parasites are the eternal rivals of the MC—although the modern world's developed sanitation and health systems are more capable of extinguishing these infections, gut parasites are still capable of modulating the surrounding immune environment to evade detection. Secretions by *Acanthocheilonema viteae* (ES-62) were capable of suppressing IL-33/ST2-mediated signaling in peritoneal-derived murine MCs; MCs of different tissue residency (specifically bone marrow-derived mucosal MCs) were not as suppressed from the worm byproduct alone, highlighting the tissue specificity of MCs [50]. ES-62 was also shown to be protective against fatal pathology in a chronic OVA/alum asthma model through inhibition of IL-33/ST2-mediated signaling. Parasitic inhibition of MCs varies by parasite and the duration of infection also dictates the immunomodulatory effects of the parasite's byproducts. Chronic *Litomosoides sigmodontis* infection suppressed intraperitoneal OVA-driven allergic responses and anaphylaxis; interestingly, OVA-IgE levels were unchanged during infection and IL-10 was not found to be involved in the protective effect against anaphylaxis [51]. During infection with *L. sigmodontis*, peritoneal MC counts were found to be decreased, peritoneal MCs harvested were less granular and also exhibited lower levels of histamine [51]. Parasite and worm byproducts elicit changes to the surrounding mucosa by directly altering MC function; such products are parasite specific and could prove therapeutic in dampening excessive MC activity in other disease states.

Though the pathogenesis of this disease is different from typical food allergies, celiac disease (CD) has become more prevalent in modern society. The disease initiates through T-cells in an antigen-specific manner against gliadin within dietary gluten and engages both the innate and adaptive immune systems to induce a proinflammatory response in gut mucosa [52]. MCs are involved in the regulation of the adaptive immune response to dietary gluten and are found in higher counts in celiacs consuming gluten; the higher counts of MCs were found to promote CD severity and progression and MCs were directly activated by digested gliadin fragments [53,54]. The gliadin-mediated activation of MCs in celiacs was also different compared to MCs from a non-celiac patient, highlighting the genetic and environmental basis for CD. Suppressing MC responses and/or replenishment with healthy MCs may slow the progression and severity of CD by restricting adaptive-innate immune signaling and shaping the mucosal environment away from a proinflammatory state.

5. Cancer

Among Paul Ehrlich's original observations on MCs are their association with cancerous tumors; MCs are potent mediators of both pro- and anti-tumor responses in a context-specific manner [55]. As a sentinel cell capable of eliciting inflammatory responses independent of the adaptive immune system, inappropriate MC activation can set the stage for a chronically inflamed environment for cancer proliferation [56]. The production of pro-inflammatory IL-6 and IL-1β can also drive this inflammation in the tumor microenvironment (TME). Recent hypotheses suggest MCs have subsets with unique cytokine profiles similar to macrophage polarization and MCs are capable of switching between the subsets in a context-specific, localized manner, in other words, "tumor educated" MCs [57]. Aggressive triple-negative (ER$^-$PR$^-$HER2$^-$) breast cancers were shown to have higher counts of infiltrating MCs and M2 macrophages mediated by higher expression of annexin A1 [58]. Such immune responses would benefit the progression of cancer through promoting chronic inflammation and wound repair pathways over cytotoxic pathways. MC activity also evolves as tumors progress and expand. In small intestinal cancers, MCs expand in benign polyps in the presence of IL-10, IL-13, and IL-33 as well as ILC2 cells. The presence of these MCs is maintained in an IL-10 dependent manner—overexpression of IL-10 greatly expanded MC populations in these polyps [59]. The presence of IL-10 in conjunction with MC chemokines and alarmins such as IL-33 explains the pro-cancer, pro-inflammatory role MCs can play in certain cancers; in the context of small bowel cancers, MC protease expression resembled MMCs but included CTMC-related mast cell proteases too [59]. When the polyps switched to an invasive phenotype, CTMCs expressing both MMC and CTMC proteases expanded, demonstrating cancer's ability to alter MC activity toward a pathogenic, pro-cancer function [59]. A mechanism behind this phenotypic switch could be a result of MC interactions with epithelial cells during an inflammatory state, specifically during wound repair. In an azoxymethane-induced colonic tumor model, MCs recruited to epithelial cells during inflammatory wound repair obtained a pro-tumorigenic role and their density in the gut was correlated with cancer grade [60]. Interestingly, the capability of MCs to resolve IL-33-mediated inflammation by damaged epithelial cells was critical in promoting tissue repair following inflammation through protease release. MCs are important in regulating and resolving inflammation within their local tissues; tumors can elicit pro-inflammatory functions in MCs to reprogram them into a pathogenic state. MCs are capable of being activated through IL-33, which illustrates how MCs respond differently to stimulation depending on the surrounding tissue state and current immune status. Additionally, MC-derived IL-6 and TGF-β1 could be considered a pro-tumorigenic threat, as these cytokines can directly contribute to the recruitment of myeloid-derived suppressor cells (MDSCs) and effector T cell polarization away from an anti-tumor T_h1 toward a T_h17 phenotype. This likely impacts the efficiency of modern biologic therapies, especially checkpoint inhibiting immunotherapies, where only about 20% of patients respond favorably. It was reported that MDSCs can enhance MC activation, which further suggests a pro-tumor positive feedback loop; however, it remains to be specifically demonstrated whether MCs can enhance MDSC function [61]. Given the presence of MCs across all tissue types, MCs are also implicated as either potential protectors or drivers of cancer. The pro-fibrotic role of MCs in wound repair and inflammation can be dysregulated within a TME and their capability to signal to MDSCs and surrounding fibroblasts can further exacerbate the conditions of the TME. Specifically, in small-bowel cancers, MCs can act as major drivers of inflammation through IL-33/ST2-mediated signaling, promoting chronic inflammation and strongly skewing toward a T_h17 immune response. Therapies aiming to disrupt MC signaling to the surrounding stroma and immune cells could enhance adaptive immune cytotoxicity and restrict MDSC-mediated activity.

The NLRP3 inflammasome not only contributes to gut-related inflammatory disorders but the resulting chronic inflammation also increases the risk of developing colorectal cancer [62,63]. The NLRP3 inflammasome is largely mediated by downstream apoptosis-associated speck like protein containing a caspase recruitment domain (ASC) and caspase-1 activity. In the context of colorectal tumorigenesis, NLRP3 can play a protective role; ASC and caspase-1 were also found to be protective against tumorigenesis in mice [64]. This connection between NLRP3, bowel diseases, and cancer is multifaceted and the resulting inflammation and cytokine secretion (namely IL-18) can be protective against tumor growth [65]. However, the same cytokines produced following NLRP3 activation are also associated with exuberant inflammation and autoimmune disorders, illustrating both the protective and pathogenic effects of NLRP3. Indeed, the common mutations to NLRP3 and its downstream mediators varies across cancer types and tissue location; the data on these mutations contradicts the protective findings of NLRP3's IL-18-mediated downstream activity [66]. In addition to acknowledging the tissue specific roles of MC, careful consideration must be made when observing dysregulation of immune mechanisms across different tissue types.

6. Autoimmunity/Autoinflammation

Although MC activity alone does not constitute autoimmunity, such activity is sufficient in inducing an autoinflammatory response, in which innate immune cells are activated in response to tissue-specific stimuli [13]. These autoinflammatory diseases can contribute to the pathogenesis of other inflammatory disorders, namely through chronic inflammation. Despite this dichotomy, autoimmune disorders and autoinflammation can coalesce as diseases such as psoriasis and Crohn's disease, characterized by innate immune activation of T-cells and inflammatory cytokine production [67,68]. Given the biology of MC, their capability to induce an autoinflammatory immune environment through cytokine secretion is only bolstered by their nearly ubiquitous tissue presence and their ability to migrate into so-called immune privileged sites, such as central nervous system parenchyma; and as sentinel cells MCs are one of the first innate immune cells to be activated during an inflammatory response [69]. Consequently, pathogenic activation of MCs is capable of causing harm in privileged tissues.

MCs are hypothesized to mediate autoinflammation through NLRP3 inflammasome sensing of extracellular threats; mutations to the NLRP3 inflammasome and its mediators leads to monogenic diseases such as familial Mediterranean fever (FMF) and cryopyrin-associated periodic syndrome (CAPS) which arise from exuberant caspase-1 activity leading to downstream IL-1β secretion and subsequent inflammation [70].

Due to the ability of MCs to promote and sustain localized inflammation, therapeutic targeting of MCs in autoimmune and autoinflammatory disorders (such as rheumatoid arthritis, UC, or CD) could help to dampen the adaptive autoimmune and innate autoinflammatory responses and promote repair of the damaged tissues. Identifying the soluble factors released in the context of each disease state is critical to understanding how MCs will contribute to the promotion or protection against inflammation.

7. IL-10 and TGF-β1

Across these various disease states, MC activity appears to be enhanced, leading to prolonged inflammation and subsequent tissue damage. While most other immune cells are broadly suppressed by IL-10 and/or TGF-β1, MCs react differently. MC responses to typically immunosuppressive cytokines can instead promote MC activation and/or potentiate wound repair pathways and fibrosis (see Figure 2).

TGF-β1 has been characterized as immunosuppressive on MCs through reduced FcεRI expression at the protein level, suggesting subsequently reduced FcεRI-mediated signaling [71]. In terms of phenotypic data, the evidence is conflicting—broad suppression of MC proliferation and activation has been noted [72]. However, some papers present changes in MC inflammatory products based upon the relative differences +/-FcεRI crosslinking; this can lead to the misconception that there is suppression of response when indeed TGF-β1 alone can stimulate MC release of certain factors without concomitant activation through IgE. TGF-β1 may specifically modulate late-phase responses by MCs which could explain the lack of observed effect regarding histamine release or degranulation.

In mice, inhibition of TGF-β1 through a neutralizing antibody caused oral and esophageal inflammation, hallmarked by TGF-β1 producing MCs. Although there was no difference observed in the gut and intestines, the inflammatory response demonstrated by MCs in the mouth and esophagus highlight the role of the MC as a vanguard of innate immunity [73]. Indeed, TGF-β1 is a potent chemoattractant for MCs which implies MCs are equipped to respond; such migration may be critical for wound repair [74]. The TGF-β1-dependent effects observed here also demonstrate how MCs are critical to maintaining homeostasis through tissue-specific interactions. Under pathologic conditions, this signaling axis can skew the local immune response in the tissue. In a murine tumor model, abolishment of TGF-β1 or IL-10 through neutralizing antibodies restored the T_h1/T_h2 balance in the tissue, characterized by reduced T_h2 cytokine secretion [75].

Interestingly, these typically suppressive cytokines can promote a form of protective inflammation mediated by MC activity. In the case of TGF-β1, there is evidence that MCs can activate in response to TGF-β1 in an IgE-independent manner; regulatory T cells (T_{reg}) were found to directly enhance MC IL-6 production through surface-bound TGF-β1 and MC cytokine release is enhanced when treated with soluble TGF-β1 [76,77]. Indeed, such atypical activation paradigms potentiate the capability of MCs to impact their surroundings by polarizing toward a T_h17 environment. In the context of pathology, MCs are capable players in fronting the initial response to cellular injury by shaping the cytokine milieu of the threatened environment. While it is well-appreciated that MCs release IL-6 and T_h2-polarizing cytokines, the production of (and unique responses to) TGF-β1, IL-17, and IL-22 may reinforce T_h17-like responses. IL-17$^+$ and IL-22$^+$ MCs have been reported [78,79] in psoriatic lesions and while the role of an MC-to-$T_h17/22$ balance is not clear, the fact that these cytokines are produced by MCs is an important therapeutic consideration, since, for example, MCs can also serve to modulate dendritic cell function [80]. This interaction is also interestingly involved in reducing lung inflammation through suppression of neutrophils and promoting MC IL-6 [81]. The stimulatory response displayed by MCs in these circumstances could be the result of an evolutionary advantage to resist immunosuppression by parasites/worms; MCs may also activate to some degree in the context of wound repair. TGF-β1 stimulation of murine bone marrow-derived MCs is also sufficient in inducing mMCP-1 and mMCP-2 expression facilitated through GATA2 and Smad (2,4, potentially 3) signaling [82]. This response may prime MCs as localized protective effector cells during wound repair or during the resolution of an immune response in tissues. In addition, MC-produced IL-6 is key for clearing bacteria around a wound and allowing for repair [83]. This inflammatory response by MCs may be prompted by TGF-β1 release from the surrounding stroma during an injury, promoting an IgE-independent reaction by MCs without prior adaptive immune priming.

In the gut, IL-10 is a major regulator of homeostasis and is capable of both pro- and anti-inflammatory effects, and like mast cells, its role is context-dependent. IL-10 is critical in providing protective immune cell activation and protective inflammation involved in the development of food allergies and septic defense [46,84]. This protective inflammation is mediated by NLRP3 expression. NLRP3-deficient mice were more susceptible to the development of experimental colitis, reflected by reduced IL-1β, TGF-β, and IL-10 expression [28]. For individuals with exuberant inflammatory diseases such as Crohn's disease, defects in NLRP3 may lead to pathologic gut inflammation due to the loss of protective tissue-specific inflammation. Conversely, secreted IL-10 in response to NLRP3 activation has also been implicated as a negative regulator of NLRP3 activation; expression of NLRP3 is essential for protective inflammation but unregulated inflammation caused by NLRP3 may also be harmful [85]. In an antigen induced (methylated bovine serum albumin) arthritis model, IL-10 knockout mice displayed more severe symptoms and had higher expression levels of IL-1β, IL-33, and NLRP3 [86]. Non-lethal exposure to endotoxins such as LPS can render immune cells refractory to subsequent exposure and is characterized by reduced macrophage/monocyte cytokine (specifically TNF-α) production [87]. Development of this endotoxin tolerance in MCs has also been shown to be TLR-mediated and associated with a hyporesponsive phenotype [88]. Interestingly, endotoxin tolerance can be alternatively induced alongside TGF-β and IL-10 synthesis in monocytes in response to low levels of toxin; IL-10 suppresses NLRP3 activation during chronic exposure to LPS [85,89]. The downstream effect of NLRP3 activation regarding IL-10 expression is context specific and the timing and duration of NLRP3 activation might also explain the multifarious roles of IL-10 in inflammasome activation and regulation. Specifically, in the small intestines of IL-10-deficient mice, IL-10, TGF-β, and type 3 immune cytokines (IL-17a, IL-22, IL-23) were unaltered. However, IL-33 and IFN-γ concentrations were increased [59]. Progression of polyposis was mediated by MC and T-cell derived IL-10. MMCs expand first in response to small bowel helminth infestation and gradually shifts to CTMC-dominance during resolution of infection [90,91]. In sum, IL-10 is capable of promoting MC activation across multiple tissue types; however, its suppressive capacity must not be overlooked—IL-10 exhibits both pro- [46,59] and anti-inflammatory [84] effects in a tissue-specific and cell-specific manner. Mutations in NLRP3 and IL-10 may help to describe patient susceptibility to inflammatory disease in the gut; prolonged inflammatory diseases likely present with a defect in IL-10 signaling, as chronic stimulation of NLRP3 should engage immune-tolerizing mechanisms through paracrine and autocrine IL-10 secretion. In the context of pathologic MC disorders, dysregulation of both stimulatory and inhibitory paradigms of regulation can indeed promote exuberant MC-mediated inflammation.

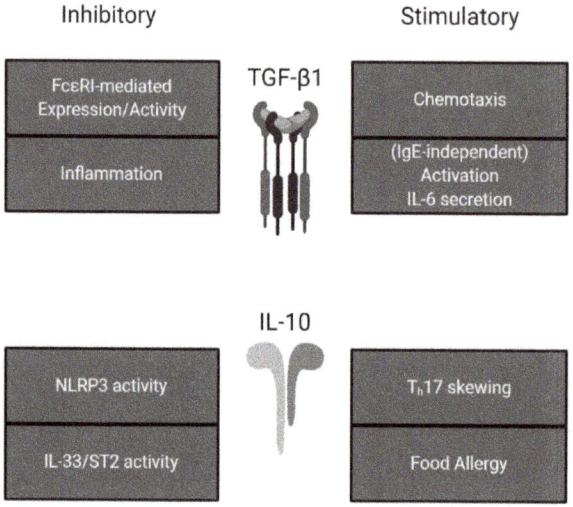

Figure 2. Effects of TGF-β1 and IL-10 on mast cell activity. TGF-β1 and IL-10 exhibit both stimulatory and inhibitory effects on mast cells. Summarized from the present review.

8. Conclusions/Summary

These alternative activation paradigms highlight the context-specific ability of MCs to mediate the surrounding stroma through cytokine secretion. IL-33 was found to synergize with SP in promoting TNF-α expression; IL-33 was shown to upregulate surface NK-1 expression [45]. MRGPRX2 has been detected in skin MCs and synovial MCs but not lung MCs, suggesting CTMCs may be more susceptible to this signaling and thus be the source of pathogenic inflammation in disease states [92].

Mutations in NLRP3 or dysregulation of signaling may coincide with TGF-β-signaling defects; overexpression of NLRP3 led to increased Smad3 phosphorylation in the kidney, suggesting a pro-fibrotic role [93]. In patients with chronic kidney disease, MCs in the kidney were found to express chymase, tryptase, renin, and TGF-β1 [94]. Expression of chymase is capable of cleaving pro-TGF-β1 into its active form as well as promoting Angiotensin-II activity [95]. The presence of these pro-fibrotic, pro-inflammatory cytokines in the kidney illustrates the context-specific functions of MCs across tissue types. Finally, prolonged activation of NLRP3 and TLR priming can render the MC refractory to future responses [85]. Altogether these observed interactions beg the question of defining an IgE-independent trained immune response in MCs, and whether such training is specific to tissues and/or pathologies.

The timing and context concerning these activation pathways also dictates the suppressive or stimulatory downstream effects. IL-33-mediated signaling on skin MCs transiently potentiates their activation but chronic exposure to the alarmin resulted in suppressed MRGPRX2 receptor expression instead [96]. Pathogenic activation of IL-33/ST2 signaling also occurs in cancer and is associated with an increase in immunosuppressive cell types and increased M2 macrophages. Tumor growth and metastasis was also increased, characterized by the presence of TGF-β^+ MDSC [97].

Ultimately, MCs are capable promoters of inflammation outside of their typical IgE-mediated role. Therapeutics targeting MC biology should respect the phenotypic differences among MCs originating from different tissues. While MCs may not be the etiologic source of disease, their ability to facilitate inflammation and positively regulate subsequent immune cell interactions/recruitment highlights their pathological capabilities when dysregulated. The fact that MCs express at least one purportedly specific receptor (MRGPRX2) and a relatively specific FcεRI emphasizes a continued interest in these cells as ripe therapeutic targets.

Funding: This research received no external funding.

Conflicts of Interest: The authors declare no conflict of interest.

References

1. Hsu, C.L.; Neilsen, C.V.; Bryce, P.J. IL-33 is produced by mast cells and regulates IgE-dependent inflammation. *PLoS ONE* **2010**, *5*. [CrossRef]
2. Joulia, R.; L'Faqihi, F.E.; Valitutti, S.; Espinosa, E. IL-33 fine tunes mast cell degranulation and chemokine production at the single-cell level. *J. Allergy Clin. Immunol.* **2017**, *140*, 497–509. [CrossRef] [PubMed]
3. Gentek, R.; Ghigo, C.; Hoeffel, G.; Bulle, M.J.; Msallam, R.; Gautier, G.; Launay, P.; Chen, J.; Ginhoux, F.; Bajénoff, M. Hemogenic Endothelial Fate Mapping Reveals Dual Developmental Origin of Mast Cells. *Immunity* **2018**, *48*, 1160–1171. [CrossRef] [PubMed]
4. Frossi, B.; Mion, F.; Sibilano, R.; Danelli, L.; Pucillo, C.E.M. Is it time for a new classification of mast cells? What do we know about mast cell heterogeneity? *Immunol. Rev.* **2018**, *282*, 35–46. [CrossRef] [PubMed]
5. Veerappan, A.; O'Connor, N.J.; Brazin, J.; Reid, A.C.; Jung, A.; McGee, D.; Summers, B.; Branch-Elliman, D.; Stiles, B.; Worgall, S.; et al. Mast cells: A pivotal role in pulmonary fibrosis. *DNA Cell Biol.* **2013**, *32*, 206–218. [CrossRef] [PubMed]
6. Lippert, U.; Artuc, M.; Grützkau, A.; Babina, M.; Guhl, S.; Haase, I.; Blaschke, V.; Zachmann, K.; Knosalla, M.; Middel, P.; et al. Human skin mast cells express H2 and H4, but not H3 receptors. *J. Investig. Dermatol.* **2004**, *123*, 116–123. [CrossRef]
7. Morse, K.L.; Behan, J.; Laz, T.M.; West, R.E.; Greenfeder, S.A.; Anthes, J.C.; Umland, S.; Wan, Y.; Hipkin, R.W.; Gonsiorek, W.; et al. Cloning and Characterization of a Novel Human Histamine Receptor. *J. Pharmacol. Exp. Ther.* **2001**, *296*, 1058–1066.
8. Hill, S.J. Distribution, properties, and functional characteristics of three classes of histamine receptor. *Pharmacol. Rev.* **1990**, *42*, 45–83.
9. Forsythe, P. Mast Cells in Neuroimmune Interactions. *Trends Neurosci.* **2019**, *42*, 43–55. [CrossRef]
10. Gupta, K.; Harvima, I.T. Mast cell-neural interactions contribute to pain and itch. *Immunol. Rev.* **2018**, *282*, 168–187. [CrossRef]
11. Kulka, M.; Sheen, C.H.; Tancowny, B.P.; Grammer, L.C.; Schleimer, R.P. Neuropeptides activate human mast cell degranulation and chemokine production. *Immunology* **2008**, *123*, 398–410. [CrossRef] [PubMed]
12. Yoshida, K.; Tajima, M.; Nagano, T.; Obayashi, K.; Ito, M.; Yamamoto, K.; Matsuoka, I. Co-Stimulation of Purinergic P2X4 and Prostanoid EP3 Receptors Triggers Synergistic Degranulation in Murine Mast Cells. *Int. J. Mol. Sci.* **2019**, *20*. [CrossRef] [PubMed]
13. Bonnekoh, H.; Scheffel, J.; Kambe, N.; Krause, K. The role of mast cells in autoinflammation. *Immunol. Rev.* **2018**, *282*, 265–275. [CrossRef] [PubMed]
14. Subramanian, H.; Gupta, K.; Ali, H. Roles of Mas-related G protein–coupled receptor X2 on mast cell–mediated host defense, pseudoallergic drug reactions, and chronic inflammatory diseases. *J. Allergy Clin. Immunol.* **2016**, *138*, 700–710. [CrossRef]
15. Tatemoto, K.; Nozaki, Y.; Tsuda, R.; Konno, S.; Tomura, K.; Furuno, M.; Ogasawara, H.; Edamura, K.; Takagi, H.; Iwamura, H.; et al. Immunoglobulin E-independent activation of mast cell is mediated by Mrg receptors. *Biochem. Biophys. Res. Commun.* **2006**, *349*, 1322–1328. [CrossRef]

16. Van Der Kleij, H.P.M.; Bienenstock, J. Significance of conversation between mast cells and nerves. *Allergy Asthma Clin. Immunol.* **2005**, *1*, 65–80. [CrossRef]
17. Garcia-Recio, S.; Gascón, P. Biological and Pharmacological Aspects of the NK1-Receptor. *Biomed. Res. Int.* **2015**, *2015*. [CrossRef]
18. Borsook, D.; Upadhyay, J.; Klimas, M.; Schwarz, A.J.; Coimbra, A.; Baumgartner, R.; George, E.; Potter, W.Z.; Large, T.; Bleakman, D.; et al. Decision-making using fMRI in clinical drug development: Revisiting NK-1 receptor antagonists for pain. *Drug Discov. Today* **2012**, *17*, 964–973. [CrossRef]
19. Karhu, T.; Akiyama, K.; Vuolteenaho, O.; Bergmann, U.; Naito, T.; Tatemoto, K.; Herzig, K.H. Mast cell degranulation via MRGPRX2 by isolated human albumin fragments. *Biochim. Biophys. Acta Gen. Subj.* **2017**, *1861*, 2530–2534. [CrossRef]
20. McNeil, B.D.; Pundir, P.; Meeker, S.; Han, L.; Undem, B.J.; Kulka, M.; Dong, X. Identification of a mast-cell-specific receptor crucial for pseudo-allergic drug reactions. *Nature* **2015**, *519*, 237–241. [CrossRef]
21. Ogasawara, H.; Furuno, M.; Edamura, K.; Noguchi, M. Novel MRGPRX2 antagonists inhibit IgE-independent activation of human umbilical cord blood-derived mast cells. *J. Leukoc. Biol.* **2019**, *106*, 1069–1077. [CrossRef] [PubMed]
22. Belanger, K.A.K.; Ameredes, B.T.; Boldogh, I.; Aguilera-Aguirre, L. The Potential Role of 8-Oxoguanine DNA Glycosylase-Driven DNA Base Excision Repair in Exercise-Induced Asthma. *Mediators Inflamm.* **2016**, *2016*. [CrossRef] [PubMed]
23. Lai, C.C.; Boguski, M.; Broek, D.; Powers, S. Influence of guanine nucleotides on complex formation between Ras and CDC25 proteins. *Mol. Cell. Biol.* **1993**, *13*, 1345–1352. [CrossRef] [PubMed]
24. Stunnenberg, H.G.; Netea, M.G.; Latz, E.; Xavier, R.J.; ONeill, L.A.J.; Natoli, G.; Mills, K.H.G.; Joosten, L.A.B. Trained immunity: A program of innate immune memory in health and disease. *Science* **2016**, *352*, 1098.
25. Latz, E.; Xiao, T.S.; Stutz, A. Activation and regulation of the inflammasomes. *Nat. Rev. Immunol.* **2013**, *13*, 397–411. [CrossRef]
26. Subramanian, N.; Bray, M.A. Interleukin 1 releases histamine from human basophils and mast cells in vitro. *J. Immunol.* **1987**, *138*, 271–275.
27. Vannier, E.; Dinarello, C.A. Histamine enhances interleukin (IL)-1-induced IL-6 gene expression and protein synthesis via H2 receptors in peripheral blood mononuclear cells. *J. Biol. Chem.* **1994**, *269*, 9952–9956.
28. Hirota, S.A.; Ng, J.; Lueng, A.; Khajah, M.; Parhar, K.; Li, Y.; Lam, V.; Potentier, M.S.; Ng, K.; Bawa, M.; et al. NLRP3 inflammasome plays a key role in the regulation of intestinal homeostasis. *Inflamm. Bowel Dis.* **2011**, *17*, 1359–1372. [CrossRef]
29. Molodecky, N.A.; Kaplan, G.G. Environmental risk factors for inflammatory bowel disease. *Gastroenterol. Hepatol.* **2010**, *6*, 339–346.
30. Baumgart, D.C.; Carding, S.R. Series Gastroenterology 1 Infl ammatory bowel disease: Cause and immunobiology. *Lancet* **2007**, *369*, 1627–1640. [CrossRef]
31. Plantinga, T.S.; Crisan, T.O.; Oosting, M.; Van De Veerdonk, F.L.; De Jong, D.J.; Philpott, D.J.; Van Der Meer, J.W.M.; Girardin, S.E.; Joosten, L.A.B.; Netea, M.G. Crohn's disease-associated ATG16L1 polymorphism modulates pro-inflammatory cytokine responses selectively upon activation of NOD2. *Gut* **2011**, *60*, 1229–1235. [CrossRef] [PubMed]
32. Smithson, J.E.; Campbell, A.; Andrews, J.M.; Milton, J.D.; Pigott, R.; Jewell, D.P. Altered expression of mucins throughout the colon in ulcerative colitis. *Gut* **1997**, *40*, 234–240. [CrossRef] [PubMed]
33. Sotolongo, J.; España, C.; Echeverry, A.; Siefker, D.; Altman, N.; Zaias, J.; Santaolalla, R.; Ruiz, J.; Schesser, K.; Adkins, B.; et al. Host innate recognition of an intestinal bacterial pathogen induces TRIF-dependent protective immunity. *J. Exp. Med.* **2011**, *208*, 2705–2716. [CrossRef] [PubMed]
34. Shea-Donohue, T.; Stiltz, J.; Zhao, A.; Notari, L. Mast Cells. *Curr. Gastroenterol. Rep.* **2010**, *12*, 349–357. [CrossRef] [PubMed]
35. Redegeld, F.A.; Yu, Y.; Kumari, S.; Charles, N.; Blank, U. Non-IgE mediated mast cell activation. *Immunol. Rev.* **2018**, *282*, 87–113. [CrossRef]
36. Cario, E.; Podolsky, D.K. Differential Alteration in Intestinal Epithelial Cell Expression of Toll-Like Receptor 3 (TLR3) and TLR4 in Inflammatory Bowel Disease. *Infect. Immun.* **2000**, *68*, 7010–7017. [CrossRef] [PubMed]
37. McGovern, D.P.B.; Hysi, P.; Ahmad, T.; van Heel, D.A.; Moffatt, M.F.; Carey, A.; Cookson, W.O.C.; Jewell, D.P. Association between a complex insertion/deletion polymorphism in NOD1 (CARD4) and susceptibility to inflammatory bowel disease. *Hum. Mol. Genet.* **2005**, *14*, 1245–1250. [CrossRef]

38. Bernstein, C.N.; Robert, M.E.; Eysselein, V.E. Rectal substance P concentrations are increased in ulcerative colitis but not in Crohn's disease. *Am. J. Gastroenterol.* **1993**, *88*, 908–913.
39. Neunlist, M.; Aubert, P.; Toquet, C.; Oreshkova, T.; Barouk, J.; Lehur, P.A.; Schemann, M.; Galmiche, J.P. Changes in chemical coding of myenteric neurones in ulcerative colitis. *Gut* **2003**, *52*, 84–90. [CrossRef]
40. Chompunud, C.; Ayudhya, N.; Roy, S.; Alkanfari, I.; Ganguly, A.; Ali, H. Identification of Gain and Loss of Function Missense Variants in MRGPRX2's Transmembrane and Intracellular Domains for Mast Cell Activation by Substance P. *Int. J. Mol. Sci.* **2019**, *20*. [CrossRef]
41. Sponheim, J.; Pollheimer, J.; Olsen, T.; Balogh, J.; Hammarström, C.; Loos, T.; Kasprzycka, M.; Sørensen, D.R.; Nilsen, H.R.; Küchler, A.M.; et al. Inflammatory bowel disease-associated interleukin-33 is preferentially expressed in ulceration-associated myofibroblasts. *Am. J. Pathol.* **2010**, *177*, 2804–2815. [CrossRef] [PubMed]
42. Koloski, N.A.; Bret, L.; Radford-Smith, G. Hygiene hypothesis in inflammatory bowel disease: A critical review of the literature. *World J. Gastroenterol.* **2008**, *14*, 165–173. [CrossRef]
43. Hunter, M.M.; McKay, D.M. Review article: Helminths as therapeutic agents for inflammatory bowel disease. *Aliment. Pharmacol. Ther.* **2004**, *19*, 167–177. [CrossRef] [PubMed]
44. Wechsler, J.B.; Szabo, A.; Hsu, C.L.; Krier-Burris, R.A.; Schroeder, H.A.; Wang, M.Y.; Carter, R.G.; Velez, T.E.; Aguiniga, L.M.; Brown, J.B.; et al. Histamine drives severity of innate inflammation via histamine 4 receptor in murine experimental colitis. *Mucosal Immunol.* **2018**, *11*, 861–870. [CrossRef]
45. Taracanova, A.; Alevizos, M.; Karagkouni, A.; Weng, Z.; Norwitz, E.; Conti, P.; Leeman, S.E.; Theoharides, T.C. SP and IL-33 together markedly enhance TNF synthesis and secretion from human mast cells mediated by the interaction of their receptors. *Proc. Natl. Acad. Sci. USA* **2017**, *114*, E4002–E4009. [CrossRef] [PubMed]
46. Polukort, S.H.; Rovatti, J.; Carlson, L.; Thompson, C.; Ser-Dolansky, J.; Kinney, S.R.M.; Schneider, S.S.; Mathias, C.B. IL-10 Enhances IgE-Mediated Mast Cell Responses and Is Essential for the Development of Experimental Food Allergy in IL-10–Deficient Mice. *J. Immunol.* **2016**, *196*, 4865–4876. [CrossRef] [PubMed]
47. Chandrasekhar, J.L.; Cox, K.M.; Loo, W.M.; Qiao, H.; Tung, K.S.; Erickson, L.D. Cutaneous Exposure to Clinically Relevant Lone Star Ticks Promotes IgE Production and Hypersensitivity through CD4 + T Cell– and MyD88-Dependent Pathways in Mice. *J. Immunol.* **2019**, *203*, 813–824. [CrossRef] [PubMed]
48. Galand, C.; Leyva-Castillo, J.M.; Yoon, J.; Han, A.; Lee, M.S.; McKenzie, A.N.J.; Stassen, M.; Oyoshi, M.K.; Finkelman, F.D.; Geha, R.S. IL-33 promotes food anaphylaxis in epicutaneously sensitized mice by targeting mast cells. *J. Allergy Clin. Immunol.* **2016**, *138*, 1356–1366. [CrossRef] [PubMed]
49. Chen, C.Y.; Lee, J.B.; Liu, B.; Ohta, S.; Wang, P.Y.; Kartashov, A.V.; Mugge, L.; Abonia, J.P.; Barski, A.; Izuhara, K.; et al. Induction of Interleukin-9-Producing Mucosal Mast Cells Promotes Susceptibility to IgE-Mediated Experimental Food Allergy. *Immunity* **2015**, *43*, 788–802. [CrossRef]
50. Ball, D.H.; Al-Riyami, L.; Harnett, W.; Harnett, M.M. IL-33/ST2 signalling and crosstalk with FcεRI and TLR4 is targeted by the parasitic worm product, ES-62. *Sci. Rep.* **2018**, *8*, 1–15. [CrossRef]
51. Kropp, L.; Jackson-Thompson, B.; Thomas, L.M.; McDaniel, D.; Mitre, E. Chronic infection with a tissue invasive helminth attenuates sublethal anaphylaxis and reduces granularity and number of mast cells. *Clin. Exp. Allergy* **2019**. [CrossRef] [PubMed]
52. Han, A.; Newell, E.W.; Glanville, J.; Fernandez-Becker, N.; Khosla, C.; Chien, Y.H.; Davis, M.M. Dietary gluten triggers concomitant activation of CD4+ and CD8+ αβ T cells and γλ T cells in celiac disease. *Proc. Natl. Acad. Sci. USA* **2013**, *110*, 13073–13078. [CrossRef] [PubMed]
53. Frossi, B.; Tripodo, C.; Guarnotta, C.; Carroccio, A.; De Carli, M.; De Carli, S.; Marino, M.; Calabrò, A.; Pucillo, C.E. Mast cells are associated with the onset and progression of celiac disease. *J. Allergy Clin. Immunol.* **2017**, *139*, 1266–1274. [CrossRef] [PubMed]
54. Strobel, S.; Busuttil, A.; Ferguson, A. Human intestinal mucosal mast cells: Expanded population in untreated coeliac disease. *Gut* **1983**, *24*, 222–227. [CrossRef]
55. Himmelweit, F. (Ed.) *The Collected Papers of Paul Ehrlich*; Elsevier: Amsterdam, The Netherlands, 1960; pp. 29–64.
56. Hanahan, D.; Coussens, L.M. Accessories to the Crime: Functions of Cells Recruited to the Tumor Microenvironment. *Cancer Cell* **2012**, *21*, 309–322. [CrossRef]
57. Varricchi; de Paulis; Marone; Galli Future Needs in Mast Cell Biology. *Int. J. Mol. Sci.* **2019**, *20*, 4397. [CrossRef]

58. Okano, M.; Oshi, M.; Butash, A.L.; Katsuta, E.; Tachibana, K.; Saito, K.; Okayama, H.; Peng, X.; Yan, L.; Kono, K.; et al. Triple-Negative Breast Cancer with High Levels of Annexin A1 Expression Is Associated with Mast Cell Infiltration, Inflammation, and Angiogenesis. *Int. J. Mol. Sci.* **2019**, *20*, 4197. [CrossRef]
59. Saadalla, A.M.; Osman, A.; Gurish, M.F.; Dennis, K.L.; Blatner, N.R.; Pezeshki, A.; McNagny, K.M.; Cheroutre, H.; Gounari, F.; Khazaie, K. Mast cells promote small bowel cancer in a tumor stage-specific and cytokine-dependent manner. *Proc. Natl. Acad. Sci. USA* **2018**, *115*, 201716804. [CrossRef]
60. Rigoni, A.; Bongiovanni, L.; Burocchi, A.; Sangaletti, S.; Danelli, L.; Guarnotta, C.; Lewis, A.; Rizzo, A.; Silver, A.R.; Tripodo, C.; et al. Mast cells infiltrating inflamed or transformed gut alternatively sustain mucosal healing or tumor growth. *Cancer Res.* **2015**, *75*, 3760–3770. [CrossRef]
61. Morales, J.K.; Saleem, S.J.; Martin, R.K.; Saunders, B.L.; Barnstein, B.O.; Faber, T.W.; Pullen, N.A.; Kolawole, F.M.; Brooks, K.B.; Norton, S.K.; et al. Myeloid-derived suppressor cells enhance IgE-mediated mast cell responses. *J. Leukoc. Biol.* **2014**, *95*, 643–650. [CrossRef]
62. Fiocchi, C. Inflammatory bowel disease: Etiology and pathogenesis. *Gastroenterology* **1998**, *115*, 182–205. [CrossRef]
63. Itzkowitz, S.H.; Yio, X. Inflammation and cancer - IV. Colorectal cancer in inflammatory bowel disease: The role of inflammation. *Am. J. Physiol. Gastrointest. Liver Physiol.* **2004**, *287*. [CrossRef] [PubMed]
64. Allen, I.C.; Tekippe, E.M.E.; Woodford, R.M.T.; Uronis, J.M.; Holl, E.K.; Rogers, A.B.; Herfarth, H.H.; Jobin, C.; Ting, J.P.Y. The NLRP3 inflammasome functions as a negative regulator of tumorigenesis during colitis-associated cancer. *J. Exp. Med.* **2010**, *207*, 1045–1056. [CrossRef] [PubMed]
65. Zaki, M.H.; Vogel, P.; Body-Malapel, M.; Lamkanfi, M.; Kanneganti, T.-D. IL-18 Production Downstream of the Nlrp3 Inflammasome Confers Protection against Colorectal Tumor Formation. *J. Immunol.* **2010**, *185*, 4912–4920. [CrossRef]
66. Moossavi, M.; Parsamanesh, N.; Bahrami, A.; Atkin, S.L.; Sahebkar, A. Role of the NLRP3 inflammasome in cancer. *Mol. Cancer* **2018**, *17*, 158. [CrossRef]
67. Christophers, E.; Metzler, G.; Röcken, M. Bimodal immune activation in psoriasis. *Br. J. Dermatol.* **2014**, *170*, 59–65. [CrossRef]
68. Graham, D.B.; Xavier, R.J. From genetics of inflammatory bowel disease towards mechanistic insights. *Trends Immunol.* **2013**, *34*, 371–378. [CrossRef]
69. Silverman, A.J.; Sutherland, A.K.; Wilhelm, M.; Silver, R. Mast cells migrate from blood to brain. *J. Neurosci.* **2000**, *20*, 401–408. [CrossRef]
70. Stojanov, S.; Kastner, D.L. Familial autoinflammatory diseases: Genetics, pathogenesis and treatment. *Curr. Opin. Rheumatol.* **2005**, *17*, 586–599. [CrossRef]
71. Gomez, G.; Ramirez, C.D.; Rivera, J.; Patel, M.; Norozian, F.; Wright, H.V.; Kashyap, M.V.; Barnstein, B.O.; Fischer-Stenger, K.; Schwartz, L.B.; et al. TGF-beta 1 inhibits mast cell Fc epsilon RI expression. *J. Immunol.* **2005**, *174*, 5987–5993. [CrossRef]
72. Gebhardt, T.; Lorentz, A.; Detmer, F.; Trautwein, C.; Bektas, H.; Manns, M.P.; Bischoff, S.C. Growth, phenotype, and function of human intestinal mast cells are tightly regulated by transforming growth factor β1. *Gut* **2005**, *54*, 928–934. [CrossRef] [PubMed]
73. Vitsky, A.; Waire, J.; Pawliuk, R.; Bond, A.; Matthews, D.; LaCasse, E.; Hawes, M.L.; Nelson, C.; Richards, S.; Piepenhagen, P.A.; et al. Homeostatic role of transforming growth factor-β in the oral cavity and esophagus of mice and its expression by mast cells in these tissues. *Am. J. Pathol.* **2009**, *174*, 2137–2149. [CrossRef] [PubMed]
74. Olsson, N.; Piek, E.; ten Dijke, P.; Nilsson, G. Human mast cell migration in response to members of the transforming growth factor-beta family. *J. Leukoc. Biol.* **2000**, *67*, 350–356. [CrossRef] [PubMed]
75. Maeda, H.; Shiraishi, A. TGF-beta contributes to the shift toward Th2-type responses through direct and IL-10-mediated pathways in tumor-bearing mice. *J. Immunol.* **1996**, *156*, 73–78. [PubMed]
76. Lyons, D.O.; Plewes, M.R.; Pullen, N.A. Soluble transforming growth factor beta-1 enhances murine mast cell release of Interleukin 6 in IgE-independent and Interleukin 13 in IgE-dependent settings in vitro. *PLoS ONE* **2018**, 1–17. [CrossRef]
77. Ganeshan, K.; Bryce, P.J. Regulatory T cells enhance mast cell production of IL-6 via surface-bound TGF-β. *J. Immunol.* **2012**, *188*, 594–603. [CrossRef]

78. Mashiko, S.; Bouguermouh, S.; Rubio, M.; Baba, N.; Bissonnette, R.; Sarfati, M. Human mast cells are major IL-22 producers in patients with psoriasis and atopic dermatitis. *J. Allergy Clin. Immunol.* **2015**, *136*, 351–359.e1. [CrossRef]
79. Lin, A.M.; Rubin, C.J.; Khandpur, R.; Wang, J.Y.; Riblett, M.; Yalavarthi, S.; Villanueva, E.C.; Shah, P.; Kaplan, M.J.; Bruce, A.T. Mast Cells and Neutrophils Release IL-17 through Extracellular Trap Formation in Psoriasis. *J. Immunol.* **2011**, *187*, 490–500. [CrossRef]
80. Dudeck, A.; Suender, C.A.; Kostka, S.L.; von Stebut, E.; Maurer, M. Mast cells promote Th1 and Th17 responses by modulating dendritic cell maturation and function. *Eur. J. Immunol.* **2011**, *41*, 1883–1893. [CrossRef]
81. Ganeshan, K.; Johnston, L.K.; Bryce, P.J. TGF-β1 Limits the Onset of Innate Lung Inflammation by Promoting Mast Cell-Derived IL-6. *J. Immunol.* **2013**, *190*, 5731–5738. [CrossRef]
82. Kasakura, K.; Nagata, K.; Miura, R.; Nakaya, H.; Okada, H.; Arai, T.; Arai, T.; Kawakami, Y.; Kawakami, T.; Yashiro, T.; et al. Cooperative Regulation of the Mucosal Mast Cell–Specific Protease Genes Mcpt1 and Mcpt2 by GATA and Smad Transcription Factors. *J. Immunol.* **2020**. [CrossRef] [PubMed]
83. Zimmermann, C.; Troeltzsch, D.; Giménez-rivera, V.A.; Galli, S.J.; Metz, M.; Maurer, M.; Siebenhaar, F. Mast cells are critical for controlling the bacterial burden and the healing of infected wounds. *Proc. Natl. Acad. Sci. USA* **2019**, *116*, 20500–20504. [CrossRef] [PubMed]
84. Mazer, M.; Unsinger, J.; Drewry, A.; Walton, A.; Osborne, D.; Blood, T.; Hotchkiss, R.; Remy, K.E. IL-10 Has Differential Effects on the Innate and Adaptive Immune Systems of Septic Patients. *J. Immunol.* **2019**, *203*, 2088–2099. [CrossRef] [PubMed]
85. Gurung, P.; Li, B.; Subbarao Malireddi, R.K.; Lamkanfi, M.; Geiger, T.L.; Kanneganti, T.D. Chronic TLR Stimulation Controls NLRP3 Inflammasome Activation through IL-10 Mediated Regulation of NLRP3 Expression and Caspase-8 Activation. *Sci. Rep.* **2015**, *5*, 1–10. [CrossRef] [PubMed]
86. Greenhill, C.J.; Jones, G.W.; Nowell, M.A.; Newton, Z.; Harvey, A.K.; Moideen, A.N.; Collins, F.L.; Bloom, A.C.; Coll, R.C.; Robertson, A.A.B.; et al. Interleukin-10 regulates the inflammasome-driven augmentation of inflammatory arthritis and joint destruction. *Arthritis Res. Ther.* **2014**, *16*, 1–10. [CrossRef] [PubMed]
87. Sanchez-Cantu, L. Endotoxin Tolerance Is Associated with Reduced Secretion of Tumor Necrosis Factor. *Arch. Surg.* **1989**, *124*, 1432. [CrossRef]
88. Espinosa-Riquer, Z.P.; Ibarra-Sánchez, A.; Vibhushan, S.; Bratti, M.; Charles, N.; Blank, U.; Rodríguez-Manzo, G.; González-Espinosa, C. TLR4 Receptor Induces 2-AG–Dependent Tolerance to Lipopolysaccharide and Trafficking of CB2 Receptor in Mast Cells. *J. Immunol.* **2019**, *202*, 2360–2371. [CrossRef]
89. Randow, F.; Syrbe, U.; Meisel, C.; Krausch, D.; Zuckermann, H.; Platzer, C.; Volk, H.D. Mechanism of endotoxin desensitization: Involvement of interhukin 10 and transforming growth factor β. *J. Exp. Med.* **1995**, *181*, 1887–1892. [CrossRef]
90. Friend, D.S.; Ghildyal, N.; Gurish, M.F.; Hunt, J.; Austen, K.F.; Stevens, R.L.; Hu, X. Reversible expression of tryptases and chymases in the jejunal mast cells of mice infected with Trichinella spiralis. *J. Immunol.* **1998**, *160*, 5537–5545.
91. Friend, D.S.; Ghildyal, N.; Austen, K.F.; Gurish, M.F.; Matsumoto, R.; Stevens, R.L. Mast cells that reside at different locations in the jejunum of mice infected with Trichinella spiralis exhibit sequential changes in their granule ultrastructure and chymase phenotype. *J. Cell Biol.* **1996**, *135*, 279–290. [CrossRef]
92. Varricchi, G.; Pecoraro, A.; Loffredo, S.; Poto, R.; Rivellese, F.; Genovese, A.; Marone, G.; Spadaro, G. Heterogeneity of human mast cells with respect to MRGPRX2 receptor expression and function. *Front. Cell. Neurosci.* **2019**, *13*. [CrossRef] [PubMed]
93. Wang, W.; Wang, X.; Chun, J.; Vilaysane, A.; Clark, S.; French, G.; Bracey, N.A.; Trpkov, K.; Bonni, S.; Duff, H.J.; et al. Inflammasome-Independent NLRP3 Augments TGF-β Signaling in Kidney Epithelium. *J. Immunol.* **2013**, *190*, 1239–1249. [CrossRef] [PubMed]
94. Zheng, J.M.; Yao, G.H.; Cheng, Z.; Wang, R.; Liu, Z.H. Pathogenic role of mast cells in the development of diabetic nephropathy: A study of patients at different stages of the disease. *Diabetologia* **2012**, *55*, 801–811. [CrossRef] [PubMed]
95. Wolf, G. Link between Angiotensin II and TGF-β in the Kidney. *Miner. Electrolyte Metab.* **1998**, *24*, 174–180. [CrossRef]

96. Wang, Z.; Guhl, S.; Franke, K.; Artuc, M.; Zuberbier, T.; Babina, M. IL-33 and MRGPRX2-Triggered Activation of Human Skin Mast Cells—Elimination of Receptor Expression on Chronic Exposure, but Reinforced Degranulation on Acute Priming. *Cells* **2019**, *8*, 341. [CrossRef]
97. Jovanovic, I.P.; Pejnovic, N.N.; Radosavljevic, G.D.; Pantic, J.M.; Milovanovic, M.Z.; Arsenijevic, N.N.; Lukic, M.L. Interleukin-33/ST2 axis promotes breast cancer growth and metastases by facilitating intratumoral accumulation of immunosuppressive and innate lymphoid cells. *Int. J. Cancer* **2014**, *134*, 1669–1682. [CrossRef]

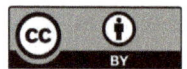

© 2020 by the authors. Licensee MDPI, Basel, Switzerland. This article is an open access article distributed under the terms and conditions of the Creative Commons Attribution (CC BY) license (http://creativecommons.org/licenses/by/4.0/).

MDPI
St. Alban-Anlage 66
4052 Basel
Switzerland
Tel. +41 61 683 77 34
Fax +41 61 302 89 18
www.mdpi.com

International Journal of Molecular Sciences Editorial Office
E-mail: ijms@mdpi.com
www.mdpi.com/journal/ijms

www.ingramcontent.com/pod-product-compliance
Lightning Source LLC
LaVergne TN
LVHW070658100526
838202LV00013B/990